A Lexicon of Psychology, Psychiatry and Psychoanalysis

Edited by Jessica Kuper

ROUTLEDGE
LONDON AND NEW YORK

First published in 1988 by
Routledge
11 New Fetter Lane, London EC4P 4EE
29 West 35th Street, New York, NY 10001

WLM 13

9 004074

Set in Linotron Baskerville
by Input Typesetting Ltd., London SW19 8DR
and printed in Great Britain
by Cox & Wyman Ltd
Reading, Berks

© *Jessica Kuper 1988*

Library of Congress Cataloging in Publication Data

A lexicon of psychology, psychiatry, and psychoanalysis/edited by
    Jessica Kuper.
        p.   cm.—(Social science lexicons)
    Includes bibliographies.
    ISBN 0–415–00233–8 (pbk.)
        1. Psychology—Dictionaries.   2. Psychiatry—Dictionaries.
    3. Psychoanalysis—Dictionaries.   I. Kuper, Jessica.   II. Series.
    BF31.L48   1988
    150'.3'21—dc19   *88–19884*

British Library CIP Data also available

Contents

A Lexicon of Psychology, Psychiatry and Psychoanalysis: the entries

Contributor List

General Editor: Jessica Kuper

Appelbaum, Paul S	Medical School, University of Massachusetts
Apter, Michael J	Dept of Psychology, University College, Cardiff
Argyle, Michael	Dept of Experimental Psychology, University of Oxford
Baddeley, Alan	MRC Applied Psychology Unit, Cambridge
Baltes, Paul B	Max Planck Institute for Human Development and Education, Berlin
Bannister, D	High Royds Hospital, Ilkley, West Yorkshire
Barron, Frank	Dept of Psychology, University of California, Santa Cruz
Beaumont, J Graham	Dept of Psychology, University of Leicester
Beer, C G	Institute of Animal Behavior, Newark College of Art and Sciences, Rutgers, The State University of New Jersey
Beisser, Arnold R	University of California, Los Angeles, Gestalt Therapy Institute
Billig, Michael	Dept of Psychology, University of Loughborough
Bliss, Eugene L	Dept of Psychiatry, University of Utah Medical Center, Salt Lake City
Boden, Margaret A	School of Social Sciences, University of Sussex
Bolen, Jean Shinoda	C J Jung Institute, San Francisco
Brislin, Richard W	Culture Learning Institute, East-West Center, Honolulu

Brown, Barrie J	Dept of Psychology, Institute of Psychiatry, University of London
Brown, Rupert J	Social Psychology Research Unit, University of Kent
Buckley, Kerry W	Northampton, Massachusetts
Canter, David	Dept of Psychology, University of Surrey
Cartwright, Rosalind D	Dept of Psychology and Social Sciences, Rush-Presbyterian-St Luke's Medical Center, Chicago
Claxton, Guy L	Centre for Science and Mathematics Education, Chelsea College, University of London
Cohen, Gillian	Human Cognition Research Laboratory, Open University, Milton Keynes
Colman, Andrew M	Dept of Psychology, University of Leicester
Coltheart, Max	Dept of Psychology, Birkbeck College, University of London
Danziger, K	Dept of Psychology, York University, Downsview, Ontario
Dietz, Park Elliot	School of Law, University of Virginia
Draguns, Juris G	Dept of Psychology, Pennsylvania State University
Duncan, John	MRC Applied Psychology Unit, Cambridge
Elbers, Ed	Dept of Psychology, University of Utrecht
Eysenck, H J	Institute of Psychiatry, University of London
Eysenck, Michael W	Royal Holloway and Bedford New College, University of London
Farr, Robert M	Dept of Social Psychology, The London School of Economics and Political Science

Feldman, Marcus W   Dept of Biological Science, Stanford University

Fielding, Guy   Dept of Communication Studies, Sheffield City Polytechnic

Fisher, S   University of Dundee

Frankel, Fred H   Dept of Psychiatry, Beth Israel Hospital, Boston

Fraser, Colin   Social and Political Sciences Committee, University of Cambridge

Friedman, William J   Dept of Psychology, Oberlin College, Ohio

Gecas, Viktor   Dept of Sociology, Washington State University, Pullman

Gibson, H B   Cambridge

Gilgen, Albert R   Dept of Psychology, University of Northern Iowa, Cedar Falls

Gilhooly, K J   Dept of Psychology, University of Aberdeen

Goethals, George W   Dept of Psychiatry, Harvard University

Gogel, Walter   Dept of Psychology, University of California, Santa Barbara

Goode, Erich   Dept of Sociology, State University of New York at Stony Brook

Grunebaum, Henry   Family Studies, The Cambridge Hospital, Cambridge, Massachusetts

Gutheil, Thomas G   Harvard University and Program in Psychiatry and the Law, Boston

Hampson, Sarah E   Oregon Research Institute

Hargreaves, David J   Dept of Psychology, University of Leicester

Harrington, David M   Dept of Psychology, University of California, Santa Cruz

Heaven, Patrick C L	School of Humanities and Social Sciences, Riverina College, Australia
Hemsley, David R	Institute of Psychiatry, University of London
Herbert, Martin	Dept of Psychology, University of Leicester
Herriot, Peter	Dept of Occupational Psychology, Birkbeck College, University of London
Howells, Kevin	Dept of Psychology, University of Leicester
Hudson, Liam	Dept of Psychology, Brunel University
Ingleby, David	Dept of Development Psychology, University of Utrecht
Jahoda, Marie	Science Policy Research Unit, University of Sussex
Jones, Alan	Dept of Senior Psychologist (Navy), Ministry of Defence (UK)
Jones, Edward E	Dept of Psychology, Princeton University
Jones, Maxwell	Wolfville, Nova Scotia
Kendall, Philip C	Dept of Psychology, Temple University, Philadelphia
Kimmel, H D	Dept of Psychology, University of South Florida
Kline, Paul	Dept of Psychology, University of Exeter
Kramer, Dierdre A	Max Planck Institute for Human Development and Education, Berlin
Kris, Anton O	Boston Psychoanalytic Institute
Landy, Frank J	Dept of Psychology, Pennsylvania State University
Lazare, Aaron	Massachusetts General Hospital, Boston
Lerner, Richard M	College of Human Development, Pennsylvania State University

Levy, Bernard S	Human Resource Institute, Brookline, Massachusetts
Liebowitz, Herschel W	Dept of Psychology, Pennsylvania State University
Lipset, David	Dept of Anthropology, University of Minnesota
Lipsitt, Lewis P	Walter S Hunter Laboratory of Psychology, Brown University, Providence, Rhode Island
McKenzie, Beryl E	Dept of Psychology, La Trobe University, Victoria, Australia
Mackintosh, N J	Dept of Experimental Psychology, University of Cambridge
Manis, Melvin	Dept of Psychology, University of Michigan, Ann Arbor
Manstead, A S R	Dept of Psychology, University of Manchester
Maratsos, Michael	Institute of Child Development, University of Minnesota
Mayes, Andrew	Dept of Psychology, University of Manchester
Melzack, Roland	Dept of Psychology, McGill University, Montreal
Mendlewicz, Julien	Erasmus Hospital, Free University, Brussels
Mensch, Ivan N	Dept of Psychiatry and Biobehavioural Sciences, School of Medicine, University of California
Moreland, Richard L	Dept of Psychology, University of Pittsburgh
Morris, Peter	Dept of Psychology, University of Lancaster
Muller-Schwarze, Dietland	College of Environmental and Forest Biology, State University of New York, Syracuse

Nemiah, John C	Beth Israel Hospital, Boston
O'Neil, W M	Emeritus Professor of Psychology, Sydney University
Parkes, Colin Murray	The London Hospital Medical College, University of London
Pollock, Alan S	Adult Outpatient Clinic, McLean Hospital, Belmont, Massachusetts
Pollock, George H	President, American Psychoanalytic Association
Pope, Harrison G	The Mailman Research Center, Belmont, Massachusetts
Rabbitt, Patrick	Dept of Psychology, University of Manchester
Rangell, Leo	University of California, Los Angeles
Ray, William J	Dept of Psychology, Pennsylvania State University
Richardson, John T E	Dept of Human Sciences, Brunel University, Uxbridge
Ritvo, Edward R	Center for Health Sciences, School of Medicine, University of California, Los Angeles
Roth, Loren H	Western Psychiatric Institute and Clinic, University of Pittsburgh
Rushton, J Philippe	University of Western Ontario, London, Ontario
Sayers, Janet	Dept of Psychology, University of Kent
Sexton, Virginia S	Dept of Psychology, St John's University, Jamaica, NY
Shallice, Tim	MRC Applied Psychology Unit, Cambridge
Sharaf, Myron	Dept of Psychiatry, Harvard University
Singer, Jerome L	Dept of Psychology, Yale University

Spiegel, David	Dept of Psychiatry, School of Medicine, Stanford University
Spielberger, Charles D	Center for Research in Behavioral Medicine and Community Psychology, University of South Florida, Tampa, Florida
Stone, Alan A	Harvard Law School, Harvard University
Stone, Karen	Belmont, Massachusetts
Stotland, Ezra	Society and Justice Program, University of Washington, Seattle
Strauss, John S	Dept of Psychiatry, Medical School, Yale University
Switzky, Harvey N	Dept of Learning, Development and Special Education, Northern Illinois University, De Kalb, Illinois
Talbott, John A	The Payne Whitney Psychiatric Clinic, The New York Hospital
Tarullo, Louisa B	Cambridge, Massachusetts
Thayer, H S	Dept of Philosophy, City University of New York
Tischler, Gary L	Yale Psychiatric Institute, New Haven
Vaillant, George E	Dartmouth Medical School, Hanover, New Hampshire
Valentine, E R	Dept of Psychology, Royal Holloway and Bedford New College, University of London
Vondracek, Fred W	College of Human Development, Pennsylvania State University
Walker, S F	Dept of Psychology, Birkbeck College, University of London
Watson, Andrew S	Dept of Psychiatry and Dept of Law, University of Michigan, Ann Arbor
Weale, R A	Institute of Ophthalmology, University of London

Wexler, Kenneth	School of Social Sciences, University of California, Irvine
Wong, Normund	Director, Karl Menninger School of Psychiatry, Menninger Foundation, Topeka, Kansas
Wortis, Joseph	Editor, *Biological Psychiatry*, Brooklyn, New York
Yates, Aubrey J	Dept of Psychology, University of Western Australia, Nedlands
Zaleznik, Abraham	Harvard University School of Business Administration

Abnormal Psychology

Abnormal psychology may be viewed as the scientific study of abnormalities of behaviour and experience, their determinants and correlates. However, the complexity of any such definition is well illustrated by the instructions for authors in the *Journal of Abnormal Psychology*, which includes as a topic falling within the journal's area of focus 'normal processes in abnormal individuals'. It is apparent that a consideration of the use of the word abnormal in this context is necessary.

It is common to distinguish at least three definitions of psychological abnormality. (1) *The statistical definition.* It is dependent upon a knowledge of the relative frequencies of certain behaviours, experiences, traits, etc., in the population; the extremes of the distributions are defined as abnormal. There are several problems with this approach: (i) Even if one restricts oneself to those dimensions studied extensively in experimental and social psychology, it is apparent that much of the population is likely to be abnormal in at least some respects. (ii) Abnormalities of relevance to adjustment may not lie solely in terms of the absolute levels of particular variables, but also in the way in which different measures covary. (iii) Abnormally high scores on measures such as those of ability would not be regarded as abnormal in the sense of a psychological aberration. (iv) The interpretation placed on statistical abnormality, for example, a high score on an anxiety questionnaire, is highly dependent on context, for instance, whether or not the subject faced an identifiable stressful experience. It should be noted that this last point applies equally to the definitions of abnormality discussed below. (2) *The social definition* of psychological abnormality indicates that behaviours seen as violating the rules of social functioning are classified as abnormal. It is clear that standards of social behaviour vary according to the social reference group. There is obviously a partial overlap with statistical definitions of abnormality in that conformity to standards defines normal social behaviour. (3) *The medical definition* of psychological abnormality suggests that it be defined in terms of specific symptoms which indicate the presence of an underlying disordered state. However, the majority of problems of adjustment which result in intervention have no clear organic basis. Although guidelines for what constitutes symptoms have been developed (e.g., Wing *et al.*, 1974) and can result in their reliable assessment, it is apparent that the designation even of such symptoms as hallucinations as psychological impairment may be dependent on social and cultural factors (Al-Issa, 1977).

Shapiro (1975) has argued that the field of psychopathology consists largely of those psychological phenomena requiring intervention. He suggests that they have at least one of the following four characteristics: they are distressing to the person concerned and/or to his associates; they are disabling; they are socially inappropriate in the context of the patient's subculture; they are inconsistent with reality. Research in abnormal psychology may be viewed as an attempt to describe and explain such phenomena in terms of concepts and theories derived from the scientific investigation of animal and human behaviour. Within abnormal psychology it is common to distinguish several models, or overall ways, of conceptualizing the area of study: the biological, emphasizing the biological bases of abnormality; the cognitive-behavioural; and the social. However, these are best seen as complementary approaches, reflecting different levels of analysis. Most of the phenomena of psychopathology are amenable to, and indeed require, analysis at all three levels.

A number of research strategies in abnormal psychology may be distinguished. (1) Group comparisons based on psychiatric classification. Despite frequent criticisms of this method of classification, the resultant groupings form the basis of much research in abnormal psychology. Such studies aim to test

deductions from hypotheses concerning the nature and determinants of the disorder. (2) Studies examining the correlates and properties of an objectively defined aspect of abnormal behaviour or experience. (3) Experimentally induced pathological behaviour: here psychopathology is modelled and reproduced in the laboratory either with animal or human subjects.
(4) Analogue studies: these involve the investigation of naturally occurring but non-clinical forms of statistically abnormal behaviour patterns, such as fear of spiders, which are seen as similar on critical dimensions to those phenomena requiring intervention.

David R. Hemsley
Institute of Psychiatry
University of London

References
Al-Issa, I. (1977), 'Social and cultural aspects of hallucinations', *Psychological Bulletin*, 84.
Shapiro, M. B. (1974), 'The requirements and implications of a systematic science of psychopathology', *Bulletin of the British Psychological Society*, 28.
Wing, J. K., Cooper, J. E. and Sartorius, N. (1974), *The Measurement and Classification of Psychiatric Symptoms*, London.
See also: *mental disorders*.

Activation and Arousal

The terms activation and arousal have often been used interchangeably to describe a continuum ranging from deep sleep or coma to extreme terror or excitement. This continuum has sometimes been thought of as referring to observed behaviour, but many psychologists have argued that arousal should be construed in physiological terms. Of particular importance in this connection is the ascending reticular activating system, which is located in the brain-stem and has an alerting effect on the brain.

Some question the usefulness of the theoretical constructs of activation and arousal. On the positive side, it makes some sense to claim that elevated arousal is involved in both motivational and emotional states. It appears that individual differences in personality are related to arousal levels, with introverts being characteristically more aroused than extroverts (H. J. Eysenck, 1967). In addition, proponents of arousal theory have had some success in predicting performance effectiveness on the basis of arousal level. In general, performance is best when the prevailing level of arousal is neither very low nor very high. Particularly important is the fact that there are sufficient similarities among the behavioural effects of factors such as intense noise, incentives and stimulant drugs to encourage the belief that they all affect some common arousal system.

On the negative side, the concepts of activation and of arousal are rather amorphous. Different physiological measures of arousal are often only weakly correlated with one another, and physiological, behavioural and self-report measures of arousal tend to produce conflicting evidence. Faced with these complexities, many theorists have suggested that there is more than one kind of arousal. For example, H. J. Eysenck (1967) proposed that the term arousal should be limited to cortical arousal, with the term activation being used to refer to emotional or autonomic arousal.

It may be desirable to go even further and identify three varieties of arousal. For example, a case can be made for distinguishing among behavioural, autonomic and cortical forms of arousal (Lacey, 1967). Alternatively, Pribram and McGuinness (1975) argued for the existence of stimulus-produced arousal, activation or physiological readiness to respond, and effort in the sense of activity co-ordinating arousal and activation processes.

In sum, the basic notion that the behavioural effects of various emotional and motivational manipulations are determined at least in part by internal states of physiological arousal is plausible and in line with the evidence. However, the number and nature of the arousal dimensions that ought to be postulated remains controversial. In addition, there is growing suspicion that the effects of arousal on behaviour are usually rather modest and indirect. What appears to happen is that people respond to non-optimal levels of arousal (too low or too high) with various strategies and compensatory activities designed to minimize the adverse effects of the prevailing level of arousal (M. W. Eysenck, 1982). Thus, the way in which performance is maintained at a reasonable level despite substantial variations in arousal needs further explanation.

Michael W. Eysenck
Royal Holloway and Bedford New College
University of London

References
Eysenck, H. J. (1967), *The Biological Basis of Personality*, Springfield, Ill.
Eysenck, M. W. (1982), *Attention and Arousal: Cognition and Performance*, Berlin.
Lacey, J. I. (1967), 'Somatic response patterning and stress: some revisions of activation theory', in M. H. Appley and R. Trumbull (eds), *Psychological Stress*, New York.
Pribram, K. H. and McGuinness, D. (1975), 'Arousal, activation, and effort in the control of attention', *Psychological Review*, 82.

See also: *nervous system*.

Adler, Alfred (1870–1937)
Born in Vienna in 1870, Alfred Adler trained as an ophthalmologist and first practised general medicine before becoming a psychiatrist and a charter member of Freud's inner circle. An energetic, articulate man and a prolific writer, Adler was soon made the titular president of the first Psychoanalytic Society. Unlike Freud, Adler was a political and social activist; in retrospect it seems that at least some of their conflicts were due to this basic difference. Adler is best known for originating the concept of the inferiority complex and of understanding personality in terms of the compensatory struggle to achieve superiority. Although Adler did in fact formulate these reductionistic and mechanistic theories, he also had other, much more subtle, ideas about human nature.

Adler disagreed with Freud's emphasis on biological and sexual factors; instead he gave primary importance to social, interpersonal, and hierarchical relationships. Adler believed that man is motivated by his expectations of the future: 'The final goal alone can explain man's behaviour.' Human behaviour is not determined by childhood experiences themselves, but by the 'perspective in which these [experiences] are regarded'. The final goal of the individual determines the perspective in which he views these important early experiences. This conception of behaviour, motivated by a particular perspective and by ideas about the future, is described as 'idealistic positivism'. It is compatible with, if not identical to, many strands of contemporary psychological, philosophical and social theory (for example, existential theories). Idealistic positivism de-emphasizes the importance of the unconscious and transforms Freud's conception of psychic determinism.

Adler rejected the idea that a human being is simply a product of environment and heredity. He posited a creative self, which makes something of hereditary abilities and interprets environmental impressions, thus constituting a unique individual personality and life-style. While Adler, the first defector from Freud's circle, is today ignored by most psychologists and psychiatrists, in his Individual Psychology can be found the beginnings of contemporary humanistic psychology. Adler's views suggested the great importance of methods of childrearing and education. According to Adler, physical infirmity, rejection, and pampering were the factors most likely to result in a pathological style of life. He helped establish child-guidance clinics in association with the Viennese school system, and became a major advocate of the child-guidance movement.

Alan A. Stone
Harvard University

Further Reading
Adler, A. (1924 [1920]), *The Practice and Theory of Individual Psychology*, London. (Original German edn, *Praxis und Theorie der Individual-Psychologie*, Munich.)

Ansbacher, H. L. and Ansbacher, R. R. (eds) (1956), *The Individual Psychology of Alfred Adler: A Systematic Presentation in Selections from his Writings*, New York.

Hall, C. S. and Lindzey, G. (1978), *Theories of Personality*, 3rd edn, New York.

Orgler, H. (1973), *Alfred Adler, The Man and His Work*, New York.

Sperber, M. (1970), *Alfred Adler, oder das Elend der Psychologie*, Vienna.

Aesthetics

The study of aesthetics, which concerns the creation and appreciation of beauty, forms part of philosophy as well as psychology, with points of contact with sociology, biology and anthropology. It could very loosely be described as the scientific study of the arts, although there are two reasons why some might disagree with this description. First, the scientific approach is not one that is universally acceptable; the distinction has been made between 'speculative' and 'empirical' aesthetics, and some areas of philosophy, art history and art criticism come into the former category. Speculative aesthetics is concerned with high-level questions such as the nature of beauty, or the meaning of art works, whereas empirical aesthetics involves the scientific study of the component processes of appreciation. Thus, the second point of disagreement might be about what constitutes a work of art: some of the experimental stimuli used in empirical aesthetics have little in common with real-life music, painting, poetry or sculpture.

Psychologists, along with other social scientists, have adopted the empirical approach; indeed, the field of experimental aesthetics is one of the oldest branches of psychology. One of the founding fathers of the discipline was the German physicist, physiologist and philosopher Gustav Theodor Fechner. Fechner's extensive studies in the field of psychophysics led him towards the problems of aesthetics, and he published his *Vorschule der Ästhetik (Prolegomenon to Aesthetics)* in 1876. Fechner's explicit aim was to found what he called an 'aesthetics from below'; he was primarily concerned with the elementary mechanisms of likes and dislikes, and he used experimental techniques that have a great deal in common with those employed in modern experimental psychology. One such technique, for example, was the 'method of choice', in which subjects were required to select the stimulus they liked best out of several that were presented to them. Fechner hoped to work up from this fairly rudimentary and basic starting point to the more complex questions of aesthetics.

He attempted, for example, to test the early theory of the 'aesthetic mean', in which beauty was considered to be associated with the absence of extremes, by assessing people's preferences for different colours, visual patterns, and auditory stimuli. He presented subjects with rectangles of different shapes in order to test the famous 'golden section' hypothesis that the ratio of 0.62 between the lengths of the longer and the shorter sides may constitute a 'divine proportion' with special aesthetic properties. Though Fechner's early efforts along these lines gave experimental aesthetics a firm methodological footing, the findings over the next few decades (Valentine, 1962) were generally inconsistent. No conclusive evidence was obtained concerning the 'aesthetic mean' or 'golden section' theories, for example, and interest in experimental aesthetics consequently declined.

In the mid-1960s, however, psychologist Daniel Berlyne coined the term 'new experimental aesthetics' to describe a branch of research that was taking a different approach to the old problems: its theoretical basis is in biology (Berlyne, 1971). Two major features of the new approach are its emphasis on *arousal* as the main determinant of aesthetic response, and on what Berlyne calls 'collative variables'. This theory holds that art objects produce pleasure by manipulating the level of arousal, attention or excitement of the observer; they do this by means of their collative properties, such as their complexity, surprisingness or familiarity. In other words, the observer collates information from different properties of the stimulus, and the resulting level of arousal will determine the likelihood of his exploring that stimulus. Berlyne further proposes that the 'hedonic value', or pleasantness, of a stimulus is related to the subject's level of arousal according to an inverted-U-shaped curve; pleasantness is greatest for stimuli that produce an intermediate level of arousal. It is the emphasis on collative variables of form, and on the potential for integration with other areas of psychology (such as motivation, exploration and play), that distinguishes the new from the old experimental aesthetics. Although some researchers would dispute the details of Berlyne's theoretical formulation, the new experimental aesthetics is nonetheless healthy and flourishing. Three broad lines of development can be distinguished:

(1) This relates directly to Berlyne's concern with collative variables; there is a growing amount of research which manipulates them, as well as considerably greater sophistication in the scaling, grouping and quantification of experimental stimuli. Multidimensional scaling techniques, for example, provide a means of operationalizing the concept of artistic style, such that real-life art works can be scaled for use as experimental stimuli. The application of information theory to aesthetic objects, begun in the 1950s, continues to provide objective measures of properties such as 'information content' and 'redundancy'. Multivariate computer content analysis has been used to assess the melodic originality of themes in classical music, for example. It may well be this kind of advance that will throw most light on questions about the nature of 'goodness of form', which were raised long ago by the Gestalt psychologists.

(2) This involves the investigation of observer characteristics. One area of research, for example, is exploring the relationship between personality factors such as extraversion/introversion and aesthetic judgement. Another concerns variables of cognitive style, such as tolerance for ambiguity. A third growing area of research that comes loosely under this heading is that on the development of aesthetic sensitivity in children. Most prominent in this field is Howard Gardner's *Project Zero* team at Harvard University which has investigated a wide variety of children's reactions to different art forms.

(3) Possibly the most difficult research area concerns the relationship between affect and cognition: that is, how does the emotional aspect of an aesthetic response interact with the

thought processes involved? This kind of question was originally addressed by Freud in his psychoanalytic studies of the artistic process, and it is only in the 1980s that researchers such as Pavel Machotka and Robert Zajonc are turning to it once more. Endeavours such as these suggest that empirical research is now beginning to tackle some of the complex problems of speculative aesthetics; a *rapprochement* between the two may one day be possible.

David J. Hargreaves
University of Leicester

References
Berlyne, D. E. (1971), *Aesthetics and Psychobiology*, New York.
Fechner, G. T. (1876), *Vorschule der Ästhetik*, Leipzig.
Valentine, C. W. (1962), *The Experimental Psychology of Beauty*, London.

Further Reading
Gardner, H. (1973), *The Arts and Human Development*, New York.
Winner, E. (1982), *Invented Worlds*, Cambridge, Mass.
See also: *activation and arousal*.

Ageing

The study of age-related changes in cognitive processes has received fresh impetus as the proportion of elderly people in the population of Western societies continues to increase. It is important that these changes should be recognized, understood and taken into account so as to enable the elderly to cope with a modern environment and continue living a full life of work and leisure activities.

The researcher tries to isolate and identify the effects of normal ageing on cognitive abilities. Changes caused by the ageing process are confounded with associated changes in physical health, in life-style, in motivation and personality. Poor performance may be the product of sensory deficits, anxiety or lack of interest rather than mental deterioration. When old and young are compared, tests may be contaminated by cohort effects. Just as intelligence tests may be criticized for not being 'culture-fair', they can also be criticized for not being 'cohort-fair'. The educational and life experience of the generations are different and have shaped different sorts of ability. Experimental research on ageing seeks to disentangle these confounding variables and focus on the effects of age alone.

Many mental abilities do show some deterioration with age, but others are unimpaired. Individual differences tend to increase, with some individuals deteriorating while others preserve their intellect intact. In general, little decline is observable before the mid-sixties. Traditional psychometric testing has yielded age norms for performance on batteries of standard intelligence tests. The results led to a distinction between 'crystallized' (or age invariant) intelligence and 'fluid' (age sensitive) intelligence. Tests which measure intellectual attainment, such as vocabulary, verbal ability and factual knowledge, show little age effect. Tests measuring ability to manipulate or transform information such as backward digit span, or digit-symbol substitution and some tests of spatial reasoning, generally reveal a decline. These tests, however, give little insight into the changes in the underlying mechanisms that cause some abilities to be impaired and others to be preserved.

Psychologists turned, therefore, to the experimental techniques developed in the study of perception, attention, learning and memory, and applied these to the problem of ageing. The information processing approach allows complex tasks to be decomposed so that the defective component can be identified. So, for example, experimental studies of memory indicate that the process of retrieval is relatively more affected by ageing than encoding or storage (Burke and Light, 1981); and studies of mental arithmetic show that the capacity of working memory, the 'holding store', is the vulnerable component (Wright, 1981). Common factors such as a diminished rate of information processing and a diminished capacity of working memory are seen to underlie performance decrements on many tasks. The pattern of deficit can be interpreted in terms of theoretical distinctions, like that between attentional processes (ones that require conscious monitoring) and automatic processes (ones that are highly practised, rapid and unconscious). Attentional processes are more likely to be age-impaired, while automatic processes are often unaffected.

One problem that arises when complex tasks are studied is that of distinguishing between age differences in strategy and in capacity. Defective performance may result from failure to employ the right strategy rather than from reduced capacity. Where strategies are implicated, the age difference may be eliminated by remedial training. When a capacity limitation is the cause, the age difference can only be removed by restructuring the task so as to make it less demanding. The current trend in ageing research is to study performance in real-world situations with emphasis on the practical and applied aspects. For this more applied approach it is clearly very important to discover how far the difficulties old people experience in their daily lives can be overcome by training in appropriate strategies, and how far it is necessary to modify the environment to suit their capacities.

Gillian Cohen
Open University

References
Burke, D. M. and Light, L. L. (1981), 'Memory and aging: the role of retrieval processes', *Psychological Bulletin*, 90.
Wright, R. E. (1981), 'Aging, divided attention and processing capacity', *Journal of Gerontology*, 36.

Further Reading
Kausler, D. H. (1982), *Experimental Psychology and Human Aging*, New York.
See also: *intelligence and intelligence testing; life-span development; memory.*

Aggression and Anger

Biological/instinctual, psychoanalytic, ethological, social learning and cognitive theorists have all attempted to further our understanding of aggression, often spurred by a stated concern about humans' capacity to inflict suffering on others and by fears for the future of the species. While most would accept that some progress has been made, the actual achievements of social scientists to date are thought by some to be limited. The reasons for these limitations are of interest in themselves. Marsh and Campbell (1982) attribute lack of progress to a number of factors, including the difficulties in studying aggression, both in laboratory and naturalistic settings, and the compartmentalization of the academic world, such that researchers fail to cross the boundaries dividing psychology from sociology, physiology and anthropology, or even the subdivisions within psychology itself.

There are, however, two even more basic problems which have inhibited progress. The first is the difficulty in arriving at any generally acceptable definition of aggression, and the second is the related problem of the over-inclusiveness of the theories themselves. An important starting point in providing an adequate definition is to distinguish aggression from anger and hostility. Anger refers to a state of emotional arousal, typically with autonomic and facial accompaniments. A person may be angry without being behaviourally destructive and vice versa. Hostility refers to the cognitive/evaluative appraisal of other people and events. It would be possible to appraise a particular group in society in very negative terms without their eliciting anger or overt aggression, though in most cases cognition and affect will be intimately linked (see below).

Aggression itself refers to overt behaviour, though precisely what sort of behaviour should be labelled aggressive is controversial. Bandura (1973) proposes cutting through the 'semantic jungle' in this area by restricting the term to acts resulting in personal injury or destruction of property, while accepting that injury may be psychological as well as physical. There then remain problems in defining what is injurious and in dealing with 'accidental' aggression (where injury is inflicted but not intended) and 'failed' aggression (as when a person tries to shoot another person but misses). In general, the definition of an act as aggressive involves a social judgement on the part of the observer. For this reason, injurious acts may not be labelled as aggressive when socially prescribed (for example, capital punishment) or when they support values the observer endorses (for example, a parent beating a child to instil godfearing virtue). In this sense, labelling a behaviour as aggressive inevitably has a social and political dimension to it.

The second difficulty lies in the breadth of activities addressed by most theories. Stabbing another person in a fight, battering a baby, being abusive in a social encounter and waging warfare may all be behaviours that meet the definition of aggression, but they are also disparate activities with little obvious functional unity. This should, but often does not, preclude attempts to provide general theories which would account for them all. Many different theories are likely to be required to account for these different forms of aggressive behaviour.

In recent years the utility of one particular distinction has become apparent – that between 'angry' and 'instrumental' or what some have called 'annoyance-motivated' and 'incentive-motivated' aggression (Zillman, 1979). The former is preceded by affective arousal. The person is in an emotional, physiologically activated state, often induced by environmental frustration of some sort. In instrumental aggression, on the other hand , the aggressive act is used as a way of securing some environmental reward and emotional activation may not be present, as in the case of someone using violence to rob a bank. The two classes are not entirely independent in that environmental reinforcement is also involved in angry aggression, though the reward obtained is likely to be that of inflicting pain or injury itself.

The many sources of instrumental aggression have been well documented in psychological research. That some aggressive behaviour is indeed learned socially because it is effective in securing environmental rewards or because aggressive models for imitation exist is now widely accepted (for a review see Bandura, 1973). The powerful effects of pressures towards obedience to authority in producing cruelty have also been shown in laboratory investigations. Recent years, however, have witnessed a renewal of interest in angry forms of aggression and it is on this work that I shall focus for the remainder of this article.

Angry aggression is an important feature of much of the violence which causes social concern. Studies of homicide, for example, suggest that the violent act is often a response to intense anger arousal. The violent person is often described as in a 'fury' or a 'rage', directed in many cases at a person with whom they have an intimate relationship (a wife or husband). Anger may also be involved in less obvious forms of violence. There is evidence, for example, that many rapes show features of angry aggression. A substantial number of rapists are in an angry/frustrated state preceding the assault and appear to be motivated to hurt and degrade the victim rather than to obtain sexual relief (Groth, 1979).

Research on Anger
Until very recently much less attention has been directed by social scientists at the affect of anger than at its direct behavioural manifestations. Anger has been widely discussed by philosophers and poets but rarely by the experimental psychologist. The recent renewed interest in this phenomenological aspect of aggression stems in part from a general reconsideration of the emotions within psychology and also from developments in the field of cognition and its relationship to affect.

Anger seems to have four components – the environment, cognition, emotional/physiological arousal, and behaviour itself, and these components interact reciprocally in a complex fashion (Noveco, 1978). The first two of these elements, in particular, have been the focus for recent experimental investigation. Anger and angry aggression are generally preceded by a triggering environmental event. There are a number of theories of what kind of event is likely to be important (the frustration-aggression theory, for example). In a recent review, Berkowitz (1982) has argued persuasively that environmental events elicit aggression to the extent that they are *aversive*. Thus the absence of reward where it is expected or the blocking of goal-directed activity provoke aggression because they are unpleasant. Experiencing failure, being insulted, unjustly treated or attacked share the property of aversiveness and are capable, therefore, of producing anger and aggression. Berkowitz suggests that both humans and animals are born with a readiness to flee or to fight when confronted by an aversive stimulus. Which reaction will occur will depend on learning experiences (flight, for example, may have been found to be more effective) and on the nature of the particular situation (a situation where the person has expectations of control may make fight more likely). Consistent with Berkowitz's thesis that aversiveness is critical are a number of laboratory and naturalistic studies showing, for example, that pain is a potent elicitor of angry aggression. Unpleasant smells, 'disgusting' visual stimuli and high temperatures have also been found to lower the threshold for aggression, though in the latter case the relationship is curvilinear.

Diary studies of what makes people angry in everyday life confirm the importance of aversive/frustrating events but also suggest a feature of anger not always apparent in laboratory studies – that it is predominantly elicited by *interpersonal* events. Other people, rather than things or impersonal occurrences, make us angry. James Averill (1982) found that people reported becoming mildly to moderately angry in the range of several times a day to several times a week and that only 6 per cent of incidents were elicited by a non-animate object. The frustrating person in over half the episodes was someone known and liked – friends and loved ones are common sources of aversive experiences!

The second component of anger currently receiving attention is the cognitive processing of social and internal events. The concerns of cognitive theorists are typically with how people appraise, interpret and construct the social environment. Attribution theory has been a major force in cognitive theorizing and attributional processes are now widely acknowledged to be relevant to angry aggression. Such processes are best viewed as mediating the emotional and behavioural responses to the aversive/frustrating events described above. The power of attributions can be appreciated by considering the differing emotional and behavioural consequences of various attributions for an event such as being knocked off one's bicycle on the way home from work. This painful and aversive occurrence might be attributed by the cyclist to his own inadequacies ('not looking where I was going') or to chance ('given the number of cars and bicycles it is inevitable some people are knocked down'). Neither of these attributions is, intuitively, likely to produce an aggressive response. Suppose, however, that the attribution was made that the car driver had deliberately intended to knock me off my bicycle. The threshold for aggression, at least towards the driver, might be expected to be considerably lowered by such an appraisal. Attributions of 'malevolent intent' of this sort have been shown to be important for anger and aggression (see Ferguson and Rule, 1983).

The third and fourth components of anger are affective/physiological arousal itself and the aggressive act which may or may not follow anger arousal. Anger is undoubtedly accompanied by autonomic activation (increases in blood pressure, heart rate, respiration and muscle tension and so on), but it is still unclear whether the pattern of activation can be discriminated from arousal caused by other emotions. Most experiences of anger in everyday life are not followed by physical aggression. Averill (1982) found that less than 10 per cent of angry episodes induced physical aggression. What he called 'contrary reactions', activities opposite to the instigation of anger, such as being very friendly to the instigator, were twice as frequent as physical aggression. Anger may produce a range of other reactions – the previous learning experiences of the individual are clearly important in determining whether frustration and anger are responded to with withdrawal, help-seeking, constructive problem-solving or what Bandura (1973) has called 'self-anaesthetization through drugs and alcohol'.

The reciprocal bi-directional influence between the components of anger is something that has been stressed by Novaco (1978). Cognitions may induce anger and aggression, but behaving aggressively may activate hostile cognitions and also change the environment in such a way as to make the person even more frustrated. Hostile appraisals of other people

are often self-fulfilling. Untangling the complex interrelationships between these environmental, cognitive, physiological and
behavioural component processes will be the major task for
future aggression researchers.

Kevin Howells
University of Leicester

References
Averill, J. R. (1982), *Anger and Aggression: An Essay on Emotion*,
New York.
Bandura, A. (1973), *Aggression: A Social Learning Analysis*,
Englewood Cliffs.
Berkowitz, L. (1982), 'Aversive conditions as stimuli to
aggression', in L. Berkowitz (ed.), *Advances in Experimental
Social Psychology* 15, New York.
Ferguson, T. J. and Rule, B. G. (1983), 'An attributional
perspective on anger and aggression', in *Aggression:
Theoretical and Empirical Reviews Vol. 1*, New York.
Groth, A. N. (1979), *Men Who Rape*, New York.
Marsh, P. and Campbell, A. (1982) (eds), *Aggression and
Violence*, Oxford.
Novaco, R. W. (1978), 'Anger and coping with stress', in J.
P. Foreyt and D. P. Rathjen (eds), *Cognitive Behavior
Therapy*, New York.
Zillman, D. (1979), *Hostility and Aggression*, Hillsdale, N.J.
See also: *activation and arousal; attribution theory; emotion; stress.*

Altruism

For thousands of years philosophers have been intrigued by the
problem of altruism, whether considering its status as a virtue,
or debating its part in human nature. Seventeenth- and eigh-
teenth-century British philosophers in particular, including
Bentham, Hobbes, Locke, Mill, Sidgwick and Smith, argued at
length about the psychological genuineness of human benevol-
ence. It was the French philosopher, Auguste Comte, however,
who originated the term, placing it in opposition to egoism. He
believed the purpose of an advanced society was to foster the

love of humanity, and that positivistic science, especially the discipline of sociology (a term he also coined), would produce this new set of values. More recently, behavioural scientists from several disciplines have examined the concept of altruism more objectively (Rushton and Sorrentino, 1981).

The definition of altruism is a matter of controversy. Some define it in terms of underlying motivations such as empathy or intention, while others prefer definitions in terms of behavioural effects such as 'that which benefits others'. One advantage of the behavioural definition is that it finesses the endless and fruitless debate as to whether such a thing as 'true' altruism exists. Defining altruism behaviourally does not, of course, preclude looking for the underlying motivation. It also allows the concept to be applied to animals.

In regard to motives, a number of internal mediators have been suggested. Among these are role-taking ability, empathic emotion, guilt, ideas of justice, personal values and social norms. There has been much research and model building on these hypothesized processes (Rushton and Sorrentino, 1981). Many of these models suggest that there are genuinely altruistic motivations, at the very least in the sense that internal standards prevail over immediate egoism.

Where does altruism originate? Three major developmental theories are (1) sociobiology, (2) cognitive development, and (3) social learning.

(1) Sociobiologists suggest that altruism is part of the inherited nature of human beings, arising from evolutionary history. Evidence for this view comes from studies of (a) animals, and (b) behaviour genetics. In regard to (a), altruism has been found in other species that, like our own, live in social groups. Social insects such as ants, bees and wasps, through to birds, dogs, porpoises and chimpanzees, all demonstrate altruism – in parental care, mutual defence, rescue behaviour, co-operative hunting and food sharing (Wilson, 1975). Sociobiologists view altruism as having evolved to help propagate genes. The altruist is helpful to kin, who share genes and thereby increase the number of reproductively successful offspring they raise. In so doing he helps to propagate his

own genes. In this view altruism serves the 'selfish' biological purpose of propagating DNA, and is expected to follow lines of genetic similarity. In regard to (b), twin studies have found that individual differences in altruism, empathy, kindness and nurturance, as measured by paper-and-pencil questionnaires, have a substantial genetic component (Rushton, 1984).

(2) Researchers following in the cognitive developmental tradition of Piaget (1932) have documented the increments with age in children's capacity to (a) role-take the needs and perspectives of others, and (b) make moral judgements concerned with increasing ethical altruism. Both of these are seen as developing in a series of stages over the life span, invariant in sequence, hierarchical in nature, and universal across cultures. Many individuals, however, are said never to reach the higher levels of role-taking or moral reasoning due to 'developmental arrest'. This theory, therefore, essentially sees altruistic behaviour as based on maturationally unfolding cognitive development. In its support are the findings that individual differences in both role-taking ability and level of moral reasoning are predictive of altruistic behaviour, and that all three increase with age.

(3) The social learning theory approach, as its name suggests, stresses the importance of social conditioning in the development of altruism. Four processes in particular have been well researched: (a) classical conditioning; (b) response-contingent reinforcement and punishment; (c) observation of others; and (d) verbal socialization, including attributional labelling. Learning theorists have applied these procedures to understand the way in which socialization occurs through the educational system, the family, the peer group, and the mass media (Rushton, 1980). For example, if one of the main ways in which people learn is by observing others, then it follows that people should learn a great deal from viewing others on television. It is now fairly well documented that television has the power to alter the norms of appropriate behaviour.

A different orientation to altruism has come from personality theorists who have investigated whether there is a 'trait' of altruism, that is, whether some people are consistently more altruistic than others. The answer appears to be 'yes'. Evidence suggests that the likelihood of people being altruistic can be predicted from the manner in which they endorse or respond to items on paper-and-pencil measures of empathy, moral judgement, social responsibility, and moral knowledge. Altruists also appear to be consistently more honest, persistent, and self-controlled than non-altruists, and are likely to have strong feelings of personal efficacy. As already mentioned, some of this individual difference variance is inherited.

The effects on altruism of many social variables have been examined (Rushton and Sorrentino, 1981). One that has been much researched is the size of a group helping in an emergency. It is found that bystanders are more likely to offer help in an emergency if they are alone than if they are with others; the presence of others reduces helping, possibly through diffusing people's sense of responsibility. Another variable related to altruism is mood: good moods increase altruism whereas bad moods decrease it. Perhaps connected both with group size and mood is the apparent negative relation between altruism and population density: altruism is more frequent in small towns than in suburbs and more in the suburbs than in big cities. Finally, altruism has been related to friendship and similarity. In children, altruism and friendship sociograms overlap, and studies of adults have shown that they are more likely to help members of their own race or country than members of other races or foreigners. People also feel more empathic with, and help, those they perceive as similar to themselves.

Altruism has usually been viewed as an unqualified virtue. However, research is beginning to show that this is not always the case. Kindness can have unintended negative consequences. In some circumstances it can lead to a lowered self-concept, a feeling of helplessness and resentment in the recipient. Some have also argued that institutionalized altruism, such as occurs in the social welfare system, robs the individual of feelings of initiative or responsibility.

J. Philippe Rushton
University of Western Ontario

References
Piaget, J. (1932), *The Moral Judgment of the Child*, London.
Rushton, J. P. (1980), *Altruism. Socialization, and Society*, Englewood Cliffs, N.J.
Rushton, J. P. (1984), 'Sociobiology: toward a theory of individual and group differences in personality and social behavior', in J. R. Royce and L. P. Moss (eds), *Annals of Theoretical Psychology* vol. 2, New York.
Rushton, J. P. and Sorrentino, R. M. (eds) (1981), *Altruism and Helping Behavior: Social, Personality and Developmental Perspectives*, Hillsdale, N.J.
Wilson, E. O. (1975), *Sociobiology: The New Synthesis*, Cambridge, Mass.
See also: *empathy and sympathy*.

Analytical Psychology (Jungian Psychology)

C. G. Jung described his approach to psychotherapy as analytical psychology, differentiating it from Freud's psychoanalysis, and Adler's individual psychology. Jung's psychology takes into account a person's age, psychological type, and a 'collective unconscious'. This collective unconscious is distinct from the 'personal unconscious', with its forgotten or repressed contents. It is a common human inheritance, which gives everyone a propensity to respond emotionally to archetypal myths and images, to have dreams with universal symbols, and to respond instinctually.

Jung described four stages in analytical treatment: (1) confession (abreaction or catharsis); (2) elucidation (interpretation); (3) education: and (4) transformation (individuation).

(1) All therapies, the religious confessional, and initiation rituals have in common the first stage, catharsis, which Jung described as 'not merely the intellectual recognition of the facts with the head, but their confirmation by the heart and actual release of suppressed emotion'.

(2) Jung considered the second stage, elucidation or interpretation, as the main emphasis of Freudian psychoanalysis. It is a necessary stage if the patient becomes fixated on the analyst in a transference neurosis. Since transference is an unconscious

process, a transference neurosis (or psychosis) can arise in any therapeutic situation. Although Jungian analysis does not foster transference, when it does arise in the analysis, transference interpretations are a necessary stage in the work.

(3) The stage of education, in which the analyst appeals to the patient's understanding of his symptoms and provides social education, was Adler's emphasis in psychotherapy. Jung saw this third stage as an effort by the analyst to help his patient learn how to adapt as a 'normal human being' in the everyday world. If a patient in Jungian analysis has a neurosis or psychosis that has made him unfit for normal life, then the direction of therapy at some point might include this stage.

(4) The fourth stage – transformation or individuation – was Jung's contribution to the analytic process. In this stage, the patient discovers his uniqueness, connects with an inner source of meaning that Jung called the Self, and shifts the centre of his personality from the ego to the Self.

The transformation stage takes place through a dialectical process or dialogue between analyst and patient. The process involves conscious attitudes and unconscious elements in the personalities of both people; as a result, both are deeply affected. A personal analysis is a prerequisite for any analyst undertaking this work.

Jung maintained that,

> The personalities of the doctor and patient are often infinitely more important for the outcome of the treatment than what the doctor says or thinks (although what he says and thinks may be a disturbing or a healing factor not to be underestimated). For two personalities to meet is like mixing two different chemical substances: if there is any combination at all, both are transformed.

Jean Shinoda Bolen
C. J. Jung Institute
San Francisco

Further Reading

Jung, C. G. (1966), *The Practice of Psychotherapy*, vol. 16 of the Collected Works of C. G. Jung, New York.

Mattoon, M. A. (1981), *Jungian Psychology in Perspective*, New York.

See also: *Jung; unconscious.*

Anorexia Nervosa

Anorexia nervosa probably represents a weight phobia – the fear of obesity. Once a rare disorder, it is now common in affluent countries where the cultural mandate for females is a slim figure. Characteristic patterns in families of anorexics include parental expectations of perfection, at least as seen through the eyes of the affected young person.

The average patient – over 90 per cent are female – aged seventeen or eighteen, weighs 123 pounds prior to the onset of the disorder. She begins a voluntary diet, loses control and drops to seventy-nine pounds, although extreme cases go below sixty pounds. To facilitate a loss of weight, patients radically reduce their calorie intake, but many also induce vomiting, over-exercise, or take cathartics. Some periodically go on eating binges when self-control is temporarily lost.

The physiological disturbances resulting from these disordered eating habits lead to physical distress with eating and disruption of the ordinary experience of satisfaction. This situation reinforces the anorexic process. Patients continue to perceive themselves as fat despite the reality; this distortion of body image is probably a function of the phobic process, which magnifies the feared object. The malnutrition leads to an amenorrhea, constipation, hypotension, bradycardia and anaemia. However, some patients display a remarkable energy despite their wasted appearance and in fact engage in compulsive exercise.

Why does a small fraction of the dieting population lose control and develop this syndrome? Many are troubled adolescents, who regard slimness as a key to happiness, attractiveness, and a sense of inner worth. Most are diligent, perfectionist and compliant; these traits may make them more susceptible to cultural mandates for slimness. Finally, as a group they are excellent hypnotic subjects, which may contribute to the phobia. Therapy involves realimentation, usually by behavioural tactics. However, the fear of obesity tends to linger, remaining a formidable problem. Some therapists maintain that comprehensive treatment requires involving the family in an effort to deal with underlying causes of the disorder.

Eugene L. Bliss
University of Utah

Further Reading
Bliss, E. A. and Branch, C. H. H. (1960), *Anorexia Nervosa: Its History, Psychology and Biology*, Hoeber, N.Y.
Dally, P., Gomez, J. and Isaacs, A. J. (1979), *Anorexia Nervosa*, London.
Gross, M. (ed.) (1982), *Anorexia Nervosa*, Lexington, Mass.

Anxiety

The term anxiety is currently used in psychology and psychiatry to refer to at least three related, yet logically different, constructs. Although most commonly used to describe an unpleasant emotional state or condition, anxiety also denotes a complex psychophysiological process that occurs as a reaction to stress. In addition, the concept of anxiety refers to relatively stable individual differences in anxiety proneness as a personality trait.

Anxiety states can be distinguished from other unpleasant emotions such as anger, sorrow or grief, by their unique combination of experiential, physiological and behavioural manifestations. An anxiety state is characterized by subjective feelings of tension, apprehension, nervousness and worry, and by activation (arousal) and discharge of the autonomic nervous system. Such states may vary in intensity and fluctuate over time as a function of the amount of stress that impinges on an individual. Calmness and serenity indicate the absence of anxiety; tension, apprehension and nervousness accompany moderate levels of anxiety; intense feelings of fear, fright and panic are indicative of very high levels of anxiety.

The physiological changes that occur in anxiety states include: increased heart rate (palpitations, tachycardia), sweating, muscular tension, irregularities in breathing (hyperventilation), dilation of the pupils, and dryness of the mouth. There may also be vertigo (dizziness), nausea, and muscular skeletal disturbances such as tremors, tics, feelings of weakness and restlessness. Individuals who experience an anxiety state can generally describe their subjective feelings, and report the intensity and duration of this unpleasant emotional reaction.

Anxiety states are evoked whenever a person perceives or interprets a particular stimulus or situation as potentially dangerous, harmful or threatening. The intensity and duration of an anxiety state will be proportional to the amount of *threat* the situation poses for the individual and the persistence of his interpretation of the situation as personally dangerous. The appraisal of a particular situation as threatening will also be influenced by the person's skills, abilities and past experience.

Anxiety states are similar to fear reactions, which are generally defined as unpleasant emotional reactions to anticipated injury or harm from some external danger. Indeed, Freud regarded fear as synonymous with 'objective anxiety', in which the intensity of the anxiety reaction was proportional to the magnitude of the external danger that evoked it: the greater the external danger, the stronger the perceived threat, the more intense the resulting anxiety reaction. Thus, fear denotes a process that involves an emotional reaction to a perceived danger, whereas the anxiety state refers more narrowly to the quality and the intensity of the emotional reaction itself.

The concept of anxiety-as-process implies a theory of anxiety as a temporally-ordered sequence of events which may be initiated by a stressful external stimulus or by an internal cue that is interpreted as dangerous or threatening. It includes the following fundamental constructs or variables: stressors, perceptions and appraisals of danger or threat, anxiety state and psychological defence mechanisms. Stressors refer to situations or stimuli that are objectively characterized by some degree of physical or psychological danger. Threat denotes an individual's subjective appraisal of a situation as potentially dangerous or harmful. Since appraisals of danger are immediately followed by an anxiety state reaction, anxiety as an emotional state is at the core of the anxiety process.

Stressful situations that are frequently encountered may lead to the development of effective coping responses that quickly eliminate or minimize the danger. However, if a person interprets a situation as dangerous or threatening and is unable to cope with the stressor, he may resort to intraphsychic manoeuvres (psychological defences) to eliminate the resulting anxiety state, or to reduce its level of intensity.

In general, psychological defence mechanisms modify, distort or render unconscious the feelings, thoughts and memories that would otherwise provoke anxiety. To the extent that a defence mechanism is successful, the circumstances that evoke the anxiety will be less threatening, and there will be a corresponding reduction in the intensity of the anxiety reaction. But defence mechanisms are almost always inefficient and often maladaptive because the underlying problems that caused the anxiety remain unchanged.

While everyone experiences anxiety states from time to time, there are substantial differences among people in the frequency and the intensity with which these states occur. Trait anxiety is the term used to describe these individual differences in the tendency to see the world as dangerous or threatening, and in the frequency that anxiety states are experienced over long periods of time. People high in trait anxiety are more vulnerable to stress, and they react to a wider range of situations as dangerous or threatening than low trait anxiety individuals. Consequently, high trait anxious people experience anxiety state reactions more frequently and often with greater intensity than do people who are low in trait anxiety.

To clarify the distinction between anxiety as a personality trait and as a transitory emotional state, consider the statement: 'Mr Smith is anxious.' This statement may be interpreted as meaning either that Smith is anxious *now*, at this very moment, or that Smith is *frequently* anxious. If Smith is 'anxious now', he is experiencing an unpleasant emotional state, which may or may not be characteristic of how he generally feels. If Smith experiences anxiety states more often than others, he may be classified as 'an anxious person', in which case his average level of state anxiety would generally be higher than that of most other people. Even though Smith may be an *anxious person*, whether or not he is *anxious now* will depend on how he interprets his present circumstances.

Two important classes of stressors have been identified that appear to have different implications for the evocation of anxiety states in people who differ in trait anxiety. Persons high in trait anxiety are more vulnerable to being evaluated by others because they lack confidence in themselves and are low in self-esteem. Situations that involve psychological threats (that is, threats to self-esteem, particularly ego-threats when personal adequacy is evaluated), appear to be more threatening for people high in trait anxiety than for low trait anxious individuals. While situations involving physical danger such as imminent surgery generally evoke high levels of state anxiety persons high or low in trait anxiety show comparable increases in anxiety state in such situations.

Individuals very high in trait anxiety, for example, psycho-neurotics or patients suffering from depression, experience high levels of state anxiety much of the time. But even they have coping skills and defences against anxiety that occasionally leave them relatively free of it. This is most likely to occur in situations where they are fully occupied with a non-threatening task on which they are doing well, and are thus distracted from the internal stimuli that otherwise constantly cue state anxiety responses.

Charles D. Spielberger
University of South Florida

Further Reading

Freud, S. (1936), *The Problem of Anxiety*, New York.
Lazarus, R. S. (1966), *Psychological Stress and the Coping Process*, New York.

Levitt, E. E. (1980), *The Psychology of Anxiety*, Hillsdale, N.J.

Spielberger, C. D. (1972), 'Anxiety as an emotional state', in C. D. Spielberger (ed.), *Anxiety: Current Trends in Theory and Research*, 2 vols, New York.

Spielberger, C. D. (1979), *Understanding Stress and Anxiety*, London.

See also: *activation and arousal; emotion; stress.*

Aptitude Tests

Aptitude tests are standardized tasks designed to indicate an individual's future job proficiency or success in training. Some tests have been specifically developed for this purpose (for example, name and number comparison tests for selecting clerical workers), whilst others have been borrowed from educational, clinical and research use (for example, Cattell's 16 Personality Factor Questionnaire). Tests may be administered to an individual or to a group. The main types now in use are of intellectual, spatial, mechanical, perceptual and motor abilities, and of interests and personality traits.

Tests must be shown to be job-relevant, the most persuasive evidence usually being the demonstration of a relationship between pre-entry tests scores and later training or job performance ('predictive validity'). For example, Flanagan (1948) showed in one study that none of the very low scorers (grade 1) on a pilot aptitude test battery graduated from pilot training, as against some 30 per cent of average scorers (grade 5) and over 60 per cent of the very high scorers (grade 9). Ghiselli (1973) concluded that aptitude tests are generally better at predicting training success rather than job proficiency, but that for every type of job there is at least one type of test which gives a moderate level of prediction. Combining tests into a battery would tend to improve prediction.

It was generally accepted until recently that a test had to show predictive validity in each specific instance of use, but many psychologists now believe that validity can be generalized given an adequate specification of the test and of the job. Thus, an organization need no longer rely solely on its own research, since evidence from a number of organizations can be collected to serve as a national or international data-base.

The financial benefit to an organization from test use depends on other factors besides validity, notably on how selective it can be when choosing job applicants and the nature of the job (variation in performance in monetary terms). The reductions in costs or increase in profits can be impressive: Schmidt *et al.* (1979) estimated that the selection of computer programmers using a programmer aptitude test could produce productivity gains of some 10 billion dollars per year for the US economy.

The 1970s saw, particularly in the US, increasing criticism of aptitude tests in personnel selection because of alleged unfairness to minority groups. Some of the specific instances raised in the law courts indicated that the necessary validation research had not been carried out; test use was therefore potentially unfair to all applicants and disadvantageous to the organization. There remains much debate on how fairness can best be estimated and how test use should be modified to maximize it.

Most tests have until now been paper-and-pencil, with only a small proportion involving other types of material or apparatus. Future developments are likely to include the production of computerized versions of existing tests and of new tests designed to benefit from computer technology, for example, tests involving the display of dynamic material on the visual display unit.

Alan Jones
Department of Senior Psychologist (Navy)
Ministry of Defence (UK)

References

Flanagan, J. C. (1948), *The Aviation Psychology Program in the Army Air Forces*, Report No. 1, Washington D. C. Ghiselli, E. E. (1973), 'The validity of aptitude tests in personnel selection', *Personnel Psychology*, 26.

Schmidt, F. L., Hunter, J. E., McKenzie, R. C. and Muldrow,

T. W. (1979), 'Impact of valid selection procedures on work-force productivity', *Journal of Applied Psychology*, 64.

Artificial Intelligence

Workers in artificial intelligence (AI) try to write programs enabling computers to carry out complex information-processing tasks requiring flexibility and context-sensitivity.

Examples of such tasks include: noticing a creature moving in the shadows, attending to it, and recognizing it as a robin (and, sometimes, mistaking it for a chaffinch); understanding speech, even in noisy conditions; having a conversation about people's plans and motives, and interpreting their behaviour in terms of specific purposes; understanding a piece of written text well enough to be able to answer questions about it, or to translate it sensibly into a foreign language; seeing an analogy, and using it to help solve a problem; making a medical diagnosis, and prescribing medicine appropriately; playing chess, backgammon, or poker – and learning to play better; picking up a delicate object and packing it into a box; assembling a structure out of Meccano parts, where the diagrammed instructions have been lost.

Each of these can already be achieved by AI-systems – but only to a limited extent. Intelligence normally requires considerable knowledge, and the ability to locate the relevant items quickly. It is very difficult to make knowledge fully explicit, and to formulate principles of inference that will use it sensibly. Existing AI-systems are restricted to a narrow domain. A program that can see cannot hear, and one that can read cannot play chess; a program that can play chess cannot play draughts, or understand English (except possibly descriptions of chess-moves); and one that can summarize news stories about earthquakes cannot understand letters about the first cuckoo of spring. The robot which can see, hear, touch, speak, plan, move and manipulate *in a wide variety of contexts* is still only science fiction.

AI-workers differ in their aims. Some hope to develop a general theory of intelligence, applicable to Martians, men and machines. Others are primarily interested in human intelligence: they try to write programs that process information in ways like those used by the human mind. Still others see AI as technology: they want computer systems that will be useful to the public (the military, the medic, the man-in-the-street), not caring whether their programs solve problems in the way that we do.

AI has had a short history, but already promises to change everyday life as much as the Industrial Revolution did. It grew out of the work on digital computers in World War II (with anticipations by Turing in the 1930s and Babbage in the nineteenth century). It received its name in 1956 (though many AI-workers prefer to use the blander 'knowledge-engineering'). Through the 1960s and 1970s, interest in AI gradually increased, but even in 1980 most educated people had not heard of it. The media suddenly became aware of it when, in the early 1980s, the Japanese announced their 'Fifth Generation Computer' project. This was an ambitious ten-year national plan, lavishly funded by government and industry. It aimed to develop large parallel-processing machines, and intelligent software, enabling computers of the 1990s to understand Japanese and other natural languages, to interpret the speech of many different individuals, to act as intelligent assistants in a wide variety of tasks, and to provide advanced problem-solving and sensori-motor abilities for mobile domestic and industrial robots.

It remains to be seen whether the plan will succeed. Most people grossly underestimate the difficulties involved: one of the prime lessons of AI is the previously unrecognized richness and subtlety of 'common sense'.

Specialist expertise is a different matter: 'expert systems' are already on the market. They offer consultant advice on technical matters like medical diagnosis, tax laws, oil prospecting and genetic engineering. They are rule-based programs, incorporating the theoretical knowledge and 'rules of thumb' of the experienced person. They can offer explanations of their advice to the user (who may decide to reject it), and can be incrementally improved by accepting new information (for example, that a certain drug should not be prescribed for specific types of patient). A few of these programs already give more reliable advice than all but the very best human experts (and one or two outperform us all).

But 'expert systems' are not infallible, any more than human specialists are. In general, AI programs are not foolproof systems guaranteed to reach the right answer, nor is their reasoning 'objective' in an absolute sense. *Any* finite intelligent system living in a complex and changing world would be liable to mistakes, for intelligence is a matter of making sensible decisions *without* having all the evidence. One can do this only on the basis of one's expectations, or previous knowledge – which will sometimes prove inadequate. Moreover, programs designed to answer similar questions will give different answers if they use different models, or representations, of the world (and of ways of reasoning about the world). These representations – like those inside human heads – can be more or less veridical, more or less sensible. They are subjective and questionable rather than objective and infallible. In principle, the conclusions of a computer program are open to challenge just as a person's are.

It is often remarked that 'a program can do only what the programmer tells it to do'. Certainly, everything the program does is done because of some instruction – either written by the programmer or generated by other instructions written by the programmer. But the chains of inference made by a program can be so complex that a human cannot follow them, and many programs can accept unforeseen information (from teletype, camera or microphone). Consequently, computers can surprise us. A complex program cannot be guaranteed to do *all* and *only* what the programmer had in mind when writing it. This is true even if there are no mistakes in the program.

This points a warning about the social impact of AI. Already there are large programs whose behaviour no one person fully understands. Quite apart from clear misuse (such as 'Big Brother' applications), there is a danger that human responsibility for decisions might be insidiously undermined. And some social effects of changes in employment patterns may be highly unfortunate, at least in the transitional phase.

But AI has a rehumanizing potential also. It could provide many useful tools, and do many boring, dirty or dangerous jobs. It could free our time for interacting with other people (family, friends and the clients of 'service industries'). It could lead to a greater valuation of emotional life, in contrast to the unemotionality of (most) programs. And it could even encourage an 'image of man' that is humanist rather than mechanist: already, it has confirmed the irrelevance of IQ-tests to the understanding of intelligence, and made *mind* respectable again after the arid years of behaviourism.

Margaret A. Boden
University of Sussex

Further Reading
Waltz, D. L. (1982), 'Artificial Intelligence', *Scientific American*, vol. 247.
Boden, M. A. (1977), *Artificial Intelligence and Natural Man*, New York.
Feigenbaum, E. A. and McCorduck, P. (1983), *The Fifth Generation*, Reading, Mass.
Feigenbaum, E. A. and Barr, A. (eds) (1981 and 1982), *The Artificial Intelligence Handbook*, 3 vols, London.
See also: *intelligence and intelligence testing; mind.*

Associationism
The concept of the association of ideas is as old as Aristotle, but its use as the basic framework for a complete account of mental life is essentially British, beginning with John Locke and ending with Alexander Bain. There were some near contemporary continental associationists and some Scottish philosophers who made considerable but subsidiary use of the concept. They were not as thoroughgoing, or perhaps as single-minded, as the group recognized as British Empiricists.

Locke, Berkeley and Hume used associationism to provide support for the empiricist epistemology they were developing in opposition to Descartes's basically rationalist view. They maintained that knowledge and belief derived from, and could only be justified by, reference to sensory experience, as distinct from the innate ideas and necessary truths argued for by Descartes. They also held that such sense-based experience could be divided into elementary units such as sensations (experiences brought about by the impact of external objects on the senses), images (re-evoked or remembered sensations) and feelings (affective values attached to sensations and images). This resort to atomistic elements was probably made in the belief that such experiences were incorrigible and hence beyond dispute; what I experience on one occasion is not corrected by what I experience on comparable occasions, even though the series may build up a web of experience. This web or set of patterned knowledge is built up as the separate ideas become associated or linked in synchronous groups or chronological chains.

British associationism reached its peak as a psychological system when a series of thinkers, David Hartley, James Mill, John Stuart Mill and Bain, concentrated on erecting a free-standing theory of mental life and not just a psychological foundation for an epistemology.

It is important to note the growing positivist sensationism of the three early philosophers. Locke had assumed a mind or self on which external objects made an impact through the senses; Berkeley accepted the mind or self but denied that we could have any direct knowledge of external objects (all we could directly know were our 'ideas'); Hume went further and claimed that the so-called mind or self was no more than the passage of our 'ideas'.

Hartley, a physician rather than a philosopher, tried to give sensations, images, feelings and their associations a neurophysiological basis. He suggested that the impact of external objects on the senses set up vibrations in the sensory nervous apparatus and that these were experienced as sensations. Images were the result of later minor vibrations, which he called 'vibratiuncles', induced by associated sensations or images. James Mill, an historian and political theorist, abandoned Hartley's premature and rather fantastic neurophysiology but developed the psychological thinking on more systematic and positivistic lines. His treatment was strictly atomistic and mechanical. John Stuart Mill and Alexander Bain softened these tendencies, arguing for 'mental compounds' in the chemical sense as well as for 'mental mixtures' in which the totality was no more than the sum of the associated elements.

There was much disagreement over the 'laws' or conditions of the association of 'ideas'. It was universally accepted that frequency and contiguity (two or more 'ideas' often occurring together or in close succession) constituted a basic condition, for example 'table' and 'chair' are said to be associated because these two 'ideas' are frequently experienced in conjunction. (Some modern learning theories would call this assumption into question.) In addition to this basic law, some associationists added one or more qualitative laws, such as the 'law of similarity' governing the association of 'dark' and 'black', the 'law of contrast' 'dark' and 'light', and the 'law of cause and effect', 'boiling' with sustained 'heat'. Bain added a 'law of effect' which claimed that an experience followed by another became associated if the latter satisfied a need related to the former; this was given a prominent place in later S-R learning theory.

Though claiming to be based on observation or sensory experience, British associationism was based largely on common sense and anecdotal evidence. Later, von Helmholtz, Wundt, Ebbinghaus, Kulpe, G. E. Muller and others developed experimental methods to provide a sounder empirical basis for somewhat revised associationist theorizing.

W. M. O'Neil
University of Sydney

Further Reading
Peters, R. S. (ed.) (1953), *Brett's History of Psychology*, London.

Attachment

Attachment refers to the tie between two or more individuals; it is a psychological relationship which is discriminating and specific and which bonds one to the other in space and over enduring periods of time. Researchers and clinicians have been particularly concerned with two types of attachment: parental attachment (which sadly, in the literature, usually means *maternal*) and infantile attachment.

It is widely agreed that the infants of many vertebrate species become psychologically attached to their parents; human babies first acquire an attachment to their mothers and (usually a little later) significant others during the second half of their first year of life.

Proximity seeking (for example, following) is commonly interpreted as an index of infant-to-parent attachment; other indicators include behaviour in 'strange situations' and activities such as differential smiling, crying and vocalization, as well as protest at separation. Multiple criteria are used to specify attachment phenomena because of individual differences in the way attachment is organized and manifested – differences that seem to be related to variations among mothers in their infant-care practices. Indeed, because the child's attachment system is, in a sense, the reciprocal of the parents', it may be preferable to speak of, say, the mother and young child as forming a single, superordinate attachment system. The delicate and complementary intermeshing of their respective, individual attachment repertoires is such that it is not possible to describe one fully without also describing the other.

There is little agreement on the nature of this powerful motivational process: a plethora of explanatory ideas have been put forward, in the name of learning theory (Gerwitz, 1972; Hoffman *et al.*, 1973), psychoanalysis (Freud, 1946) and ethology (Ainsworth, 1973; Bowlby, 1969). Bowlby – to take one example – sees attachment behaviour as the operation of an internal control system. Children are biologically predisposed to form attachments. It could be said that they are genetically programmed to respond to social situations and to display forms of behaviour (smiling, crying, clinging, and so on) from the beginning of life up to and beyond the point in time when they make a focused attachment to parental figures. What is new, then, when the infant becomes attached is not the display of new forms of behaviour or new intensities of social responses, but a pattern of organization of these responses in relation to one significant person. Virtually all the elements in the child's behaviour repertoire become capable of being functionally linked to a controlling system or plan, which is hierarchical in its organization and target-seeking in its effect. The 'target' is defined as the maintenance of proximity to the care-giver, and the hierarchical nature of the organization is revealed in the fact that a particular response can serve a number of different functions in maintaining this proximity.

Bowlby's conceptualization of attachment seems to offer fruitful ways of looking at the concept; it suggests new ways in which attachment systems can be compared. Instead of thinking of children as simply being more or less attached, their attachment systems can be compared according to the nature of the favoured strategies they employ, how strongly they are established, the degree of elaboration of alternative strategies, and the nature of their setting, that is, the closeness of the proximity they are set to maintain.

The preoccupation with the allegedly decisive influence of the mother on the infant's development, and the foundational significance of the first attachment has had salutary effects: highlighting the psychological needs of the young child and humanizing substitute child-care arrangements. The cost was a professional ideology, particularly rampant in the 1950s, whereby mothers were inculpated in the causation of psychopathology varying from infantile autism to juvenile delinquency. Rutter (1972), among others, has been instrumental in producing a more balanced view of the role of attachment and maternal care in the development of normal and abnormal behaviour.

Mother-to-infant attachment is usually referred to as maternal bonding. The widespread belief that in some mammalian species, including our own, mother-to-infant bonding occurs rapidly through mother-infant skin-to-skin contact during a short duration critical period after birth, has been challenged. The ethological support for the bonding doctrine, derived from early experiments with ewes and goats ('olfactory imprinting'), has not stood the test of time. Nor has evidence from human longitudinal studies comparing mothers who, after giving birth to a baby, have either been separated from it or have been allowed extended skin-to-skin contact with it, supported a 'sensitive' period, 'ethological' explanation. The impact of the doctrine upon the thinking of practitioners in obstetric, paediatric and social work fields has been considerable, particularly in relating bonding failures (allegedly due to early separation experiences) to serious problems such as child abuse. These clinical applications have also been challenged. It seems more likely that exposure learning, different forms of conditioning, imitation and cultural factors, all influence the development of mother-to-infant (and, indeed, father-to-infant) attachments and involve a process of learning gradually to love an infant more strongly – a process characterized by ups and downs, and one which is often associated with a variety of mixed feelings about the child.

Martin Herbert
University of Leicester

References

Ainsworth, M. D. S. (1973), 'The development of infant-mother attachment', in B. M. Caldwell and H. N. Ricciuti (eds), *Review of Child Development Research, Vol. III*, Chicago.

Bowlby, J. (1969), *Attachment and Loss*, Vol. I. *Attachment*, New York.

Freud, A. (1946), 'The psychoanalytic study of infantile feeding disturbances', *Psychoanalytic Study of the Child*, 2.

Gerwitz, J. L. (1972), 'Attachment, dependence, and a distinction in terms of stimulus control', in J. L. Gewirtz (ed.), *Attachment and Dependency*, Washington, D.C.

Hoffman, H. S. and Ratner, A. M. (1973), 'A reinforcement model of imprinting: implications for socialization in monkeys and men', *Psychological Review*, 80.

Rutter, M. (1972), *Maternal Deprivation Reassessed*, Harmondsworth.

Further Reading

Klaus, M. H. and Kennell, J. N. (1976), *Maternal Infant Bonding*, Saint Louis.

Rajecki, D. W., Lamb, M. E. and Obmascher, P. (1978), 'Toward a general theory of infantile attachment: a comparative review of aspects of the social bond', *The Behavioural and Brain Sciences*, 3.

Sluckin, W., Herbert, M. and Sluckin, A. (1983), *Maternal Bonding*, Oxford.

See also: *Bowlby; separation and loss.*

Attention

All behaviour is a matter of selecting a particular course of action among many alternatives. In experimental psychology, many different aspects of this selectivity are studied under the heading of 'attention'.

Perhaps the most characteristic example concerns the limit on how much we can see, hear or do at one time. The driver of a car may stop speaking when the demands of the traffic situation increase. A student daydreaming in a lecture may 'wake up' to discover he has taken no notes. Difficulties in doing several things at once, and the associated need to select between competing alternatives ('paying attention'), were already under experimental study in the nineteenth century. Helmholtz showed that if a page of text is briefly illuminated in a dark room, it may be impossible to read more than a small part, but possible to choose *which* part at will (and without moving the eyes). The publication of Broadbent's *Perception and Communication* in 1958 established selective perception of this type as a core topic in the modern development of 'information processing' psychology.

Some workers propose that limits on our ability to do several things at once reflect the existence of a unique psychological resource, limited in supply and called upon (to various extents) by all the different activities we can perform: listening to a conversation, playing the piano, solving a puzzle, and so on. Doing two things at once causes trouble if the total resource demand exceeds the total supply. Connections are often made between the 'attentional' resource and consciousness, since there seem definite limits to the number of things we can be conscious of at one time. A frequent idea is that well-practised activities may require rather little of this resource, in line with the experience that they are sometimes performed unconsciously and with little disturbing influence on whatever else we are doing.

Others take a different view. Many different psychological operations are involved in the control of behaviour: orientation of receptors towards chosen objects; perceptual recognition of visual, auditory and tactile patterns; operations performed upon spatial, verbal and other internal representations; control of speech and other movements, and so on. Such processes are separable in several senses. For example, they may take place in different anatomical areas of the brain. A strong possibility, among the multiplicity of psychological operations involved in the multiplicity of different actions we can perform, is that there are many different ways in which simultaneous tasks can interfere and interact with one another. Thus there may be many different reasons for our limited ability to do several things at once.

Other aspects of selectivity have different bases. A thing may not be done because there are better alternatives for the purpose at hand, because the person is drunk, sleepy or bored, and so on. Though these different aspects of selectivity may all be studied under the heading of attention, it is of course questionable how much they have in common. Sometimes when we say that a person 'paid attention' to one thing and not to another, we mean little more than that, for whatever reason, one thing was done while the other was not. As a whole, experimental psychology attempts to understand the underlying process in the selection of appropriate activity.

John Duncan
MRC Applied Psychology Unit,
Cambridge

Reference
Broadbent, D. E. (1958), *Perception and Communication*, London.

Further Reading
Allport, D. A. (1980), 'Attention and performance', in G.
    Claxton (ed.), *Cognitive Psychology: New Directions*, London.
Kahneman, D. (1973), *Attention and Effort*, Englewood Cliffs,
    N.J.
See also: *sensation and perception*.

Attitudes

In a classic article published nearly fifty years ago, Gordon
Allport (1935) contended that the attitude concept was 'the
most distinctive and indispensable concept in contemporary
social psychology'. While this confident assertion may perhaps
be more debatable in the 1980s, the study of attitudes continues
to occupy the attention of many researchers.

Attitudes are predominantly a matter of affective evaluation.
They represent the evaluations (positive or negative) that we
associate with diverse entities, for example, individuals, groups,
objects, actions and institutions. Attitudes are typically assessed
through a direct inquiry procedure in which respondents are
essentially asked to indicate their evaluative reaction (like-
dislike, and so on) to something or someone. A number of
indirect (disguised) measurement procedures have also been
developed (Kidder and Campbell, 1970), but these are sometimes difficult to apply and have not been widely utilized.

Some theorists contend that attitudes should not be defined
solely in affective (or evaluative) terms, suggesting instead that
attitudes are normally found in combination with 'related'
cognitive and behavioural components. Thus, people who *like*
unions will usually hold characteristic beliefs; they may believe,
for example, that union activities have often been treated
unfairly in the press. In addition, people with pro-union attitudes will often *act* accordingly, by joining a union, or by
purchasing union goods in preference to those produced by non-
unionized labour. Despite the plausibility of these assertions,
however, they have not gone unchallenged; in particular, the

relationship between attitudes and behaviour has often proven to be weak or nonexistent.

Rather than defining attitudes such that associated beliefs and behaviours are included as essential components (by definition), contemporary researchers have preferred to focus on the evaluative aspect of attitudes, to judge from the assessment procedures they have developed, and have gone on to study *empirically* (1) the relationship between attitudes and beliefs, and (2) the relationship between attitudes and behaviour.

(1) *Attitudes and beliefs.* A commonsensical approach suggests that our attitudes, pro or con, derive from our beliefs. For example, if we learn that a newly-opened store offers excellent service, superior goods and low prices, we are likely to evaluate it positively. Advertising campaigns are often based on an implicit model of this type; they may attempt to change our beliefs about a product or institution by telling us of the good qualities it possesses, in the hope that this will ultimately influence our attitudes and buying behaviour.

While it is clear that attitudes can be influenced by changes in belief (as outlined above), there is also evidence for the reverse proposition. That is, attitudes may not only be influenced by beliefs, but they may also contribute to the things that we believe (Rosenberg *et al.*, 1960). In one study, for example, respondents were led (through direct post-hypnotic suggestion) to accept a new position with respect to foreign aid. Subsequent inquiry indicated that these hypnotically-induced attitudes were accompanied by a spontaneous acceptance of new beliefs that had not been mentioned during the induction procedure, beliefs that were supportive of the respondents' new views. Other studies suggest that attitudes may also play a type of filtering role, influencing the extent to which we accept new information that bears on the validity of our attitudes (Lord, Ross and Lepper, 1979).

(2) *Attitudes and behaviour.* Attitudes are generally thought to influence behaviour. People who favour a given candidate or political position are expected to vote for that person, or to provide other concrete support (for example, in the form of donations), in contrast to those who hold relatively negative

views. Despite the seeming obviousness of this proposition, however, many studies have found only weak, unreliable relations between attitudes and everyday behaviour. Part of the difficulty here derives from the fact that behaviour is often dependent on situational factors that may override the influence of the individual's preferences. Despite the fact that someone holds extremely positive views towards organized religion, he may nonetheless be unresponsive to requests for financial donations to his church if he has recently lost his job. Similarly, a hotel clerk may override his personal prejudices and politely serve patrons of diverse ethnic origins, if this is what his job requires. On the other hand, there is now persuasive evidence that attitudes may be more substantially associated with everyday actions if we take a broader view of behaviour, tracking the individual's reactions in a wide range of settings rather than just one. For example, although religious attitudes (positive-negative) may be weakly associated with financial contributions to the church, a more clearcut linkage between religious attitudes and religious behaviour may be observed if a composite behavioural index is employed, one that takes account of such matters as weekly religious observance, observance during holiday celebrations, saying Grace before meals, and so on (Fishbein and Ajzen, 1974). Attitudes may also be effectively related to overt actions if they are action-oriented and are measured with appropriate specificity. Thus, church donations may be related to people's attitudes toward the concrete act of 'donating to the church', as contrasted with their general attitude towards 'organized religion'.

One of the most firmly established phenomena in contemporary attitude research is the fact that behaviours may have a causal impact on attitudes, rather than simply reflecting the actor's previously-held views. This proposition has been supported in a wide range of experiments. In a classic study by Festinger and Carlsmith (1959), some respondents were led to describe a certain laboratory activity as 'interesting', despite the fact that they actually regarded it as rather dull. People who had enacted this form of counter-attitudinal behaviour for a modest (one-dollar) incentive subsequently rated the dull laboratory task in relatively favourable terms, compared to those who had not been required to produce counter-attitudinal statements. Other researchers have employed a procedure in which a person who was supposed to be 'teaching' something to another, seemingly punished the learner with electric shocks whenever he made an error. Subsequent inquiry revealed that people who had served as 'teachers' in this type of situation became increasingly negative to their 'pupils' as a consequence.

The continuing vitality of the attitude construct may derive, in part, from the seemingly universal importance of evaluation (Osgood, 1964). We are apparently disposed to respond evaluatively to the people, objects, events and institutions that we encounter. These evaluative (attitudinal) reactions, their origins, correlates and consequences, continue to constitute a fertile domain for academic and applied research.

Melvin Manis
University of Michigan and
Ann Arbor Veterans Administration Medical Center

References

Allport, G. W. (1935), 'Attitudes', in C. Murchison (ed.), *A Handbook of Social Psychology*, Worcester, Mass.

Festinger, L. and Carlsmith, J. M. (1959), 'Cognitive consequences of forced compliance', *Journal of Abnormal and Social Psychology*, 58.

Fishbein, M. and Ajzen, I. (1974), 'Attitudes toward objects as predictive of single and multiple behavioral criteria', *Psychological Review*, 81.

Kidder, L. H. and Campbell, D. T. (1970), 'The indirect testing of social attitude', in G. I. Summers (ed.), *Attitude Measurement*, Chicago.

Lord, C. G., Ross, L. and Lepper, M. R. (1979), 'Biased assimilation and attitude polarization: the effects of prior theories in subsequently considered evidence', *Journal of Personality and Social Psychology*, 37.

Osgood, C. E. (1964), 'Semantic differential technique in the comparative study of cultures', *American Psychologist*, 66.

Rosenberg, M. J., Hovland, C. I., McGuire, W. J., Abelson, R. P. and Brehm, J. W. (1960), *Attitude Organization and Change*, New Haven.

Further Reading

Petty, R. E. and Cacioppo, J. T. (1981), *Attitudes and Persuasion: Classical and Contemporary Approaches*, Dubuque, Iowa.

McGuire, W. J. (1969), 'The nature of attitudes and attitude change', in *The Handbook of Social Psychology*, 2nd edn, vol. 3, Reading, Mass.

See also: *authoritarianism and the authoritarian personality; cognitive dissonance; prejudice; semantic differential.*

Attribution Theory

Attribution theory is concerned with the study of perceived causation. All developments of this theory stem from Heider's influential work (Heider, 1958) in which he proposed that naive explanations of behaviour distinguish between personal (dispositional) and impersonal (situational) causes, a distinction that has been a central theme in subsequent theorizing.

Early developments of attribution theory emphasized the rational and exhaustive nature of attribution processes. Jones and Davis's (1965) theory of correspondent inferences specified when dispositional or personal attributions will be made: when observed behaviour is considered intentional and corresponds to the inferred disposition, particularly those behaviours which result in distinctive and socially undesirable outcomes. Kelley (1967) proposed that attributions are governed by the principle of covariation: an effect will be attributed to personal or impersonal factors depending on with which of these factors it covaries.

More recently, irrational biases in attribution have been emphasized. Jones and Nisbett (1971) noted the tendency for actors to attribute their behaviour to situational factors, whereas observers attribute behaviour to dispositional factors. For example, if I trip over the cat, it is because the cat got in the way, but if someone else does it is because that person is clumsy. Ross (1977) has proposed a more basic bias, the fundamental attribution error, which refers to the pervasive tendency for people to explain behaviour in dispositional terms, underestimating the importance of situational factors.

The enthusiasm for documenting the naive psychologist's attribution errors rather than accuracies might seem misplaced, but biases in attribution are believed to be evidence of the useful short cuts in human thinking which usually help make people such efficient information processors.

Sarah E. Hampson
Oregon Research Institute

References
Heider, F. (1958), *The Psychology of Interpersonal Relations*, New York.
Jones, E. E. and Davis, E. E. (1965), 'From acts to dispositions: the attribution process in person perception', in L. Berkowitz (ed.), *Advances in Experimental Social Psychology*, Vol. 2, New York.
Jones, E. E. and Nisbett, R. E. (1971), *The Actor and the Observer: Divergent Perceptions of the Causes of Behavior*, Morristown, N.J.
Kelley, H. H. (1967), 'Attribution theory in social psychology', in L. Berkowitz (ed.), *Advances in Experimental Social Psychology*, Vol. 10, New York.
Ross, L. (1977), 'The intuitive psychologist and his shortcomings: distortions in the attribution process', in L. Berkowitz (ed.), *Advances in Experimental Social Psychology*, Vol. 10, New York.

Further Reading
Harvey, J. H., Ickes, W. and Kidd, R. E. (eds) (1981), *New Directions in Attribution Research*, Vol. 3, Hillsdale, N.J.
See also: *personal construct theory*.

Authoritarianism and the Authoritarian Personality

Soon after the end of the Second World War, a group of social scientists in the US, under the leadership of T. W. Adorno, sought to identify the factors giving rise to anti-Semitism. They hoped that by identifying the causes, they would be in a position to prevent a repetition of the holocaust. Their research led to the publication of the now classic volume, *The Authoritarian Personality* (Adorno *et al.*, 1950). They viewed the concept of authoritarianism as consisting of the following (Sanford, 1956):

(1) Conventionalism: rigid adherence to conventional middle-class values.

(2) Authoritarian Submission: submissive, uncritical attitude toward idealized moral authorities of the in-group.

(3) Authoritarian Aggression: tendency to be on the look out for, and to condemn, reject and punish people who violate conventional values.

(4) Anti-intraception: opposition to the subjective, the imaginative, the tenderminded.

(5) Superstition and Stereotypy: belief in mystical determinants of the individual's fate; the disposition to think in rigid categories.

(6) Power and Toughness: preoccupation with the dominance-submission, strong-weak, leader-follower dimension; identification with power figures; exaggerated assertions of strength and toughness.

(7) Destructiveness and Cynicism: generalized hostility, vilification of the human.

(8) Projectivity: disposition to believe that wild and dangerous things go on in the world; the projection outward of unconscious emotional impulses.

(9) Sex: ego-alien sexuality; exaggerated concern with sexual 'goings on', and punitiveness toward violators of sexual mores.

The publication of *The Authoritarian Personality* generated voluminous social psychological research, which mainly supported the view that authoritarians are raised in homes characterized by strict discipline. Their parents typically endeavour to keep them subordinate, conforming, and dependent, and in later life these same children manifest conservative, domineering, rigid and prejudiced attitudes.

Some research has been critical of *The Authoritarian Personality*

(Christie and Jahoda, 1954). Doubts were expressed concerning the validity and reliability of the primary measuring instrument (the F scale). It was noted that the F scale elicits in the respondent the tendency to agree with the items regardless of content (this refers to acquiescence). Perhaps most important of all, it was shown that the F scale was unable to predict actual authoritarian *behaviour*. As such, it is little more than a measure of *attitudes*. If social psychology is to contribute to explaining human behaviour, our measuring instruments must be able to predict the behaviour we are seeking to explain.

More recently Ray (1976) developed the Directiveness Scale, which is well able to predict dominant behaviour, a key characteristic of authoritarianism. Ray's scale is regarded as a starting point for the construction of a behaviour inventory encompassing not only dominance, but rather all aspects of authoritarianism.

Patrick C. L. Heaven
Riverina College, Australia

References
Adorno, T. W., Frenkel-Brunswik, E., Levinson, D. J. and Sanford, N. (1950), *The Authoritarian Personality*, New York.
Christie, R. and Jahoda, M. (1954), *Studies in the Scope and Method of 'The Authoritarian Personality'*, Glencoe, Ill.
Ray, J. J. (1976), 'Do authoritarians hold authoritarian attitudes?', *Human Relations*, 29.
Sanford, N. (1956), 'The approach of the authoritarian personality', in J. L. McCary (ed.), *Psychology of Personality: Six Modern Approaches*, New York.

Further Reading
Altemeyer, B. (1982), *Right-Wing Authoritarianism*, Winnipeg.
See also: *attitudes; prejudice*.

Autism

In psychiatry generally, the term autism refers to apparent withdrawal from the outside world, self-absorption, and lack of communication with others. In childhood, the syndrome of autism is a severely incapacitating developmental disability which appears prior to thirty months of age. It occurs in approximately five out of every 100,000 births and is four times more common in boys than in girls. It has been found throughout the world in families of all racial, ethnic and social backgrounds. No known factors in the psychological environment of a child have been shown to cause autism.

The symptoms, expressive of neuropathology, include:
(1) Disturbances in the rate of appearance of physical, social and language skills.
(2) Abnormal responses to sensations. Any one or a combination of sight, hearing, touch, pain, balance, smell, taste, and the way a child holds his body are affected.
(3) Speech and language are absent or delayed, while specific thinking capabilities may be present. Immature rhythms of speech, limited understanding of ideas, and the use of words without attaching the usual meaning to them are common.
(4) Abnormal ways of relating to people, objects and events.

Autism occurs by itself or in association with other disorders which affect the function of the brain, such as viral infections, metabolic disturbances (PKU), epilepsy, and Fragile X syndrome. On IQ testing of autistic people, approximately 60 per cent have scores below 50, 20 per cent between 50 and 70, and only 20 per cent greater than 70. Most show wide variations of performance on different tests and at different times. Autistic people live a normal life span. Since symptoms change, and some disappear with age, periodic re-evaluations are necessary to respond to changing needs. Multiple incidences in a family are common. The severe form of the syndrome may include the most extreme forms of self-injurious, repetitive, highly unusual and aggressive behaviours. Such behaviours may be persistent and highly resistant to change, often requiring unique management, treatment or teaching strategies.

Special education programmes using behavioural methods and designed for specific individuals have been shown to be most helpful. Psychotropic medication may be used to reduce temporarily injurious behaviour. Supportive counselling may help families with autistic members, just as it helps families who have members with other severe permanent disabilities.

Edward R. Ritvo
University of California,
Los Angeles

Further Reading
Ritvo, E. R. (ed.) (1976), *Autism, Current Research and Management*, New York.
Ritvo, E. R. and Freeman, B. J. (1978), 'National Society for Autistic Children definition of the syndrome of autism', *Journal of the American Academy of Child Psychiatry*, 17.

Aversion Therapy

Aversion therapy is an attempt by a clinician to suppress undesirable behaviour by punishing it with unpleasant (aversive) stimulation. Punishment, of course, is also delivered by the natural environment (as in the painful consequences of falling or touching hot objects) and in other social contexts (as in a schoolmaster's use of caning or a mother's painting a bitter substance on her child's hands to inhibit nail-biting or thumb-sucking). But random and arbitrary punishments are not aversion therapy, and the result of such punishments is often paradoxical. In aversion therapy, a trained clinician designs a treatment protocol based on the needs and particular behavioural problem of an individual patient.

Like other behaviour therapy techniques, aversion therapy has ancient antecedents but derives its scientific rationale and some of its technical principles from the experimental psychology of learning. Nonetheless, leading authorities on learning (notably E. L. Thorndike, J. B. Watson and B. F. Skinner) have thought that positive reinforcement would be more effective, and that aversive techniques would have only temporary effects that would not generalize beyond the treatment setting. Subsequent research has shown that the duration of effect can be increased by simultaneously rewarding desired behaviours and through 'booster sessions', and that generalization can be increased by having multiple therapists deliver the aversive stimulation in multiple settings.

The delivery of unpleasant stimulation distinguishes aversion therapy from those punishment techniques that remove a reward, such as 'timeout' (removal to a less rewarding setting) or 'response cost' (removal of money, tokens, points or other sources of pleasure). Aversive stimuli that have been used clinically include reprimands (expressions of disapproval), tastes (for example, concentrated lemon juice, pepper sauce or shaving cream), odours (aromatic ammonia and so on), sounds (loud noises of interrupted music), sights (light, flashes of interrupted television), tactile sensations (tickling, hand-slapping, snaps with a rubber band, spanking or electric shock), and more generalized discomfort (forced exercise, drug-induced nausea and vomiting, or even paralysis with neuromuscular blocking agents). When the form of aversive stimulation is unpleasant mental imagery, the technique is known as covert sensitization.

Many studies have shown that aversion therapy can produce complete suppression of a behaviour. It has been used with partial or apparently complete success in the treatment of tics, bruxism, stuttering, bedwetting, rumination of vomitus, smoking, alcoholism, obsessive thoughts, fetishism, sexual masochism, transvestism, exhibitionism and homosexuality, as well as in treating self-injurious, aggressive and other behaviour problems among autistic children and among schizophrenic and mentally retarded individuals.

There have also been untoward side effects, for example, with children, expressions of fear or distress, emergence of, or increases in, other undesirable behaviours, suppression of desirable behaviours, and increases in the target behaviour in settings where it is unpunished. In general, adverse reactions have occurred when insufficient attention has been given to rewarding desired behaviour; these reactions have been of brief duration and are quickly responsive to treatment.

Inappropriate, excessive or capricious administration of aversive stimulation has led to scandals, lawsuits and prohibitions. Documented abuses and fear-arousing portrayals (as in Stanley Kubrick's film, *A Clockwork Orange*) have rendered aversion therapy highly controversial and have also fuelled the public's fear of non-aversive behaviour therapies and of electro-convulsive therapy (ECT), which some lay people mistake for an aversive technique.

As with other powerful treatments, a judicious decision to use aversion therapy should take into consideration the possible alternative treatments, the documented effectiveness and risk of the proposed technique for the purpose, the degree of pain or discomfort the treatment would entail, the danger of the target behaviour to the patient (and, in some situations, to others), the ability and freedom of the patient to consent knowingly to this treatment and to terminate its use, and the availability of safeguards against abuse. With incompetent patients and in residential institutions, it is essential that the treatment plan be reviewed, both by other clinicians and by an independent human rights committee, and that the treatment process be monitored continually

Park Elliott Dietz
University of Virginia

Further Reading
Axelrod, S. and Apsche, J. (eds) (1983), *The Effects of Punishment on Human Behavior*, New York.
Rachman, S. and Teasdale, J. (1969), *Aversion Therapy and Behavior Disorders: An Analysis*, Coral Gables, Florida.

Behaviourism
Behaviourism is mainly a twentieth-century orientation within the discipline of psychology in the United States. The behavioural approach emphasizes the objective study of the relationships between environmental manipulations and human and animal behaviour change, usually in laboratory or relatively controlled institutional settings. Emerging as a discrete movement just prior to World War I, behaviourism represented a vigorous rejection of psychology defined as the introspective study of the human mind and consciousness. Early behaviou-

rists eschewed the structuralism of Wundt and Titchener, the functional mentalism of James, Dewey, Angell and Carr, and the relativism and phenomenology of Gestalt psychology.

John B. Watson is credited with declaring behaviourism a new movement in 1913; but the foundations of the development extend back to the ancient Greeks and include empiricism, elementism, associationism, objectivism and naturalism. The direct antecedents of behaviourism during the late nineteenth and early twentieth centuries were: the studies of animal behaviour and the functional orientation inspired by Darwin's theory of evolution; the conditioning research of Russian physiologists Ivan Pavlov and Vladimir Bekhterev emphasizing stimulus substitution in the context of reflexive behaviour; and the puzzle box studies of American psychologist Edward Thorndike concerned with the effects of the consequences of behaviour on response frequency. The two predominant and often competing theoretical-procedural models of conditioning research have been classical conditioning derived from the work of Pavlov and Bekhterev, and Skinner's operant conditioning.

While it is generally claimed that behaviourism as a distinct school ceased to exist by the 1950s, behaviourism as a general orientation has gone through the following overlapping periods: classical behaviourism (1900–25), represented by the work of Thorndike and Watson; neo-behaviourism (1920s–40s), an exciting time when the theories of Clark Hull, Edward Tolman, Edwin Guthrie and Burrhus F. Skinner competed for pre-eminence; Hullian behaviourism (1940s–50s) when Hull's complex hypothetico-deductive behaviour theory appeared most promising; Skinnerian behaviourism (1960s–mid-1970s) during which time operant conditioning techniques, emphasizing the control of behaviour implicit in the consequences of behaviour, afforded the most powerful methodologies; and finally cognitive behaviourism (1975–present) when the limits of a purely Skinnerian approach to behaviour change became increasingly apparent, and cognitive perspectives, such as social learning theories, seemed necessary to account for behaviour change.

A behavioural orientation has been central to twentieth-century psychology in the United States primarily because of a strong faith in laboratory research and experimental methodologies; an interest in studying the process of learning; a preference for quantitative information; the elimination from the discipline of ambiguous concepts and investigations of complex and therefore difficult to describe private (subjective) experiences; and, since the late 1950s, a very conservative approach to theory building.

While each of the major behavioural programmes from Thorndike's to Skinner's failed to provide a comprehensive account of behaviour change, the behavioural orientation has led to the development of behaviour-control methodologies with useful application in most areas of psychology. In addition, the movement has inspired precision and accountability in psychological inquiry.

Behavioural methodologies have, of course, been employed by psychologists in countries other than the United States, particularly those with strong scientific traditions such as Britain and Japan. Behavioural assumptions have also influenced other social sciences, especially sociology and political science. But because laboratory animal research is central to the behavioural orientation, behaviourism as a major movement only developed in psychology.

Albert R. Gilgen
University of Northern Iowa

Further Reading
Marx, M. H. and Hillix, W. A. (1979), *Systems and Theories in Psychology*, New York.
See also: *behaviour therapy; cognitive-behavioural therapy; conditioning, classical and operant; Hull; Pavlov; Skinner; Watson.*

Behaviour Therapy

The movement that has come to be known as behaviour therapy (or behaviour modification) arose shortly after the end of World War II, having its origins independently in the United States,

Britain and South Africa. In Britain, behaviour therapy developed mainly out of dissatisfaction with the traditional role of the clinical psychologist who worked within a medical model which likened 'mental disease' to 'bodily disease', except that the former was a disease of the mind rather than the body. There was also dissatisfaction with the psychodynamic approach that viewed patients' symptoms as indicators of some underlying conflict requiring for their resolution in-depth analysis, and with the diagnostic (testing) approach resulting in patients being labelled, but without any obvious consequent implications for therapy.

To replace these traditional approaches, it was proposed that psychologists make use of the entire body of knowledge and theory that constituted psychology as a scientific discipline and in which only the psychologist was an expert. In practice, the aim was to be achieved by stressing experimental investigation of the single case (that is, the presenting patient), in which the precise nature of the patient's problem was to be elucidated by systematic investigations. Behaviour therapy was simply the extension of this method to attempts to modify the maladaptive behaviour by similar controlled experimental procedures. In the United States, behaviour therapy developed mainly out of the efforts to apply the principles of operant conditioning to the description and control of human behaviour, especially, in its early stages, the bizarre behaviours of psychotics. In South Africa, the impetus for behaviour therapy came largely from the work of Wolpe. His reciprocal inhibition theory, developed from studies of animal neuroses, underlay the technique of systematic desensitization which was applied to the treatment of phobias with great success, and served more than anything else to bring behaviour therapy to notice as a significant new way of approaching the therapy of maladaptive behaviours.

Between 1950 and 1970 behaviour therapy developed rapidly, its achievements being critically reviewed in three simultaneous publications (Bandura, 1969; Franks, 1969; Yates, 1970). Although Eysenck's definition of behaviour therapy as 'the attempt to alter human behaviour and emotion in a beneficial manner according to the laws of modern learning theory'

(Eysenck, 1964) has been very widely accepted, Yates (1970) has stressed that behaviour therapy is a much broader endeavour than Eysenck's definition suggests, since, in principle, the whole body of the knowledge and theory that constitutes psychology is available to the behaviour therapist when dealing with a presenting patient. But for some behaviour therapists, the development of techniques that 'work' is more important than the use of theory and the experimental method, even though the best-known technique of all (Wolpe's systematic desensitization) was based on specific theoretical considerations. Justification for a technique-oriented approach, however, stems in part from the demonstration that flooding, a technique directly contradicting Wolpe's theory, appears to be as effective as systematic desensitization in the therapy of phobias. There are few other standard techniques available, one notable successful example being the bell-and-pad method of treating enuresis (bedwetting).

The rapid growth of behaviour therapy has led to its application to a far wider range of problems than could earlier have been envisaged (Yates, 1981). In its early stages behaviour therapy was mainly concerned with the investigation of individuals, either alone or in hospital settings. Now it is widely used by professional social workers, in marital therapy, in the design of social communities, in crime prevention and the treatment of criminals, to name but a few areas. The approach has been utilized in the control of littering, energy consumption and refuse disposal; in community aid to the disadvantaged (such as persuading low-income parents to have their children accept dental care). A good indication of the vastly expanded range of behaviour therapy can be gained by perusing successive volumes of the *Journal of Applied Behavior Analysis* (1968+), *Progress in Behavior Modification* (1975+) and the *Annual Review of Behavior Therapy* (1969+).

An important development over the past ten years has been the attempt to reconcile behaviour therapy with psychodynamic psychotherapy and even to integrate them. Yates (1970) had argued that the two approaches differed so fundamentally in their theories about the genesis and maintenance of abnormalities of behaviour that any reconciliation and integration was impossible. However, such moves had started as early as 1966 and by 1980 had achieved considerable progress (Yates, 1983). The strength of the movement is indicated by the appearance of a symposium in *Behavior Therapy* (1982, 13: articles by Kendall, Goldfried, Wachtel and Garfield). While admitting the strength of the evidence in favour of a reconciliation and integration, a fundamental difficulty remains, namely, the relationship between theory and therapy which makes it difficult, if not impossible, for agreement to be reached on the appropriate therapy for disorders such as enuresis and stuttering; this consequently undermines the apparent integration achieved in relation to more complex disorders such as anxiety (Yates, 1983).

Behaviour therapy has become as prominent an approach to the explanation and treatment of disorders of behaviour in the second half of this century as psychoanalysis was in the first half. There seems no doubt that it has fundamentally and irrevocably altered the framework within which disorders of behaviour are viewed. Its greatest virtue is perhaps its relative open-endedness and therefore its capacity for change and self-correction in the light of empirical evidence. It seems unlikely that it will suffer the fate of many of its predecessors, which became prematurely frozen within a rigid conceptual and methodological framework.

Aubrey J. Yates
University of Western Australia

References
Bandura, A. (1969), *Principles of Behavior Modification*, New York.
Eysenck, H. J. (1964), 'The nature of behaviour therapy', in H. J. Eysenck (ed.), *Experiments in Behaviour Therapy*, London.
Franks, C. (1969), *Behavior Therapy: Appraisal and Status*, New York.
Yates, A. J. (1970), *Behavior Therapy*, New York.

Yates, A. J. (1981), 'Behaviour therapy: past, present, future
    – imperfect?', *Clinical Psychology Review*, 1.
Yates, A. J. (1983), 'Behaviour therapy and psychodynamic
    psychotherapy: basic conflict or reconciliation and
    integration?', *British Journal of Clinical Psychology*, 22.

Further Reading
Kazdin, A. E. (1978), *History of Behavior Modification:
    Experimental Foundations of Contemporary Research*, Baltimore.
Wachtel, P. L. (1977), *Psychoanalysis and Behavior Therapy:
    Toward an Integration*, New York.
Wolpe, J. (1958), *Psychotherapy by Reciprocal Inhibition*, Stanford.
See also: *aversion therapy; behaviourism; cognitive-behavioural
    therapy; conditioning, classical and operant.*

Bereavement

The term bereavement covers any situation in which people
experience the loss of an object to which they were attached.
In a narrow sense it is taken to refer to the loss by death of a
loved person, but in its wider sense can cover many other losses.

Bereavement includes grief, the psychological reaction of the
individual, and mourning, the social expression of grief
(although this term has also been ambiguously used for the
process of grieving).

Burton's claim that grief is 'the model, epitome and chief
cause of melancholia' (1621) is echoed in Freud's classical
paper, 'Mourning and melancholia' (1917), but it was Lindemann's study of 101 bereaved people that gave rise to the
first, and arguably the best, systematic description of 'The
symptomatology and management of acute grief' (1944). More
recently, John Bowlby (1980) and sociologist Peter Marris
(1974) have classified the nature of grief and the central place
which it must play in our understanding of the human reaction
to social change.

Grief is a process of psychological change through which the
individual tends to pass from (1) a phase of numbness or dis-
belief, to (2) pining and yearning for the lost object, to
(3) disorganization and despair, and followed by (4) a phase

of reorganization and recovery. These phases are not clear-cut and the griever moves back and forth across them as each reminder of the loss evokes another pang of grief (Bowlby and Parkes, 1970).

During this process the individual can be seen as engaging in a struggle between competing motivations:

(a) to search for and recover the lost object;

(b) to find some way of minimizing or avoiding the pain of grief;

(c) to revise and relearn basic assumptions about the world that have been invalidated by the loss.

How these competing urges are expressed depends upon a wide range of individual and social factors, hence the confusing diversity of the manifestations of mourning reported by anthropologists (Rosenblatt *et al.*, 1976). Nevertheless, a common pattern can be discerned and has given rise to ritual observances which often seem to provide social support and a frame of reference for the bereaved, a *rite de passage*.

Because grief is so painful and because some patterns of grieving are more painful than others, it is not surprising to find that many bereaved people come to regard themselves, and to be regarded by others, as sick. While there may be some justification for regarding certain complications of grieving as pathological, the wholesale medicalization of mourning has created fresh problems for the mourner. Some bereaved people readily use alcohol or medically-prescribed drugs in order to suppress the 'symptoms' of grief and cling to mourning as a 'sick role'.

The breakdown in developed countries of extended family networks, together with disillusionment with the belief systems and loss of many of the rituals attending bereavement, has added to the plight of the bereaved, as has the increased mechanization and alienation of our systems of medical care which effectively remove the dying person from his family and deprive the family of the opportunity to care. Consequently, grief is often complicated by bewilderment, avoidance, anger and guilt. But the pendulum is now swinging, with the emergence of hospices, bereavement counselling, self-help (or mutual help) groups and a resurgence of neighbourhood and family support for the bereaved.

Colin Murray Parkes
The London Hospital Medical School
University of London

References
Bowlby, J. (1980), *Loss: Sadness and Depression*, vol. III of *Attachment and Loss*, London.
Bowlby, J. and Parkes, C. M. (eds) (1970), 'Separation and loss', in E. J. Anthony and C. Koupernik (eds), *The Child in his Family*, vol. I, New York.
Lindemann, E. (1944), 'The symptomatology and management of acute grief', *American Journal of Psychiatry*, 101.
Marris, P. (1974), *Loss and Change*, London.
Rosenblatt, P. C., Walsh, R. P. and Jackson, D. A. (1976), *Grief and Mourning in Cross-Cultural Perspective*, New Haven.

Further Reading
Parkes, C. M. (1972), *Bereavement: Studies of Grief in Adult Life*, London.
See also: *attachment; Bowlby; separation and loss*.

Biological Psychiatry

The long history of psychiatry reflects a constant conflict between philosophical idealism, with its insistence on the primacy of ideas, and materialism, with its emphasis on the biological substrate. In the US a psychological approach – notably in the form of psychoanalysis – was dominant in the 1940s. A counter movement developed to restore the medical, and especially neurological, dimensions of psychiatry. It called itself biological psychiatry, and its basic assumption was that the psychoses reflected actual derangements of brain function, and should be studied and treated by neurological as well as psychological means. The movement was initiated by Johannes Maargaard Nielsen, a Los Angeles neurologist, who founded a

Society of Biological Psychiatry in 1946. Though a behavioural scientist like the late Horsley Gantt, a pupil of Pavlov, was a president of the American Society of Biological Psychiatry, that society tended to focus on physiological research and paid relatively little attention to the more general scientific study of behaviour. This has perpetuated and reinforced the notion that biological psychiatry is limited to physiology, but its development has served to stimulate the use of scientific and experimental methods in psychiatric research, and has fostered a preference for systematic data collection and analysis over the use of anecdotal case histories and appeals to unvalidated theories.

Shock treatment. The physiological approach to psychiatric disorder received enormous impetus with the promulgation of the insulin shock treatment of schizophrenia by Manfred Sakel in the 1930s. Sakel, a general physician, had observed that deep insulin coma (due to low blood sugar), if terminated promptly, had a beneficial effect on some forms of psychotic excitement. He then elaborated a systematic application of the principle for the treatment of schizophrenia, with the sponsorship and support of Professor Poetzl of the University of Vienna. Since it was the first effective treatment of schizophrenia, and the most significant advance in psychiatry since the discovery of the fever treatment of general paresis by Wagner-Jauregg, it won wide acclaim. Sakel was invited to the US where he resided until his death in 1957 (Wortis, 1959).

In spite of the initial resistance of the psychiatric establishment, insulin treatment was almost universally accepted, and paved the way for the next big discovery, Meduna's convulsive treatment. Like insulin shock, this treatment was based mainly on empirical observation, and its mode of action, as with insulin shock, is still not understood. Initially Meduna induced convulsions by injection of stimulants, but this was soon superseded by the use of an electrical stimulus applied to the scalp. The term 'shock' was used in connection with the insulin treatment because the occurrence of unconsciousness from insulin overdosage was regarded as a dangerous complication in the treatment of diabetics, and the warning word seemed appropriate. Later, the use of a brief electric stimulus to induce a fit was also called a shock, but the term, however, has unfortunately been unduly alarming, since in neither of these treatments does the patient subjectively experience any shock.

Lobotomy. Another treatment that gained wide acceptance in this period was pre-frontal lobotomy, based on the observation of Moniz in 1936 that brain lesions which interrupted thalamo-cortical pathways relieved anxiety and tension, and ameliorated some psychoses (Freeman and Watts, 1950). The price for this amelioration, however, was a loss of significant brain function, with a blunting of personality and increased impulsivity. As a result the treatment has fallen largely into disfavour.

The new psychopharmacology. Though insulin treatment is time-consuming and expensive, and electroshock causes memory difficulties, all these treatments still have some applicability, especially electroconvulsive therapy. But in the past three decades they have been largely supplanted by a wide range of new psychopharmacological agents. The first of these, chlorpromazine, was developed in 1951 by Laborit, in France, and is a non-hypnotic sedative with a selective action on the lower brain centres that regulate emotion. It proved to be remarkably effective in schizophrenia and related psychoses. A variety of stimulants are now also available to relieve depression: a profusion of new drugs are now used for many minor and major disorders. Most recently nutritional therapy has been added to this armamentarium (Pfeiffer, 1975).

The remarkable technologies that now allow us to explore the chemistry of neurotransmission (Krieger, 1983), to measure metabolism within the human brain by computerized radiography, to insert genes into living cells, and to study ultramicroscopic structures, all hold much promise, and may soon uncover the causes of mental illness.

Psychotherapy. The rigorous experimental methodology that has been demanded of all these new treatments has also affected psychotherapy. The first of the psychotherapeutic schools to publish controlled studies with strict experimental design and statistical analysis was behavioural therapy, derived from Pavlovian conditioning. In the more recent period, however, all schools of psychotherapy, including psychoanalysis, have been made aware of the need to subject their methods and their claims to the same scientific rigour of biological psychiatry. At the same time there is always the danger that a crude and uncritical application of physical treatment modalities can lead to new excesses. Psychiatrists, as always, need to be alert to the whole range of physiological, psychological and social factors involved in psychiatric disorders.

Joseph Wortis
State University of New York
Stony Brook

References

Freeman, W. and Watts, J. W. (1950), *Psychosurgery*, Springfield, Ill.

Krieger, D. T. (1983), 'Brain peptides: what, where and why', *Science*, 222.

Pfeiffer, C. C. (1975), *Mental and Elemental Nutrients*, New Canaan.

Wortis, J. (1959), 'The history of insulin shock treatment', in M. Rinkel (ed.), *Insulin Treatment in Psychiatry*, New York.

Wortis, J. (1983), 'Johannes Maargaard Nielsen', *Biological Psychiatry*, 18.

See also: *electroconvulsive therapy; genetic aspects of mental illness; nervous system; physiological psychology; psychopharmacology.*

Birth Order

The extensive research on birth order may reflect the relative ease with which it can be assessed, or perhaps its intuitive appeal as a source of individual differences in behaviour. For whatever reasons, psychologists have studied the effects of birth order on many variables, including physical and mental health, intelligence and achievement, personality, and social relations. They have been especially interested in the effects on intelligence and personality.

The relationship between birth order and intelligence was first discussed by Sir Francis Galton, who noted that prominent

English scientists were usually the first-born or only children in their families. Galton suggested that the special attention that these scientists received from their parents during childhood may have enhanced their intellectual development. Galton's work stimulated many other psychologists to study the effects of birth order on intelligence. Unfortunately, this later research often suffered from serious methodological problems and rarely reflected any clear theoretical perspectives. The observed effects of birth order on intelligence were sometimes positive and sometimes negative, and never very strong. In fact, some of the best research showed that those effects disappeared entirely when other relevant variables such as family size were taken into account. Many psychologists now believe that there is no real relationship at all between birth order and intelligence.

Alfred Adler was the first to discuss the relationship between birth order and personality. On the basis of his clinical experiences, Adler suggested that birth order can influence a child's relationships with other family members and thereby affect his adult personality. For example, the pampering that last-born children often receive from their parents and siblings could cause them to became lazy, unambitious and insecure as adults. Adler's work led other psychologists to investigate the relationship between birth order and personality, but much of this research was also plagued by methodological problems and theoretical ambiguities. Although many significant birth order effects were reported, they were often difficult to interpret and were rarely replicable. Only a few birth order effects were both sensible and reliable, and those seemed to be mediated by other variables. For example, several studies showed that first-borns were more dependent and conforming than others, yet this relationship was severely attenuated when differences in social class were taken into account. These and other research findings persuaded many psychologists that birth order and personality are essentially unrelated.

There are clearly some good reasons to be dismayed by the current status of research on the psychological effects of birth order. Indeed, some experts have recommended that such research be abandoned altogether. An alternative recommendation, more difficult but less extreme, might be to improve the quality of birth order research until it yields more meaningful results. At a methodological level, more attention should be given to such variables as family size, social status, and parental characteristics, all of which may be correlated with birth order and therefore involved in its effects. Birth order itself could also be measured in a more precise way by taking into account not only the ordinal position of the child in the family, but also the ages and sexes of his siblings. At a theoretical level, more formal theories are needed to generate clear and testable hypotheses about birth order effects. Such theories should ideally place birth order within the context of other family variables to which it is related. One approach that seems promising in this regard is the confluence model of intellectual development proposed by Zajonc and his colleagues (Zajonc and Markus, 1975; Zajonc, Markus and Markus, 1979). This theory and others like it should help to clarify the current confusion regarding birth order effects.

Richard Moreland
University of Pittsburgh

References

Zajonc, R. B. and Markus, G. B. (1975), 'Birth order and intellectual development', *Psychological Review*, 82.
Zajonc, R. B., Markus, H. and Markus, G. B. (1979), 'The birth order puzzle', *Journal of Personality and Social Psychology*, 37.

Further Reading

Adams, B. N. (1972), 'Birth order: a critical review', *Sociometry*, 35.
Ernst, C. and Angst, J. (1983), *Birth Order: Its Influence on Personality*, Berlin.
Falbo, T. (1977), 'The only child: a review', *Journal of Individual Psychology*, 33.

Schooler, C. (1972), 'Birth order effects: not here, not now!',
Psychological Bulletin, 78.
See also: *Adler; intelligence and intelligence testing*.

Bowlby, John E. (1907–)

John Bowlby is best known for his pioneering research on the
development and nature of mother-child attachment and for
his long association with the child family psychiatry service at
the Tavistock Clinic in London. Born on 26 February 1907 in
London into a medical family, he was educated at Dartmouth
and Trinity College, Cambridge. In 1937, he was appointed
staff psychiatrist at the London Child Guidance Clinic. Later
during the Second World War he served as consultant
psychiatrist in the RAMC (1940–5) in the rank of Lieutenant
Colonel. In 1946 he joined the Tavistock Clinic as chairman of
the Department for Children and Parents, where he remained
until his retirement in 1972.

Bowlby is both a prolific writer and controversial figure. His
many publications include *Personal Aggressiveness and War* in
1938, *Forty Four Juvenile Thieves* in 1946, *Maternal Care and Mental
Health* (written for the World Health Organization) in 1951,
Child Care and the Growth of Love in 1953 and, perhaps most
extensive and authoritative, his three volumes in the series
Attachment and Loss published between 1969 and 1980.

Bowlby received many academic and national honours in his
years of work with disturbed children and their families
including an honorary D.Sc at Cambridge in 1977 and the
Distinguished Scientific Contribution Award for research into
child development in 1981. Well before this latter honour,
however, Bowlby's research and clinical work into early separation, mother-child attachment, and childhood disturbance had
had a widespread impact on all the mental health and welfare
professions, in particular child psychiatry and social work,
although in later years the methodological basis for Bowlby's
theory of maternal deprivation was subjected to criticism and
debate, with new evidence and more thorough analysis
suggesting alternative explanations for his earlier work. His

influence on professionals of all kinds working with disturbed
children and their families has been acknowledged world-wide.

Barrie J. Brown
Institute of Psychiatry
University of London

See also: *attachment; bereavement; separation and loss.*

Bruner, Jerome Seymour (1915–)

Jerome Seymour Bruner was educated at Duke University and
Harvard, where he received his doctorate in psychology in 1941.
During the Second World War, he studied public attitudes and
the effects of propaganda in the US Office of War Information
and, later, in the Psychological Warfare Division of the Supreme
Headquarters of the Allied Expeditionary Forces. After the war
he returned to Harvard and became professor of psychology in
1952.

At Harvard, he and George Miller founded the Center for
Cognitive Studies in 1960. Between 1972 and 1980, Bruner was
professor of psychology at the University of Oxford. He
returned to the United States in 1980 as Director of the New
York Institute for the Humanities, New York University.

Much of Bruner's work deals with the nature and function
of human cognition. His early work with Leo Postman on visual
perception and recognition led to a major research programme
concerned with categorization, identification, and concept
formation (Bruner, Goodnow, & Austin, 1956). In explicit
contrast to the dominant behaviourist ethos of North American
psychology at the time, Bruner and his colleagues emphasized
the strategic, goal-driven nature of much of human thinking,
and the fact that human beings systematically select or abstract
from the potential information contained within their environment. Inevitably, Bruner became interested in the differences
between people in their strategies for acquiring concepts and
their subsequent performance in cognitive tasks. This work
represents an early but significant landmark in the development
of 'cognitive psychology': the systematic investigation through

laboratory experimentation of human thinking, reasoning, and remembering, and of the different types of mental processes and representations which underlie such faculties.

Most of Bruner's subsequent work has applied cognitive psychology to the study of human development, and has moved from laboratory-based research to more naturalistic methods of inquiry. In 1959 he chaired an interdisciplinary meeting on science education in primary and secondary schools in which he and other psychologists considered a wide range of serious pedagogical issues concerning curriculum development and teaching skills, as well as more general questions of human learning and the growth of knowledge. His report of the meeting (Bruner, 1960) is very much a personal account of the potential contribution of research in cognitive psychology to the practical problems of schoolroom learning.

Bruner took up many of these issues during the 1960s in essays about the biological, developmental, and cultural constraints upon the growth of human knowledge and intelligence. He emphasized that course design and instructional practice should be based on a proper understanding of the nature of cognitive development and should exploit the learners' active participation in the educational process (Bruner, 1966, 1971, 1973). He also explored the origins of intellectual capabilities in infancy and early childhood, stressed the role of organization and discovery in the acquisition of complex skills, and considered the role of language and culture in mediating the development of children's thought.

However, the political events of that decade, particularly the student protest in the United States and Europe, caused Bruner to consider whether educational reform was inhibited by deeper, structural characteristics of Western society and especially by the preschool impact of social class divisions upon children's goals and aspirations. He was involved in establishing the Head Start programme in the 1960s and with other efforts to explore and improve the quality of children's preschool care in the United States. In the United Kingdom, Bruner undertook a commissioned study of the provision of care for preschool children through nursery schools, play-groups, day-care centres, and child-minders. Here, too, he was concerned both with the research findings themselves and the practical applications: how they might be effectively disseminated to those responsible for the provision of preschool care and also to the practitioners themselves (Bruner, 1980).

While in Oxford, Bruner carried out several experimental studies of prelinguistic communication in infants as well as a longitudinal investigation of the acquisition of language in young children. In other respects, however, Bruner's time in Oxford seems to have been less successful. His colleagues were unsympathetic to his suggestions that empirical psychology should not restrict itself solely to the study of problems which were open to formal experimental investigation.

Bruner has not only been concerned with the intellect but also with the artistic or intuitive side of human nature. He sought to link the growth of knowledge through science and education to its expression in art and literature (Bruner, 1962). He has tried to provide an integrated account, which incorporates both the scientific and the humanistic conceptions of human intelligence. This is a major theme of his most recent books (Bruner, 1984, 1986).

John T. E. Richardson
Brunel University, Uxbridge

References

Bruner, J. S. (1960), *The Process of Education*, Cambridge, Mass.

Bruner, J. S. (1962), *On Knowing: Essays for the Left Hand*, Cambridge, Mass.

Bruner, J. S. (1966), *Toward a Theory of Instruction*, Cambridge, Mass.

Bruner, J. S. (1971), *The Relevance of Education*, New York.

Bruner, J. S. (1973), *Beyond the Information Given*, New York.

Bruner, J. S. (1980), *Under Five in Britain*, London.

Bruner, J. S. (1983), *Child's Talk: Learning to Use Language*, New York.

Bruner, J. S. (1984), *In Search of Mind: Essays in Autobiography*, New York.

Bruner, J. S. (1986), *Actual Minds, Possible Worlds*, Cambridge, Mass.

Bruner, J. S., Goodnow, J. J. and Austin, G. A. (1956), *A Study of Thinking*, New York.

Character Disorders

Although omitted from the latest diagnostic and statistical manual of the American Psychiatric Association (APA), the term character disorder is used mainly by dynamic psychiatrists to describe a situation in which elements of a person's character interfere with his everyday functioning. We must first examine character to understand its disorders.

Character may be described as that durable and persisting set of defences used by the individual in adapting to the world. Of central importance in character formation are the internalization of the parents and other identifications with moral precepts and codes. Analytically-trained psychiatrists refer to the embodiment of the person's parentally-inspired internal code as the super-ego or conscience.

A second essential element of the concept of character is that it is considered 'the way one is', or 'that's who I am'; in dynamic terms, character is experienced as ego-syntonic (consistent with one's self-concept) as opposed to ego-alien (inconsistent with one's self-concept). The term ego-alien can describe neurotic symptoms. For example, a person with a compulsive character may accept, even take pride in, the description of himself as meticulous, while a person with the neurotic compulsion to wash his hands constantly may chafe against this symptom, wish to be free of it, be ashamed of it, and see it as definitely not a part of his rational self.

The step from character to character disorder involves the impact of character traits or character structure on a person's daily life functioning; when the elements of the person's character become an interference, or take a destructive form, we speak of character disorders. A troubling psychiatric confusion is that the terms 'character' and 'personality' are often used as though synonymous. However, some use the term personality to refer to the outward presentation of an individual, his 'face' towards the world, rather than referring to the intra-psychic structure. (The psychopath or sociopath, which many consider the most significant 'character disorder', is discussed separately.)

Among the other commonly recognized character disorders is depressive character, not uncommonly seen in persons for whom the depressed state is a way of life. Chronic pessimism, decreased self-esteem and pervasive sadness are its hallmarks.

Besides meticulousness, the compulsive character is marked by an addiction to orderliness, cleanliness, and scrupulousness, as well as a tendency to adhere to the 'letter of the law'. A frequent concomitant is isolation of affect which constricts the range of emotional responsivity, often compensated by prominence of intellectual functioning.

The passive-aggressive character is most readily identified through understanding of his most common habitat, the bureaucracy. In this character structure, deep hostility is expressed through delay, passivity, obstructionism and procrastination. The French refer to the passive-aggressive bureaucrat as a '*petit fonctionnaire*', the minor functionary whose power is both realized and expressed by his capacity to keep one waiting.

The narcissistic character is recognized by an extreme love of and need for adulation and admiration from those around him, coupled with what the layman terms egotism, a self-obsessed attitude. The craving for applause is addictive in its power and pervasiveness; this entity is thus not uncommonly seen in professional performers.

The schizoid character, in contrast, might be described as the withdrawn, 'cool' loner who has approached the problem of dealing with the world by withdrawing from it, at least in emotional attachments and investments. The subject's emotional inaccessibility, which may be frustrating to others, is used to defend the individual from the anxiety that might otherwise attend social interaction.

Thomas G. Gutheil
Harvard University
Program in Psychiatry and the Law, Boston

Further Reading
Cleckley, H. (1955), *The Mask of Sanity*, St Louis, Missouri.
McCord, W. and McCord, J. (1964), *The Psychopath*,
    Princeton.
Reich, W. (1945), *Character Analysis*, New York.
Vaillant, G. (1975), 'Sociopathy as human process', *Archives
    of General Psychiatry*, 32.
See also: *depressive disorders; neuroses; obsessive-compulsive disorders;
    personality; psychopathic personality; psychosis.*

Clinical Psychology

Clinical psychology is one of the speciality areas of applied psychology, together with such other specialities as industrial, physiological, measurement and developmental psychology. The science and profession of clinical psychology, as one of the mental health disciplines, utilizes the principles of psychology to: (1) understand, diagnose and treat psychological problems; (2) teach and train students in these principles and their applications; and (3) conduct research in human behaviour as well as function as consumer of research advances as a means of upgrading the delivery of health care.

The two World Wars and the major development of public schools in the United States between the wars vastly accelerated the growth of clinical psychology, first as purely a psychological or 'mental' test application in assessing intellectual and other psychological responses and capabilities, and then, after the Second World War, expanding into other roles, in the psychotherapies as well as in research and training and in formal graduate programmes in clinical psychology. In the US alone, it has been estimated that during the Second World War 16 million military candidates and recruits were given psychological tests for classification and assignment to duties. In the First World War psychologists did psychometric assessment only; in the Second World War they also carried out treatment responsibilities for mentally ill personnel, together with psychiatrists, social workers, nurses, and technicians.

Two major developments after the Second World War furthered the growth of clinical psychology in the US – the establishment of the National Institute of Mental Health and its support for training and research; and the decision of the Veterans Administration to fund training for clinical psychology as one of the disciplines in mental health, to assess and treat veterans with psychological illness. There followed the accreditation, by the American Psychological Association (APA), of doctoral training programmes (130 in 1982) and internship programmes (211 in 1982) in professional psychology (clinical, counselling, school and, more recently, professional-scientific psychology); and certification and licensing by states.

Two other standards organizations developed, the first in 1947 and thus growing during the great 'spurt' years of the past 35 years; and the second initially an outgrowth of the former. The American Board of Professional Psychology (ABPP) was established in 1947 by the Council of Representatives of the American Psychological Association 'to define the standards, conduct examinations, grant diplomas, and encourage the pursuit of excellence in professional psychology' (1980). The four fields of specialization are clinical, counselling, industrial and organizational, and school; and, shortly, neuropsychology.

In 1957, there were in the APA 15,545 Life Members, Fellows and Associates, of whom 1,907 Fellows and Associates were in the Division of Clinical Psychology. A quarter century later there were 52,440 Fellows, Members and Associates; nearly 4,600 of whom were in the Division of Clinical Psychology and more than 7,400 in four closely related Divisions – Community, Psychotherapy, Health and Clinical Neuropsychology (however, many APA members belong to several Divisions so that there is considerable overlap among these members). At the present time there are over 2,600 ABPP Diplomates of whom more than 1,800 are in the speciality of Clinical, and nearly 14,000 registrants in the National Register.

Two recent directions have both moved clinical psychology toward a reintegration with other fields of psychology and have created new specialities within clinical psychology. Health psychology has drawn to it scientists and professionals from other domains of psychology, principally clinical, social, physiological and learning or cognitive areas. This field was initially a research area and increasingly has become an applied field. The second direction represents an interesting cycle in the history of clinical psychology. As noted above, psychological or 'mental' tests have had a prominent 90-year role in the history and development of clinical psychology. After the Second World War, primarily in the US, graduate programmes decreased their commitment to teaching assessment methods, and their graduates increasingly turned to psychotherapy as a principal activity. Then, research training support, litigation over the effects upon individuals of toxic and other industrial and environmental pollutants, and mounting interest in psychological changes in disease and accident victims and in the elderly all contributed to bringing assessment again into prominence, especially neuropsychological assessment; and there now are local, state, regional, national and international societies of neuropsychologists.

Ivan N. Mensh
University of California, Los Angeles

Further Reading

American Board of Professional Psychology (1980), *Directory of Diplomates*, Washington DC.

Cattell, R. B. (1983), 'Let's end the duel', *American Psychologist*, 38.

Council for the National Register of Health Science Providers in Psychology (1981), *National Register of Health Service Providers in Psychology*, Washington DC.

Mensh, I. N. (1966), *Clinical Psychology: Science and Profession*, New York.

Cognitive-Behavioural Therapy

Cognitive-behavioural interventions are an attempt to preserve the demonstrated efficiencies of behavioural therapy within a less doctrinaire context and to incorporate the cognitive activities of the client in the efforts to produce therapeutic change (Kendall and Hollon, 1979). Based upon current data (Smith,

1982), cognitive-behavioural therapy is a dominant force in psychotherapy, ranking with psychoanalysis and just behind eclecticism as a major theoretical and applied framework.

Basic to the cognitive-behavioural approach is a set of principles captured briefly as follows: (1) Client and therapist work together to evaluate problems and generate solutions (e.g., collaborative empiricism). (2) Most human learning is cognitively mediated. (3) Cognition, affect, and behaviour are causally interrelated. (4) Attitudes, expectancies, attributions and other cognitive activities are central in producing, predicting, and understanding behaviour and the effects of therapy. (5) Cognitive processes can be integrated into behavioural paradigms, and it is possible and desirable to combine cognitive treatment strategies with enactive and contingency management techniques (Kendall and Bemis, 1984; Mahoney, 1977).

Within the boundaries of these fundamental principles, the actual implementation of the cognitive-behavioural therapies varies. The major strategies within cognitive-behavioural therapy include: (1) Cognitive-behaviour therapy of depression; (2) Rational-emotive therapy; (3) Systematic rational restructuring; (4) Stress inoculation, and (5) Self-control training with children.

(1) Cognitive-behavioural therapy of depression (Beck, Rush, Shaw and Emery, 1979) is structured, active, and typically time-limited. Learning experiences are designed to teach clients to monitor their negative thinking, to examine the evidence for and against their distorted (negative) thinking, to substitute more reality-oriented interpretations for negative thinking, and to begin to alter the dysfunctional beliefs and life style associated with negative thinking. Behavioural strategies such as self-monitoring of mood, activity scheduling, graduated task assignments, and role-playing exercises are integrated with more cognitive procedures such as focusing on changing negative thinking, reattribution, and decentering.

(2) Rational-emotive therapy (RET) offers both a theoretical and therapeutic system consistent with cognitive-behavioural therapy (Ellis, 1980). In RET, events do not cause emotional and behavioural consequences; private beliefs do. When the

individual's beliefs (salient assumptions) are inaccurate/ irrational and are framed in absolutistic or imperative terms, maladjustment is likely to result. RET teaches clients to identify and change the illogical notions that underlie their distressing symptoms.

(3) Systematic rational restructing (SRR) is a derivative of RET which offers a clear description of the procedures of treatment. SRR offers specific techniques for modifying anxiety and irrational beliefs and is implemented in four stages: (a) presenting the rationale for the treatment to the clients; (b) reviewing the irrationality of certain types of beliefs and assumptions; (c) analysing the client's problems in terms of irrational thinking and undesirable self-talk; (d) teaching the client to modify self-talk and irrationality (e.g., Goldfried, 1979).

(4) Stress-inoculation (Meichenbaum, 1977) is a three-stage intervention which focuses on teaching cognitive and behavioural skills for coping with stressful situations. In the educational phase, clients are taught a conceptual framework for understanding stress in cognitive terms. The second phase, skills training, teaches clients cognitive (imagery, changing irrational self-talk) and behavioural (relaxation, breathing) skills. In the final stage, clients practise the new skills in stressful situations.

(5) Focusing on children, self-instructional training is designed to teach thinking skills (Kendall and Braswell, 1985). Especially relevant for children who lack foresight and planning (e.g., impulsive, nonself-controlled, hyperactive/attention disorder), self-instructional procedures involve rehearsal of overt, then covert, self-guiding verbalizations. Using tasks and role-plays, the therapist and child practise thinking out loud. Behavioural contingencies are also implemented.

Cognitive-behavioural therapies are consistent with therapeutic integration, where varying resources are tapped as sources of effective treatment. In one sense they are prototypic of integration: performance-based behavioural treatments with a focus on the cognitive representation/meanings of events and the merits of thinking — in other words, thought and action in psychotherapy.

Philip C. Kendall
Temple University

References
Beck, A. T., Rush, A. J., Shaw, B. F. and Emery, G. (1979), *Cognitive Therapy of Depression*, New York.
Ellis, A. (1980), 'Rational-emotive therapy and cognitive behaviour therapy: similarities and differences', *Cognitive Therapy and Research*, 4.
Goldfried, M. R. (1979), 'Anxiety reduction through cognitive-behavioral intervention', in P. C. Kendall and S. D. Hollon (eds), *Cognitive-Behavioral Interventions: Therapy, Research, and Procedures*, New York.
Kendall, P. C. and Bemis, K. M. (1984), 'Thought and action in psychotherapy: the cognitive-behavioral approaches', in M. Hersen, A. E. Kazdin and A. S. Bellack (eds), *The Clinical Psychology Handbook*, New York.
Kendall, P. C. and Braswell, L. (1984), *Cognitive-Behavioral Therapy for Impulsive Children*, New York.
Kendall, P. C. and Hollon, S. D. (eds) (1979), *Cognitive-Behavioral Interventions: Theory, Research and Procedures*, New York.
Mahoney, J. M. (1977), 'Reflections on the cognitive-learning trend in psychotherapy', *American Psychologist*, 32.
Meichenbaum, D. (1977), *Cognitive-Behavior Modification: An Integrative Approach*, New York.
Smith, D. (1982), 'Trends in counseling and psychotherapy', *American Psychologist*, 37.
See also: *behaviour therapy*.

Cognitive Dissonance

The theory of cognitive dissonance, which gained prominence in social psychology during the 1960s and 1970s, was first proposed by Leon Festinger (1957) and later refined and elaborated by Brehm and Cohen, Aronson, and Wicklund and Brehm

(1976). The elements in the theory are the cognitions (items of knowledge or belief) that a person may hold at a given time. Between any pair of cognitions, one of the following relations is assumed to exist: consonance (one of the cognitions follows from the other), dissonance (one cognition follows from the negation of the other), or irrelevance (neither cognition follows from the other or from its negation). The 'follows from' criterion refers to psychological, rather than to logical, implication. Thus, for example, the pair of cognitions *I voted for a socialist candidate in the last election* and *I believe in socialism* are consonant because the second follows psychologically from the first; this is evident from the fact that, given the first cognition, an observer would normally expect the second rather than its negation to be more likely.

The dissonance relation, which is of special importance in the theory, is held to be a motivating state of tension, in many ways like hunger or thirst, and the theory's main assumption is that dissonance tends to generate dissonance-reducing behaviour. Three methods of reducing dissonance are possible: changing one of the dissonant cognitions, decreasing the perceived importance of the dissonant cognitions, and adding further (justifying) cognitions. A familiar example is the dissonance normally experienced by people who hold the cognitions *I smoke cigarettes* and *cigarette smoking damages one's health*. It may be difficult to change the first cognition, which is behaviourally anchored, but research has confirmed that many smokers reduce the dissonance by changing the second – that is, by debunking the evidence linking cigarette smoking with health risks – and by adding further (justifying) cognitions, such as *I smoke only mild brands* and *there will soon be a cure for lung cancer*.

Despite its almost tautological simplicity, cognitive dissonance theory has been shown to generate non-obvious predictions across a wide range of human behaviour. The attitudinal consequences of making free choices, of stating opinions at variance with one's true beliefs, and of resisting temptation have been illuminated by dissonance theory, and empirical research in these areas has yielded results that are broadly in line with predictions from the theory. The behaviour of end-of-the-world cultists after their prophecies have failed has also been investigated in the light of the theory.

Though undoubtedly successful, cognitive dissonance theory has been criticized for its conceptual fuzziness and for the ambiguity of the predictions that can sometimes be derived from it. The most sustained critique has come from Daryl Bem (1967) who has attempted, not altogether convincingly, to reinterpret dissonance effects in terms of a self-perception theory based on radical Skinnerian behaviourism.

Andrew M. Colman
University of Leicester

References
Bem, D. J. (1967), 'Self-perception: an alternative interpretation of cognitive dissonance phenomena', *Psychological Review*, 74.
Festinger, L. (1957), *A Theory of Cognitive Dissonance*, Stanford.
Wicklund, R. A. and Brehm, J. W. (1976), *Perspectives on Cognitive Dissonance*, Hillsdale, NJ.
See also: *attitudes; sensation and perception.*

Cognitive Science

According to Drever's (1964) *Dictionary of Psychology*, 'cognition' is 'a general term covering all the various modes of knowing – perceiving, imagining, conceiving, judging, reasoning'. It picks out those forms of abstract thinking and problem solving which are based upon the manipulation of either linguistic symbols (propositions) or iconic symbols (images). The term 'cognitive science' refers to the interdisciplinary study of information processing in human cognition. Although there are obvious precursors in the work of mathematicians such as Alan Turing and John von Neumann, of neurophysiologists such as Warren McCulloch and Walter Pitts, and of communications theorists such as Norbert Wiener and Claude Shannon, it is generally agreed that cognitive science came into being in 1956. This year marked the beginnings of genuine collaboration amongst research workers in artificial intelligence (Allen Newell and

Herbert Simon), cognitive psychology (Jerome Bruner and George Miller), and linguistics (Noam Chomsky), and Gardner (1985) has identified cognate movements in epistemology, anthropology, and the neurosciences. Kosslyn (1983) has summarized the manner in which cognitive science has taken advantage of developments in these different disciplines: 'From computer science it draws information about how computers and computer programs work; from philosophy it has adopted not only many of its basic questions and a general orientation toward the mind, but many of the fundamental ideas about information representation (e.g. 'propositions'); from linguistics it draws a basic way of thinking about mental events and theories of language; and from cognitive psychology it draws methodologies and specific findings about human information-processing abilities.'

Cognitive science has been inspired very much by insights within the discipline of psychology, and in particular has developed in step with the field of cognitive psychology. However, it is intrinsically at odds with much of mainstream cognitive psychology, which grew out of what used to be called 'human experimental psychology', and which has incorporated the behaviourist methodology which dominated research earlier this century. Cognitive science owes rather more to the 'human factors' tradition within cognitive psychology, which developed during the Second World War in order to tackle problems concerning human–machine interaction. This work led to an interest in the control mechanisms governing intelligent behaviour, to the idea of human thought and action as consisting of discrete stages of information processing, and inevitably to the use of the digital computer as a metaphor in theorizing about human cognition. Such research aims to produce general frameworks which are of direct benefit in the design and construction of complex systems but which may not be amenable to rigorous experimental evaluation (Reason, 1987). An illustration of the disparity between cognitive psychologists and cognitive scientists arises in their attitudes to introspective reports of conscious experience. Cognitive psychologists tend to be suspicious of introspective reports and sceptical of their value as empirical data, whereas in cognitive science the use and analysis of such verbal 'protocols' is widely accepted (see, for example, Ericsson and Simon, 1984). As an excellent case study within the field of cognitive science, Kosslyn (1983) has given an autobiographical account of his work on mental imagery, which combines systematic experimentation with introspectionist methodology.

Gardner (1985) has identified two 'core assumptions' in contemporary research in cognitive science. The first assumption is that to explain intelligent behaviour it is necessary to incorporate the idea of 'internal' or 'mental' representations as a distinctive and irreducible level of theoretical analysis. Indeed, theories in cognitive science are often based upon the structuralist notion that internal representations intervene between experience and behaviour. Human cognition is regarded as the symbolic manipulation of stored information, and in order to understand intelligent human behaviour, it is necessary to investigate the properties of these internal representations and of the processes that operate upon them. Nevertheless, it should be noted that sociologists have argued that descriptions of mental experience are socially constructed and are at the very least problematic as explanations of behaviour (see Woolgar, 1987).

The second 'core assumption' is that the computer is a useful model of human thought and a valuable research tool. Precisely because digital computers are artefactual systems that have been specifically designed for the symbolic manipulation of stored information, the language of computer science seems to provide a convenient and congenial means of articulating notions concerning human cognition. As Kosslyn (1983) has noted, cognitive scientists have therefore borrowed much of the vocabulary that was originally developed to talk about computer functioning and use it to talk about mental representation and processing in human beings. Indeed, the language of computer science tends to function as a theoretical *lingua franca* amongst the variety of disciplines that make up cognitive science; as Levy (1987) has put it, the computational representation of models is the 'common test-bed' of cognitive science. Of course, the contemporary digital computer may not provide the best model for characterizing human information processing, and alternative system architectures may prove to be more useful (Kosslyn, 1983): a very fashionable approach based upon the notion of parallel distributed processing is claimed to be much more appropriate for modelling human cognition because it is more akin to the known physiology of the central nervous system (McClelland, Rumelhart and Hinton, 1986). Nevertheless, the supposed functional similarity between computers and human brains provides a distinctive means of evaluating the theories of cognitive science: the computer simulation of behaviour. The point has been elegantly summarized by Kosslyn (1983): 'If the brain and computer both can be described as manipulating symbols in the same way, then a good theory of mental events should be able to be translated into a computer program, and if the theory is correct, then the program should lead the computer to produce the same overt responses that a person would in various circumstances.'

A fundamental criticism of research in cognitive science is that it has tended to view cognition in abstract terms, devoid of any personal, social, or ecological significance. As Gardner (1985) remarks, cognitive science tends to exclude (or at least to 'de-emphasize') 'the influence of affective factors or emotions, the contribution of historical and cultural factors, and the role of the background context in which particular actions or thoughts occur'. Gardner implies that this feature of cognitive science is the result of a deliberate strategic decision in order to render the problems under investigation more tractable. However, it has to be recognized that the pattern of much research within cognitive science (as in other areas of scholarly investigation) is set by existing traditions, and therefore such strategic choices have typically gone by default. The relevance of cognitive science to everyday human experience and its practical application in real-life situations will undoubtedly be enhanced by the incorporation of emotional, cultural, and contextual factors into theoretical accounts of human cognition.

John T. E. Richardson
Brunel University, Uxbridge

References

Drever, J. (1964), *A Dictionary of Psychology* (rev. H. Wallerstein), Harmondsworth.

Ericsson, K. A. and Simon, H. A. (1984), *Protocol Analysis: Verbal Reports as Data*, Cambridge, Mass.

Gardner, H. (1985), *The Mind's New Science: A History of the Cognitive Revolution*, New York.

Kosslyn, S. M. (1983), *Ghosts in the Mind's Machine: Creating and Using Images in the Brain*, New York.

Levy, P. (1987), 'Modelling cognition: Some current issues', in P. Morris (ed.), *Modelling Cognition*, Chichester.

McClelland, J. L., Rumelhart, D. E. and Hinton, G. E. (1986), 'The appeal of parallel distributed processing', in D. E. Rumelhart, J. L. McClelland and the PDP Research Group, *Parallel Distributed Processing: Explorations in the Microstructure of Cognition*, vol. 1, Cambridge, Mass.

Reason, J. (1987), 'Framework models of human performance and error: A consumer guide', in L. Goodstein, H. B. Anderson and S. E. Olsen (eds), *Tasks, Errors and Mental Models*, London.

Woolgar, S. (1987), 'Reconstructing man and machine: A note on sociological critiques of cognitivism', in W. E. Bijker, T. P. Hughes and T. Pinch (eds), *The Social Construction of Technological Systems*, Cambridge, Mass.

Comparative Psychology

Comparative psychology is a term applied nowadays only to the study of animals, and not to comparisons made between or within human cultures. There are several issues involved in the psychological study of animals, some of them resolvable by evidence, and others more questions of the purposes and strategies of the enterprise itself. It is partly a strategic question whether to try to list the peculiarities of individual species, or to search for general principles which apply to large groups of species. Cutting across this distinction is the question of whether to be satisfied with descriptions or whether to look more deeply for explanations of known or as-yet-unknown facts.

Descartes dissected animals, and had a positive influence in arguing from his knowledge of the sensory nerves that the brain is the organ of all sensation and feeling. However, he also started a mechanistic trend in the explanation of animal behaviour, by inventing the concept of the sensory-motor reflex, and he unfortunately effectively split off discussion of human psychology, seen as the experience of a uniquely human soul, from animal psychology, seen as collections of reflexes. A return to Aristotle's idea of a natural scale of life, which had persisted up until Descartes, and in which there are clear continuities between human and animal psychology, was promoted by, among others, Darwin, his collaborator Romanes, and Herbert Spencer.

In the twentieth century, several branches of comparative psychology have been influenced by the Darwinian theory of evolution. Behaviourists such as Watson and Skinner and learning theorists such as Pavlov and Thorndike reflect Darwinian theory in so far as results obtained in experiments with animals are held to have relevance for human psychology. On the other hand, these theorists and their followers ignore evolution to the extent that they neglect species differences. The inheritance of characteristics, whether physical or mental, was an axiom of Darwin's theory, and therefore it is acceptably Darwinian to propose that each animal species comes equipped with a different set of capacities, or a different set of 'species-specific behaviours'. This last term was introduced by ethologists including the 1973 Nobel Laureates, Tinbergen and Lorenz, who approached animal behaviour as biologists rather than psychologists, and catalogued such items as 'fixed action patterns' of courtship behaviour in birds, which take particular stereotyped forms in a given species. Another zoologist, E. O. Wilson, in 1975 coined the term 'Sociobiology', intended to cover complex social behaviour (even, controversially, in the human species) in relation to biological variables.

The nature-versus-nurture debate continues. It is plain that animal behaviour is not so determined by education, culture and history as is that of the human species, and that inherited and instinctual influences must play a correspondingly greater role in animal psychology. But it is a matter of factual evidence, from both field observations and laboratory experiment, that local traditions and individual accomplishments have considerably more importance in the life of birds and mammals than the inherited-clockwork-reflexes view would suggest.

Much factual data about many animal species is continually being collected, but agreed theories do not necessarily flow from the increased volume of facts. One theoretical trend in biology, which serves as a very remote level of explanation in psychology, is statistical treatment of various genetical possibilities – as applied to social behaviour this had been popularized as the 'selfish gene' theory. It has had some success in accounting for such things as the breeding strategies adopted by particular animal species – including, for example, the inbreeding avoidance which has been discovered in many wild populations. Within more strictly psychological theories, there has been a trend in the second half of the twentieth century to move away from the extreme scepticism and behaviourism of the first half. Elaborate and painstaking laboratory testing has added weight to theories which presume that psychological capacities under the headings of perception, expectancy, emotion and memory are present in at least the higher vertebrates, the mammals and birds. Specialized experimentation with monkeys and chimpanzees has confirmed that intellectual abilities of some description are present in these species, although attempts to train chimpanzees in the social and syntactical complexities of human language have had successes so limited that they would be better called failures.

Animals are widely used for investigating physiological mechanisms rather than psychological theories: for instance, for investigating the details of the eye and brain which allow for vision, or for studying the brain biochemistry which accounts for the emotional effects of tranquillizing or addictive drugs. For this and other reasons an important comparison in comparative psychology is between the human species and the rest. It was Aristotle's view that perception, memory, passion, appetite and desire, as well as pleasure and pain, belong to almost all living creatures. Modern studies would place greater restrictions on the generality of these psychological components, but for a full understanding of human youth and age, sleep and dreams, and human passion and perception, biological comparisons remain essential.

S. F. Walker
Birkbeck College, University of London

Further Reading
McFarland, D. (ed.) (1980), *The Oxford Companion to Animal Behaviour*, Oxford.
Walker, S. F. (1983), *Animal Thought*, London.
See also: *instinct*.

Conditioning, Classical and Operant

The Russian physiologist, Ivan Pavlov, was not the first scientist to investigate how animals learn, but he was certainly one of the first to undertake a systematic series of experiments intended to provide precise quantitative information on the subject, and it is to his work that we owe the term 'conditioning' to describe one form of that learning. In the course of his work on the digestive system of dogs, Pavlov had found that salivary secretion was elicited not only by placing food in the dog's mouth but also by the sight or smell of food, and that eventually a dog might start to salivate at the sight or sound of the attendant who usually provided the food. These 'psychic secretions', although initially interfering with the planned study of the digestive system, provided the basis for the study of conditional reflexes for which Pavlov is now far more famous.

Pavlov's experimental arrangement was simple. A hungry dog is restrained on a stand; every few minutes, the dog receives some meat powder, the delivery of which is signalled by an arbitrary stimulus, such as the ticking of a metronome or the flashing of a light. The food itself elicits copious salivation, which is measured by diverting the end of the salivary duct through a fistula in the dog's cheek. After a number of trials on which the delivery of food is always preceded by the ticking of the metronome, the dog does not wait for the food, but starts to salivate as soon as the metronome is sounded. Food is referred to as an unconditional stimulus because it unconditionally elicits salivation; the metronome is a conditional stimulus which comes to elicit salivation conditional on its relationship to the food. By similar reasoning, salivation to food is an unconditional response, but when the dog starts salivating to the metronome, this is a conditional response, strengthened or reinforced by the delivery of food whenever the metronome sounds, and weakened or extinguished whenever the metronome occurs without being followed by food. In translation from the original Russian, 'conditional' and 'unconditional' became 'conditioned' and 'unconditioned' and the verb 'to condition' was rapidly introduced to describe the procedure which brought about this change in the dog's behaviour.

At about the same time as Pavlov was starting his work on what is now called classical conditioning, a young American research student, Edward Thorndike, was undertaking an equally systematic series of experiments which are now regarded as providing the first analysis of operant conditioning. Thorndike was more catholic in his choice of animal to study than was Pavlov, using cats, chickens and monkeys impartially. And the impetus for his work was also different. While Pavlov was a physiologist who saw himself as studying the brain and how it controlled not only inborn but also acquired reflexes, Thorndike was concerned to study how animals learned in an objective and scientific manner in order to dispel the myths that he thought had arisen about the amazing feats of intelligence of which animals were capable, myths that owed much to a post-Darwinian desire to prove the mental continuity of man and other animals.

In a typical experiment, Thorndike would place a cat in a 'puzzle box' from which the animal could escape, and so get access to a dish of food only by performing some arbitrary response such as pressing a catch or pulling on a piece of string. Thorndike recorded the time it took the animal to perform the required response on successive trials, and observing a gradual decline in this time, interpreted the learning in terms of his celebrated 'law of effect': the reward of escaping from confinement and obtaining food strengthened the one response that was successful in achieving this, while all other responses, being followed by no such desirable effects, were weakened.

The term 'operant conditioning' was introduced by the American psychologist, B. F. Skinner, who refined Thorndike's procedure by the simple device of delivering food to the animal (via, for example, an automatic pellet dispenser) while it remained inside the box. In this apparatus, a rat could be trained to perform hundreds of responses, usually pressing a small bar protruding from one wall, in order to obtain occasional pellets of food. The response of pressing the bar was termed an 'operant' because it operated on the animal's environment, and the procedure was therefore operant conditioning, which was reinforced by the occasional pellet of food, and extinguished if pressing the bar was no longer followed by food.

Although Skinner, unlike Thorndike, took over much of Pavlov's terminology, he interpreted the learning he observed in a way much more closely related to Thorndike's analysis. For Skinner, as for Thorndike, the central feature of learning and adaptation is that an animal's behaviour should be modified by its consequences. The rat presses the bar because this response produces a particular outcome – the delivery of food; when it no longer does so, the rat stops pressing the bar, just as it will also stop if pressing the bar produces some other, less desirable outcome such as the delivery of a brief shock. And the schedules according to which the experimenter arranges these outcomes have orderly and appropriate effects on the animal's behaviour.

The law of effect, which summarizes these observations, is entirely in accord with common sense: parents hope and believe that rewarding children for good behaviour or punishing them for bad will also have appropriate effects, and when they are mistaken or disappointed we are more inclined to look for other sources of reward or to question the efficacy of their punishment than to question the underlying logic of the argument. Operant conditioning, therefore, although no doubt only one rather simple form of learning or way of modifying behaviour, is surely an important and pervasive one. It is not so immediately obvious that the process of classical conditioning identified by Pavlov is of such importance. Why does the dog start salivating at the sound of the metronome? The experimenter delivers the food regardless of the dog's behaviour (this, of course, is the precise distinction between classical and operant conditioning, for in Skinner's experiments the rat only gets food *if* it presses the bar). It has been argued that salivation does actually achieve something – for example, it makes dry food more palatable and this is why the dog learns to salivate in anticipation of food. The explanation attempts to interpret classical conditioning in operant terms, for it seeks to identify a desirable consequence of salivation responsible for reinforcing the response. But the explanation is probably false. Another popular example of classical conditioning is that of blinking by a rabbit to a flash of light which signals the delivery of a puff of air to the rabbit's eye. Since this is a classical experiment, the puff of air is delivered on every trial regardless of the rabbit's behaviour. Just as in the case of the dog's salivary response, however, it seems reasonable to argue that the rabbit's eye blink serves to protect the eye from the puff of air and is therefore reinforced by this desirable consequence. The argument implies that if the experimenter arranged that on any trial on which the rabbit blinked in anticipation of the puff of air, the experimenter cancelled its delivery altogether, the rabbit would learn to blink ever more readily. Here, after all, blinking has an even more beneficial consequence than usual: it completely cancels an aversive consequence. But in fact such a procedure significantly interferes with the conditioning of the rabbit's eye blink.

A more plausible interpretation, then, is that classical conditioning simply reflects an animal's anticipation of a particular consequence, not necessarily an attempt to obtain or avoid that consequence – this latter being the provenance of operant conditioning. Classical conditioning probably has its most important application in the area of emotions and attitudes: the anticipation of an unpleasant event may generate a variety of emotional changes, such as fear or alarm which are not necessarily under voluntary control. Voluntary behaviour, i.e., that directly affected by its consequences, is the sphere of operant conditioning.

N. J. Mackintosh
University of Cambridge

Further Reading
Davey, G. (1981), *Animal Learning and Conditioning*, London.
Gray, J. A. (1979), *Pavlov*, London.
Mackintosh, N. J. (1983), *Conditioning and Associative Learning*, Oxford.
Pavlov, I. P. (1927), *Conditioned Reflexes*, Oxford.
Schwartz, B. (1978), *Psychology of Learning and Behavior*, New York.
Skinner, B. F. (1938), *The Behavior of Organisms*, New York.
Thorndike, E. L. (1911), *Animal Intelligence*, New York.
See also: *behaviourism; learning; Pavlov; Skinner.*

Conformity

Early attempts to explain the many uniformities observable in human social behaviour in terms of either a limited number of instincts (McDougall) or some general principle of learning such as imitation or suggestion (Tarde, Le Bon) proved to be unsatisfactory because they were essentially circular explanations. Research on conformity *per se* did not commence until the question of accounting for regularities in behaviour was tackled experimentally in the laboratory.

In the 1930s Sherif investigated, under laboratory conditions, the formation and functioning of social norms. He chose a task, based on the autokinetic effect, for which there were no pre-established norms or standards which might aid his subjects in making their judgements. When a fixed point of light is viewed in an otherwise totally darkened room it will appear to move. Sherif's subjects had to estimate, in inches, the extent of this apparent movement. Individuals, making a series of such judgements alone, established their own particular norm. When several such individuals subsequently performed the task in each other's presence, a convergence in their estimates was noted, i.e. the emergence of a group norm. Other individuals, who made their initial estimates under group conditions, subsequently maintained the group norm when responding alone. It was Durkheim who had first identified the state of 'anomie' or normlessness. Sherif, by selecting the autokinetic effect, was able to investigate scientifically this social phenomenon, and he demonstrated how a social norm acts as a frame of reference to guiding individual action.

Enlightened liberals, who value the autonomy of the individual, disliked a possible implication of Sherif's findings: that humans are gullible. Asch, in the early 1950s, hoped to demonstrate individual autonomy by removing the ambiguity in the stimuli to be judged. Naive subjects in his experiment found themselves, on certain critical trials, in a minority of one when making simple judgements about the equivalence of length of lines. They were unaware of the fact that the other participants were, in reality, stooges of the experimenter who, on the pre-selected trials, were unanimous in making a wrong choice. On each trial the naive subject responded either last or last but one. On approximately two-thirds of the occasions when this conflict occurred, the naive subject remained independent. So Asch had proved his point. Or had he? It was the minority response in the Asch situation, however, that riveted people's attention i.e. yielding to the opinion of the false majority. Individuals differed quite widely in the extent to which they conformed. That naive subjects should conform on as many as a third of such occasions deeply shocked many Americans and also, one suspects, Asch himself.

The experiment had an immediate impact outside of Asch's own laboratory. Much was written, of a popular nature, about the prevalence of conformity in social life. By varying both the size and the unanimity of the false majority Asch showed that the effect depended crucially upon the majority being unanimous and that it was maximal in strength with a majority of four. Crutchfield mechanized the Asch procedure by standardizing on a group of five and substituting 'electronic' for live stooges. All five were naive subjects, each believing himself to be subject number five. This greatly increased the efficiency of data collection without significantly reducing the level of conformity. Deutsch and Gerard increased the individual's independence in the Asch situation by either increasing the salience of self to self (by requiring subjects to note down their own responses *before* hearing the responses of the others) or by decreasing the salience of self to others (with anonymous responding).

Milgram's experimental studies of obedience were as controversial in the mid 1960s as Asch's studies had been in the early 1950s. Milgram identified the conditions conducive to the carrying out of instructions coming from a legitimate source of authority (i.e. the experimenter). In response to Asch's studies, Moscovici has developed a theory of minority influence. He is concerned with identifying how it is that minorities, over time, come to influence the majority. Whilst his theory is based on laboratory evidence, Moscovici is more broadly interested in how creative individuals (like Freud, Einstein or Darwin) manage to convert the majority to their own way of thinking. He is thus more interested in studying creativity and change than in studying the maintenance of the status quo.

Robert M. Farr
London School of Economics and Political Science

References

Asch, S. E. (1956), 'Studies of independence and submission to group pressure: 1. A minority of one against a unanimous majority', *Psychological Monographs*, 70.

Crutchfield, R. S. (1955), 'Conformity and character', *American Psychologist*, 10.

Deutsch, M. and Gerard, H. B. (1955), 'A study of normative and informational social influences upon individual judgment', *Journal of Abnormal and Social Psychology*, 51.

Milgram, S. (1974), *Obedience to Authority: An Experimental View*, London.

Moscovici, S. (1976), *Social Influence and Social Change*, London.

Sherif, M. (1935), 'A study of some social factors in perception', *Archives of Psychology*, 27.

Consciousness

The behaviourists took the view that science must ignore reports of conscious experience as unreliable, and deal only with publicly observable phenomena. 'Consciousness' was, accordingly, no more amenable to scientific investigation than concepts like 'ghost' and 'soul'. Latterly a cognitive approach has become increasingly influential in psychology, and in consequence the explanation of the existence and function of consciousness is no longer a taboo subject.

A variety of empirical phenomena indicate that if there is to be a scientific understanding of human thought, consciousness cannot be dismissed as a mere epiphenomenon. On the contrary, it relates to some very central aspect of the human information-processing system. The most dramatic of these phenomena are neuropsychological observations. Thus a syndrome called blindsight has been discovered which can arise with lesions to the occipital lobe of the brain. In this condition the patient can remain completely unaware of visual stimuli presented within a certain part of the field of vision. Yet if asked to 'guess', the patient can point very accurately to where a faint light has been flashed, or to discriminate a cross from a circle. One patient, when pressed, described the experience as a 'feeling' that it was 'smooth' (the O) or 'jagged' (the X), yet he stressed that he did not 'see' anything at all (Weiskrantz *et al.*, 1974). This syndrome indicates that whatever systems are responsible for consciousness, they are not required in the performance of a task like pointing to a visual stimulus. Such a deduction would be difficult to make from phenomenological analysis of normal experience.

A better-known neurological condition, which is also relevant, is the so-called 'split brain' syndrome resulting from a rarely performed operation which attempts to control epilepsy. This involves the sectioning of the corpus callosum – the primary fibre tract joining the two cerebral hemispheres. After this operation, processing in the two separate hemispheres is relatively independent. It appears that at times each of the two processes can be sufficiently complex such that if normal people were to carry it out one would assume that they would be aware of doing so (see Levy, Trevarthen and Sperry, 1972). It is therefore plausible that in the split-brain patient the two hemispheres can give rise to two different conscious experiences at the same time.

Turning to normal human experimental psychology, it has been shown that if a meaningless pattern of jumbled lines is presented a very short time after a brief visual stimulus ('visual masking'), an observer may be unable to distinguish consciously anything about the stimulus. Yet a masked stimulus may facilitate the detection of a second stimulus, semantically related to it, which follows a second or so later (see Marcel, 1983). Thus semantic processing must be occurring without the subject being aware of it.

This third phenomenon, like the first one, shows that the relation between conscious awareness and types of cognitive operation can be intuitively surprising. A satisfactory explanation must, however, specify the relation between consciousness and the operation of the nervous system. The second phenomenon suggests that an attempt to explain awareness as some property of the physics or chemistry of the brain's material constituents is unlikely to be successful. Such phenomena have rather encouraged pyschologists to attempt to explain consciousness not as a property of the cellular composition of the brain, but of the functional system of information-processing operations upon which thought is based. Consciousness, within a phenomenological conceptual framework, is thought to correspond to certain types of information-processing operations, within a mechanistic conceptual framework. But there has been no agreement at all over what these particular information-processing operations are. One view popular in the early 1970s was that a central working memory is used in most major cognitive operations and that consciousness corresponded to its content (for example, Atkinson and Shiffrin, 1971). However, most workers in the field now believe that there are in fact a variety of temporary holding stores, and no good explanation exists as to why the diverse totality of their contents should have any special ontological status. A second alternative position is that a number of cognitive operations are occurring in parallel in normal thought, but one dominates in its ability to control future cognitive and motor operations and because it can be spoken about and remembered (Shallice, 1972). In this approach the existence of a unitary conscious experience corresponds to the functional necessity for a single dominant mainstream of thought. Yet a third approach is that the human cognitive system contains a subsystem which oversees and modulates the operation of the more routine overlearned processes whereby thought and action are basically carried out. Awareness in some sense corresponds to what occurs in the supervisory modulating system (for example, Marshall and Morton, 1978).

In these types of explanation the phenomenal distinction between conscious experience and unconscious cognitive acts is explained through differences in the underlying processing operations. Properties of conscious experience – for example, the fact that the contents in some sense control action, that they can be spoken about, or that they can be remembered – are assumed to correspond to the properties of some rather special processing system which has developed in evolution. These types of functionalist explanations are, however, still not free of philosophical problems. For instance, Block (1980) has argued that as a thought experiment one could simulate the neuronal interactions within a brain by communication between people. Each person would be instructed that if he received certain signals from a set of other people he should send a signal to yet further people. Thus the acts of an individual person would mimic the operation of an individual neuron. Of course an enormous number of people would be required – Block uses the example of the population of China – and the process would be far slower than in the brain processes being simulated. It is highly implausible that the whole population involved would acquire a unitary awareness, and so Block argues that consciousness cannot just be a property of the system of processing operations since these are isomorphic in the two situations. Yet a processing system of sufficient power could presumably develop a set of 'concepts' to describe its own internal states. If a system with a particular functional architecture tended to develop the same set of such concepts, even given a wide variety of 'environments', and if these were isomorphic with those we attribute to consciousness, this would make the functionalist approach plausible despite paradoxes like Block's. The information processing approaches discussed earlier are attempts to characterize the essence of such a system. Therefore, despite undoubted philosophical difficulties, information-processing theorizing provides for the first time a research programme through which a theory of consciousness could be produced which is solidly linked to scientific findings.

Tim Shallice
MRC Applied Psychology Unit, Cambridge

References

Atkinson, R. C. and Shiffrin, R. M. (1971), 'The control of short-term memory', *Scientific American*, 224.

Block, N. (1980), *Readings in Philosophy of Psychology*, vol. 1, Cambridge, Mass.

Levy, J., Trevarthen, C. and Sperry, R. W. (1972), 'Perception of bilateral chimeric figures following hemispheric disconnection', *Brain*, 95.

Marcel, A. J. (1983), 'Conscious and unconscious perception', *Cognitive Psychology*, 15.

Marshall, J. C. and Morton, J. (1978), 'On the mechanics of Emma', in A. Sinclair *et al.* (eds), *The Child's Conception of Language*, Berlin.

Shallice, T. (1972), 'Dual functions of consciousness', *Psychological Review*, 79.

Weiskrantz, L., Warrington, E. K., Saunders, M. D. and Marshall, J. (1974), 'Visual capacity in the hemianopic field following a restricted occipital ablation', *Brain*, 97.

Further Reading

Maudler, J. (1984), *Mind and Body: Psychology of Emotion and Stress*, New York.

Shallice, T. (1978), 'The dominant action system; an information-processing approach to consciousness', in K.

S. Pope and J. L. Singer (eds), *The Stream of Consciousness*, New York.

See also: *memory; nervous system.*

Constitutional Psychology

Constitutional psychology is, at the same time, an obvious and widely accepted feature of psychological thinking, and a controversial view held by relatively few psychologists. It may be defined as the study of the relation between, on the one hand, the morphological structure and the physiological functioning of the body and, on the other hand, psychological and social functioning. Few psychologists would disagree with the idea that bodily structure and functioning are related to one's psychosocial functioning, and in fact considerable data support this relation (see Sorell and Nowak, 1981, for a review).

The early work of Kretschmer (1921) and the later, more comprehensive research of Sheldon (1940, 1942) were criticized on conceptual, methodological, and data analytic grounds (Humphreys, 1957). The scientific community had little confidence in the strengths of association between physique type and temperament reported in this work (e.g., correlations on the order of +.8 between theoretically related physique and temperament types; Sheldon, 1941). However, more methodologically careful work has established that significant associations do exist between: (1) somatotypes (endomorphs, mesomorphs, and ectomorphs) and/or other features of the body (such as its physical attractiveness); and (2) personality or temperament characteristics theoretically related to these somatotypes (for example, viscerotonic traits, somatotonic traits, and cerebrotonic traits, respectively) or to the other bodily features (e.g., physically attractive children are more popular with peers than are physically unattractive children). But, the strengths of the association are considerably less than that reported by Sheldon; for example, correlations more typically cluster around +.3 (Walker, 1962). Moreover, research relating pubertal change (such as early, on-time, and late maturation) to psychosocial functioning has established also that significant relations exist between physiological (such as hormonal) changes or morphological characteristics and psychosocial functioning (Petersen and Taylor, 1980).

The controversy involved in constitutional psychology surrounds the explanation of the empirical relations between bodily characteristics and psychosocial functions. These explanations involve the well-known nature-nurture controversy. Only a minority of psychologists working in this area subscribe to nature-based interpretations of body-behaviour relations. Such interpretations stress that hereditary and/or other biological variables provide a common source of morphology, physiology, and psychosocial functioning. For example, the biological variables thought to provide the source of one's mesomorphic somatotype are thought also to provide the source of one's aggressive or delinquent behaviours (Hall and Lindzey, 1978). Nurture-based explanations of body–behaviour relations, which have been most popular among American psychologists (for example, McCandless, 1970), stress that environmental events (for example, socialization experiences) influence both one's bodily and one's behavioural characteristics. An example of this type of interpretation is that the socialization experiences that lead one to have a chubby body build will lead one to be dependent and/or self-indulgent (Hall and Lindzey, 1978). Finally, some interpretations propose that biological and experiential variables interact to provide a basis of one's physical, physiological, and psychosocial characteristics (see, for example, Lerner, 1982; Petersen and Taylor, 1980). A representative idea here is that children with different physical characteristics evoke differential reactions in significant others, and that these reactions feed back to children and provide a differential basis for their further psychosocial functioning; this functioning includes personality and social behaviour and also self-management behaviours (e.g., in regard to diet and exercise) which may influence their physical characteristics.

There are still no crucial or critical tests of key hypotheses derived from any of the extant interpretative positions. Indeed, data in this area, although increasingly more often theoretically-derived, are still typically open to alternative explanations. It is likely that in this area of psychology descriptive advances will continue to exceed explanatory ones for some time.

Richard M. Lerner
Pennsylvania State University

References

Hall, C. S. and Lindzey, G. (1978), *Theories of Personality* (3rd edn), New York.

Humphreys, L. G. (1957), 'Characteristics of type concepts with special reference to Sheldon's typology', *Psychological Bulletin*, 54.

Kretschmer, E. (1921), *Körperbau und Charakter*, Berlin.

Lerner, R. M. (1982), 'Children and adolescents as producers of their own development', *Developmental Review*, 2.

McCandless, B. R. (1970), *Adolescents*, Hinsdale, Ill.

Petersen, A. C. and Taylor, B. (1980), 'The biological approach to adolescence: biological change and psychological adaptation', in J. Adelson (ed.), *Handbook of Adolescent Psychology*, New York.

Sheldon, W. H. (1940), *The Varieties of Human Physique*, New York.

Sheldon, W. H. (1942), *The Varieties of Temperament*, New York.

Sorell, G. T. and Nowak, C. A. (1981), 'The role of physical attractiveness as a contributor to individual development', in R. M. Lerner and N. A. Busch-Rossnagel (eds), *Individuals as Producers of Their Development*, New York.

Walker, R. N. (1962), 'Body build and behavior in young children. I: Body build and nursery school teachers ratings', *Monographs of the Society for Research in Child Development*, 27.

Countertransference

Countertransference represents one of the most subtle and complex concepts in dynamic psychiatry. Alas for consistency, however, it is used in two quite distinct ways, each of which will be reviewed here.

(1) In the first category of definition, the term 'countertrans-

ference' refers to those feelings in the *therapist* that are stirred up unconsciously during the therapeutic process and fasten on the patient, who is thus understood to represent an important figure from the therapist's past life. In this meaning, 'counter' merely describes a vector. The issue is still transference, but since that term usually describes feelings flowing from patient to therapist, 'counter' refers here to the reverse flow. For example, the older patient might remind the younger therapist of the therapist's father, thus inhibiting the therapist from confronting the patient (where such intervention would ordinarily be necessary for the patient's good).

(2) The second major usage of the term refers to the therapist's *reaction* to the *patient's* transference. In this model, the 'counter' indicates that the therapist is responding in reaction to the stimulus provided by the patient's transferring feelings on to him. An example of this last might be that the patient transfers hostile feelings on to the therapist, and the latter, not detecting the transferential origin of these feelings, feels himself to be the subject of genuine anger and becomes angry in response.

As may be inferred from the above examples, countertransference feelings pose a problem for achievement of the realistic perceptions so essential to therapy. Because these feelings are almost unavoidable, however, they do not represent, as many novices believe, failures of technique or attitude, but rather problems requiring ongoing attention on the therapist's part. The therapist must permit their identification and resolution through introspection, self-analysis, and reality-testing.

Thomas G. Gutheil
Harvard University
Program in Psychiatry and The Law
Boston

Further Reading

Kernberg, O. F. (1965), 'Notes on countertransference', *Journal of the American Psychoanalytic Association*, 13.

Little, M. (1951), 'Countertransference and the patient's response to it', *International Journal of Psychoanalysis*, 32.

Reich, A. (1951), 'On countertransference', *International Journal of Psychoanalysis*, 32.

Winnicott, D. W. (1949), 'Hate in the countertransference', *International Journal of Psychoanalysis*, 30.

See also: *psychoanalysis; transference.*

Creativity

Creativity is the ability to bring something new into existence. It shows itself in the acts of persons. Through the creative process taking place in a person or group of persons, creative products are born. Such products may be quite diverse: mechanical inventions, new chemical processes, new solutions or new statements of problems in mathematics and science; the composition of a piece of music, or a poem, story or novel; the making of new forms in painting, sculpture, photography; the forming of a new religion or philosophical system; an innovation in law, a general change in manners, a fresh way of thinking about and solving social problems; new medical agents and techniques; even new ways of persuasion and of controlling the minds of others.

Implicit in this diversity is a common core of characteristics that mark creative products, processes, and persons. Creative products are distinguished by their originality, their aptness, their validity, their usefulness, and very often by a subtle additional property which we may call aesthetic fit. For such products we use words such as fresh, novel, ingenious, clever, unusual, divergent. The ingredients of the creative process are related functionally to the creative forms produced: seeing things in a new way, making connections, taking risks, being alerted to chance and to the opportunities presented by contradictions and complexities, recognizing familiar patterns in the unfamiliar so that new patterns may be formed by transforming old ones, being alert to the contingencies which may arise from such transformations. And in creative people, regardless of their age, sex, ethnic background, nationality, or way of life, we find certain traits recurring: an ability to think metaphorically or analogically as well as logically, independence of judgement (sometimes manifesting itself as unconventionality, rebellion, revolutionary thinking and acting), a rejection of an insufficient simplicity (or a tendency to premature closure) in favour of a search for a more complex and satisfying new order or synthesis. A certain *naïveté* or innocence of vision must be combined with stringent requirements set by judgement and experience. The act of verification is a final stage in the creative process, preceded by immersion in the problem, incubation of the process subliminally, and illumination or new vision.

The Birth of 'Creativity'

The creative aspects of Mind and of Will engaged the attention of all the major philosopher-psychologists of the late nineteenth and early twentieth centuries. Alfred Binet, the famed constructor of intelligence tests, was known first through the pages of *L'Année Psychologique* in the 1880s and 1890s as the author of widely ranging empirical studies of creativity (including research by questionnaire and interview of leading French writers) and the originator of dozens of tests of imagination (devised first as games to play with his own children). The fateful decision to exclude such occasions for imaginative play from his compendium of tasks protoypical of needed scholastic aptitudes has led to much mischief in educational application and to continuing confusion about the relationship of 'intelligence' to 'creativity'. The former as generally measured is important to certain aspects of the latter, but people of equal intelligence have been found to vary widely in creativity; and, alas, some notably creative persons have also been found notably lacking in whatever it takes to get on successfully in school.

Of the two most famous psychoanalysts, Carl Jung made the greater contribution in this field, developing especially the notions of intuition and of the collective unconscious as the sources of creation. Henri Bergson, in *Creative Evolution*, distinguished intuition from intellect as the main vehicle of the creative process in mind-in-general and in what, in retrospect, is more than mere vitalism he attributed to will, as *élan vital*, the chief motivating force of the creative process in nature. Nearly a century after Bergson's initial formulations, Gregory Bateson was writing in that same tradition, and his gradual development of 'an ecology of mind' found expression in his 1979 volume, *Mind and Nature: A Necessary Unity*.

The Modern Empirical Study of Creativity

New methods of observation and measurement have produced a marked proliferation of articles and books about creative persons, processes, and products since the Second World War. A commonly recognized milestone in the systematic research effort is an address in 1950 by J. P. Guilford who, as president of the American Psychological Association, pointed out that up to that time only 186 out of 121,000 entries in *Psychological Abstracts* dealt with creative imagination. In the following decades there was a surge of publications in the field. Studies at the University of California of highly creative contemporary writers, architects, artists, mathematicians and scientists by intensive methods of personal assessment contributed important impetus to the study of personality and creativity (work funded mostly by foundations such as Carnegie, Ford, Rockefeller, and Richardson), while the US Office of Education gave significant support to research on creativity in education. A bibliography published in the late 1960s by the Creative Education Foundation contains 4,176 references, nearly 3,000 of them dated later than 1960.

Yet this abundance of effort also produced a mixed picture of results based on psychological measurement, due mainly to inconsistencies in the choice of measures, their relative unreliability, and the equally inconsistent, somewhat unreliable, and factorially and definitionally complex criteria. Psychologists generally have restricted the term creativity to the production of humanly *valuable* novelty in an effort to exclude from consideration the relatively mundane expressions of creativity in everyday life, but this introduction of value to the definition of creativity, and the consequent invocation of historically-bound and subjective judgements to assess such value, necessarily raise theoretical and methodological questions which have bedevilled and divided students of creativity for decades. *Whose* values, for example, must be met for an act to be 'creative' – the values of the creative agent alone, or the values of a social group? And if so, which group?

Further, should the term creative be restricted to novel activities valued by connoisseurs of achievement in the 'classically creative' domains of literature, music, and the arts, or can it be applied also to novel behaviour valued by those able to recognize achievement in mathematics, science, and technology? While most creativity scholars and investigators extend 'creative' to these latter domains with few qualms, they do not generally assume that the creative processes involved in producing good literature, good music, good art and good science are the same, or that the personality and intellectual characteristics associated with creative achievement in these various domains are highly similar. And whether the term creative can be extended to novel activities of value in domains such as business, sports, teaching, therapy, parenting, and homemaking is an even more controversial question among creativity scholars.

Nor can the issue of values and standards be resolved simply by accepting as legitimate a particular domain of activity, for even within a specific domain, such as art, the question remains: whose values or standards are to be met – the values and standards of the artist who produced the piece, of other artists, of art critics, of art historians, or the audience in general? And if other artists, *which* artists; if art critics, *which* art critics; and if art historians, *which* art historians – from which schools and what eras? And if behaviour in less public domains (for example, therapy and parenting) is considered, who is to assess the novelty and effectiveness of the behaviour and how is scholarship and investigation to proceed?

Intimately related to the question of values and standards are questions concerning the nature or form of the act's impact. Several theorists, for example, have drawn distinctions between acts of 'primary' creativity – acts whose values derive from their power to transform in a basic way our perception of reality or our understanding of the universe of human experience and possibility – and acts of 'secondary' creativity – acts which merely apply or extend some previously developed meaning, principle, or technique to a new domain or instance.

While it would be comforting to be able to report that the definitional differences and distinctions reviewed here are relatively trivial compared to the core of common meaning contained within them, it is not at all clear that this is so. Whether creative individuals are identified on the basis of their achievements, or their skills and abilities, or their activities, or their personality characteristics, shapes answers to frequently asked substantive questions about creativity (for example, can creativity be taught or fostered? Can creativity be predicted? How are creativity and intelligence related?). Definitional differences and variations in emphasis have led, and will continue to lead, to many misunderstandings, misreadings, and confustions in the study of creativity. Readers of the psychological literature on creativity are therefore well advised to ascertain the conceptual perspectives and operational definitions of the scholars and investigators whose works they are examining. Thus, not only measurement unreliability in both predictors and criteria but basic definitional questions, as well as the genuine role of chance itself in both the genesis and the recognition of creativity, also have served to confound results. Overall, none the less, a strong impressionistic consensus of the sort reported at the outset of this article prevails today. And the research enterprise continues undeterred.

A critical review of the professional literature on creativity in the decade 1970–80 by F. Barron and D. Harrington in the *Annual Review of Psychology* (1981) turned up an additional 2,500 studies, produced at a steady rate of about 250 per year during that decade. Emerging new themes are creativity in women, creativity and altered states of consciousness, creativity throughout the lifespan with emphasis on the continuation of creativity in late maturity, and finally, somewhat belatedly, the social psychology of creativity: the influence of social climates and conditions facilitating creativity in the home, the classroom, the work place, and the culture itself with its enormous diversity of micro-climates and its intersection with historical and economic forces.

Frank Barron
David M. Harrington
University of California, Santa Cruz

References
Barron, F. and Harrington, D. M. (1981), 'Creativity, intelligence, and personality', *Annual Review of Psychology*, 32.
Bergson, H. (1911 [1907]), *Creative Evolution*, London. (Original French edn, *L'Evolution créative*, Paris, 1907.)

Further Reading
Albert, R. S. (1983), *Genius and Eminence: The Social Psychology of Creativity and Exceptional Achievement*, Oxford.
Barron, F. (1969), *Creative Person and Creative Process*, New York.
Ghiselin, B. (1952), *The Creative Process*, Berkeley and Los Angeles.
Koestler, A. (1964), *The Act of Creation*, New York.
Simonton, D. K. (1984), *Genius, Creativity and Leadership*, Cambridge, Mass.

Cross-Cultural Psychology

Cross-cultural psychology refers to the collective efforts of scholars in all parts of the world who do research among people who speak different languages, live in societies ranging from technologically unsophisticated to highly industrialized, and who submit to various forms of political organization. Many of the activities of these psychologists are similar to those of anthropologists, especially the emphasis on fieldwork, sensitivity to the point of view of people in the cultures under investigation, and the development of broad theories which incorporate observations made by individual researchers. Psychologists have also borrowed from anthropologists' definitions of culture. From hundreds of treatments of 'culture', key elements which have proved useful include people's conceptions about the world and the values attached to those conceptions; subjective reactions to people's view of their man-made world in the form of roles, status hierarchies, and attitudes; and symbols which provide meaning to life and which are transmitted from generation to generation.

Psychologists who undertake cross-cultural research must be willing to bear additional hardships above and beyond the difficulties of any research endeavour. Cross-cultural research involves language or dialect differences between investigator and participants, creating special problems in assuring (a) adequate and accurate communication and (b) equivalence of meaning of measuring instruments across different samples. The demands of fieldwork, including adjustment to life in another culture and time to establish one's identity among people often unfamiliar and perhaps hostile to research studies, force the development of effective skills to cope with the resulting stress.

The benefits, however, are substantial (Triandis *et al.*, 1980–1): (1) The range of independent variables available for study can be increased. For example, if a researcher is interested in the relationship between age of weaning and adult development, there is a very limited range *within* any one culture, since the norm for 'proper' weaning age is widely shared among people who have frequent contact. However, *across* cultures, the age of weaning varies widely, up to a maximum of five years. Since one variable can be related to another only if there is sufficient range in both, some studies can be done only with cross-cultural data.

(2) Variables which naturally occur together in one culture can be unconfounded, or taken apart, in another. In highly industrialized nations, it is difficult to separate the effects of age and schooling on cognitive development since virtually all children of a certain age are in school. But in other societies, some children of a given age attend school and others do not, and consequently a study of the relative contribution of the two factors can be undertaken.

(3) It is possible to test theories which are based on a clear distinction between people's competencies and their perform-

ance. One reason why researchers may not observe a competency is that people may never have had a *latent* competency challenged by a task in their everyday lives. There is the danger that the lack of behavioural evidence for the competency will be misdiagnosed as a deficit, leading to unfair charges of 'less able or intelligent'. The problem can be overcome if psychologists develop training studies in which people perform tasks that challenge their latent, but rarely used, competencies. Specifying the nature of the tasks should also be a benefit to more precise theory development, as well as to various intervention programmes, such as formal schooling.

Measurement is central to all psychological research. Probably the most central concern in measurement as applied to cross-cultural investigations is the demand for evidence that instruments are measuring relevant variables in the cultures under investigation. The demand is becoming widely accepted as a methodological *sine qua non*. The era of giving standardized tests in other cultures, without attention to cross-validation and to the construct validity of measures, is blessedly coming under intense challenges and is, one hopes, coming to an end. An alternative is the development of measures for research in another culture which assess aspects of a concept meaningful *within* that culture. For instance, Miller and her colleagues (1981), not satisfied with administering the same questionnaire in two countries and calculating mean differences, developed new measures in their investigations of the meaning of authoritarianism-conservatism in the United States and Poland. They could have administered the F-scale or the dogmatism scale in the two countries and then compared results; instead, they devised these new measures which tapped meaning unique to the United States or Poland, and they also identified a core meaning common to both countries. They found, for example, that an aspect more central to the general concept of authoritarianism-conservatism in Poland than the United States consists of items measuring a deference to hierarchical authority which is bureaucratically or legally legitimized. One of the newly-designed United States item sets focused on the endorsement of public intervention in matters ordinarily addressed elsewhere (for example, in the family or in the courts). A complete analysis of any concept, then, demands treatment of both shared aspects across cultures as well as unique aspects within each culture under investigation.

Another measurement principle in cross-cultural psychology is that direct comparisons across cultures on single measures are rarely warranted. There are too many methodological reasons why one group may score higher or lower, such as translation and/or conceptual equivalence problems, to warrant direct comparisons. An important point is that many substantive conclusions of both theoretical and practical interest can be made without direct comparison across cultures. Theoretical and practical conclusions are better made by examining the antecedents, correlates, and consequences of phenomena within cultures. Direct cross-cultural comparisons often lead to a set of score-keeping, derogatory charges of one culture high, another low on some variable. If it *is* theoretically interesting to make comparisons, it is essential to compare results consisting of patterns of multiple variables, the variables ideally measured by more than one method. Plausible rival explanations based on methodological difficulties are far more difficult to formulate, given patterns of results in contrast to single data points. Of course, substantive reasons for the patterns of variables should be specified.

Cross-cultural research has always been under threat of becoming a fringe area, separated from the mainstream of general psychology. This should not happen provided that cross-cultural researchers are careful to draw from general principles when possible and to contribute to the development of those same principles based on their data. Distinctions between cross-cultural and general psychology should diminish as more research facilities are established in various parts of the world, and as they become staffed by indigenously-trained psychologists.

Richard W. Brislin
East-West Center, Honolulu, Hawaii

References

Miller, J., Slomczynski, K. and Shoenberg, R. (1981),
  'Assessing comparability of measurement in cross-national
  research: authoritarianism-conservatism in different
  sociocultural settings', *Social Psychology Quarterly*, 44.

Triandis, H. C., Lambert, W., Berry, J., Lonner, W., Heron,
  A., Brislin, R. and Draguns, J. (eds) (1980–1), *Handbook
  of Cross-Cultural Psychology* (vols 1–6), Boston.

See also: *culture and personality*.

Culture and Personality

Culture and Personality was a psychoanalytically-oriented
subdiscipline of American cultural anthropology which sought
to relate traits of individual personality and symbolic aspects of
culture to socialization variables, that is, peculiarities of parent-
child relationships. How was individual character influenced
by culture? What were the observable processes of behaviour
by which individuals became members of their own culture?
Such questions gained prominence in the 1930s and 1940s,
when leading contributors included Bateson, Gorer, Hallowell,
Kardiner, and Kluckhohn.

The anti-eugenic and pro-relativist teaching of Franz Boas,
the immigrant German Jew and father of modern American
anthropology, is perhaps one origin of the subdiscipline. Human
behaviour was the provenance of culture and not race. The
goal was to distinguish varying cultural and psychological
processes from universal ones. Was the Oedipus complex, for
example, merely a construction whose validity was limited to
European family relationships or had it wider relevance?

Under the influence of Boas, two students, Mead and
Benedict, used vocabulary and models from developmental and
learning theories to discuss personality formation. Dubois, in
addition, employed personality assessment techniques such as
the Rorschach and word associations in her fieldwork.

Following the big wartime study of enemy national character
at Columbia University, *Research in Contemporary Cultures* (1953),
activity in this subfield began to change. Allied subfields –
medical, psychological, and cognitive anthropologies – arose

and interest in culture and personality questions was diverted into new forums.

David Lipset
University of Minnesota

Further Reading
Hsu, F. L. K. (1961), *Psychological Anthropology: Approaches to Culture and Personality*, Homewood, Ill.

Defences

The conceptualization of ego mechanisms of defence presents one of the most valuable contributions that Sigmund Freud and psychoanalysis have made to psychology. Modern psychiatrists, including non-Freudians, define defence mechanisms in a more generic sense, as innate coping styles which allow individuals to minimize sudden, often unexpected, changes in internal and external environment and to resolve cognitive dissonance (psychological conflicts). Defences are deployed involuntarily, as is the case in physiological homeostasis, and in contrast to so-called 'coping strategies'. Evidence continues to accumulate that differences in how individuals deploy defences – their unconscious coping styles – are a major consideration in understanding differential responses to environmental stress. For example, some people respond to stress in a calm, rational way, whereas others become phobic or sarcastic or emotional. These different responses are intelligible in terms of different defences.

In 1894, Sigmund Freud suggested that psychopathology was caused by upsetting affects, or emotions, rather than disturbing ideas. Freud observed that the ego's defence mechanisms can cause affects to become 'dislocated or transposed' from particular ideas or people, by processes which Freud later called dissociation, repression, and isolation. However, affects could be 'reattached' to other ideas and objects through displacement, projection and sublimation.

Freud identified four significant properties of the defences: (1) they help manage instincts and affects; (2) they are unconscious; (3) they are dynamic and reversible; and (4) although the hallmarks of major psychiatric syndromes, in most people they reflect an adaptive, not a pathological, process.

The use of defence mechanisms usually alters the individual's perception of both internal and external reality. Awareness of instinctual 'wishes' is often diminished; alternative, sometimes antithetical, wishes may be passionately adhered to. While ego mechanisms of defence imply integrated and dynamic – if unconscious – psychological processes, they are more analogous to an oppossum playing dead in the face of danger than to a reflexive eye-blink or to conscious tactics of interpersonal manipulation.

Some inferred purposes of ego mechanisms of defence are: (1) to keep affects within bearable limits during sudden changes in one's emotional life (for example, following the death of a loved one); (2) to restore psychological homeostasis by postponing or deflecting sudden increases in biological drives (such as heightened sexual awareness and aggression during adolescence); (3) to create a moratorium in which to master critical life changes (for example, puberty, life-threatening illness, or promotion); and (4) to handle unresolved conflicts with important people, living or dead.

In 1936, Freud advised the interested student: 'There are an extraordinarily large number of methods (or mechanisms, as we say) used by our ego in the discharge of its defensive functions . . . my daughter, the child analyst, is writing a book upon them.' He was referring to his eightieth-birthday present from Anna Freud; her monograph, *The Ego and the Mechanisms of Defense* (1937), is still the best single reference on the subject.

George E. Vaillant
Dartmouth Medical School, Hanover,
New Hampshire

Further Reading
Freud, S. (1964 [1894]), 'The neuro-psychosis of defence', *The Complete Works of Sigmund Freud*, vol. 3, London.

Vaillant, G. E. (1977), *Adaptation to Life*, Boston.
See also: *psychoanalysis; unconscious*.

Depressive Disorders

Depressive disorders are a heterogeneous group of conditions that share the common symptom of dysphoric mood. Current psychiatric classification divides major depressive disorders into bipolar and non-bipolar categories, depending on whether there is evidence of associated manic episodes. Less severe depressive states are categorized as dysthymic, cyclothymic, and atypical depressive disorders.

The diagnosis of a depressive disorder is made only when the intensity and duration of depressive symptoms exceed those usually provoked by the stresses of normal life. Major depressive episodes are characterized by a pervasive dysphoric mood, which may be associated with feelings of worthlessness, suicidal ideation, difficulty with concentration, inability to feel pleasure, and neurovegetative changes in appetite, sleep patterns, psychomotor activity and energy levels. In severe cases, psychotic symptoms such as hallucinations and delusions with evident depressive themes may also be present. Dysthymic disorders are conceptualized as chronic, non-psychotic conditions, of at least two years' duration, with similar symptomatology but of lesser intensity. Cyclothymic disorders involve alternating periods of dysthymic and mildly manic moods. Depressive conditions that do not clearly fit into any of these categories are designated as atypical.

Current classificatory tendencies are to group depressive disorders on the basis of their phenomonology, thus eschewing conclusions as to aetiology. Nonetheless, many experts continue to find value in differentiating between endogenous (or autonomous) and reactive, or psychotic and neurotic, conditions. However defined, the prevalence of depressive disorders is relatively high; most estimates are in the range of 7 per cent of the population suffering from a diagnosable depression each year. Lifetime incidence is thought to be 15–30 per cent, with women affected twice as often as men.

Conclusions as to aetiology remain controversial. A minority of cases have clearcut origins in medical conditions, such as viral infections, central nervous system diseases (for example, multiple sclerosis, tumours), endocrine disorders, post-partum states and nutritional deficiencies, or in the side-effects of medications, such as steroids and antihypertensives. For cases without an obvious organic basis, most experts would endorse a diathesis-stress model of causation. Some factor is believed to predispose the depressed person to experiencing the disorder, but this latent diathesis only leads to overt symptomatology when a precipitating stress occurs.

A large number of factors have been posited as inducing both the diathesis and the acute episode. Given that symptomatic depression is probably the final common pathway for a number of distinct disorders, many of these theories may be correct for separate sub-populations. The role of genetic endowment as a predisposing factor has been identified in studies that have shown a clustering of cases within families. There is evidence to suggest that pure unipolar and bipolar illnesses run in separate clusters, and that a form of dysthymic disorder may segregate in families with high incidences of alcoholism and anti-social personality disorder. Recent work has claimed to show linkage between depression and cellular antigens located on a particular chromosome.

Other theories of causation focus on the following potentially interactive factors: failures in normal personality development, losses in early life (especially death of a parent before age 17), and learned dysfunctional patterns of cognition and interpersonal behaviour.

Precipitating factors for acute episodes are often easily identifiable events, such as the loss of a parent or divorce from a spouse. In other cases, external stresses seem to be absent. Psychodynamic theorists maintain that even in these patients a seemingly minor event has been idiosyncratically interpreted as a major loss, or that something has led patients to recognize the dysfunctional nature of their existence. Freud postulated that the loss of an ambivalently regarded person is particularly likely to induce a depression because of associated difficulties in resolving grief. More biologically oriented investigators believe that some physiologic dysfunction precipitates most episodes.

Whether the cause or the result of a depressive disorder, a number of physiologic abnormalities have been associated with subgroups of depressed patients. Neurotransmitter metabolism is altered in many cases of depression. The early 'catecholamine hypothesis' pointed to evidence that a deficiency of the neuro-transmitter norepinephrine was responsible for depression, but the picture is clearly more complex than that. Various groups of depressed patients may have high, low or normal amounts of norepinephrine metabolites in blood or urine. The trans-mitters serotonin and acetylcholine have also been implicated in some studies. Although many of these findings have been replicated, a consistent theory to account for them has yet to emerge.

Other physiologic changes identified in depression include alterations in the architecture of brain-wave patterns during sleep (especially the REM phase), and in normal secretion patterns of pituitary hormones. A promising way of linking many of these abnormalities points to disturbances of the circa-dian rhythm generator in the brain-stem as a crucial defect in depression. Norepinephrine is implicated in control of the generator, which in turn can affect sleep patterns and hormone secretion rates. The peculiar observation that cases of severe depression can be successfully treated by sleep deprivation confirms the importance of this system as a locus for further study.

The natural history of depression is variable, again suggesting that we are considering a number of disorders under this general rubric. Onset of major depressive disorders can occur at any time in the life cycle, although bipolar disorders usually appear in the second or third decades of life. Untreated, these acute episodes may last for several months or even years, or may moderate somewhat and develop into dysthymic disorders. Acute episodes may be single or recurrent, and there is evidence that recurrent episodes become lengthier, with shorter inter-vening periods, as the person ages. Dysthymic disorders, especially those that appear to be related to characterologic difficulties, often begin before the age of 30. Epidemiologic studies suggest that the majority of depressive episodes are untreated, either resolving on their own, or developing into chronic disorders. An additional danger for inadequately treated patients is the risk of suicide.

Treatment of depression is as diverse as theories of aetiology. Traditional or modified forms of psychoanalysis and psycho-analytically oriented psychotherapy are often employed, although without more than anecdotal evidence of success. Enthusiasm for short-term psychotherapies in depression has been stirred by recent studies demonstrating success with time-limited interpersonal and cognitive therapies. The latter attempts to change the guilt-ridden and hopeless patterns of thought seen so frequently in depressed patients, conceptual-izing the basic disorder as one of cognition rather than of mood.

The real revolution in the treatment of depression in the last generation has occurred as a result of the development of anti-depressant medications. The tricyclic antidepressants and the monoamine oxidase inhibitors have been shown to be effective in as many as 80 per cent of major depressions, and often to be effective in dysthymic conditions. New classes of non-tricyclic drugs are now being introduced, with a major effort being made to correlate responses to particular medications with symptoma-tology and biochemical changes. The development of tech-niques for measuring blood levels of antidepressants and their metabolites has already made more precise treatment possible. Maintenance medication with antidepressants, or in the case of bipolar (and some unipolar) disorders with lithium, demon-strably decreases the frequency and intensity of recurrent episodes.

Electroconvulsive therapy (ECT) remains an important treatment, although these days it is largely reserved for life-threatening conditions, depressions refractory to drug therapy, and delusionally depressed states. Effectiveness of ECT may be as high as 90 per cent in major depressions.

In the next decade, one can look for continued changes in nomenclature of depression, as more precise ideas of aetiology are developed, and for a more careful tailoring of types of treatment to subtypes of depressive disorders.

Paul S. Appelbaum
University of Massachusetts Medical School
Worcester, Massachusetts

Further Reading
Arieti, S. and Bemporad, J. (1978), *Severe and Mild Depression*, New York.
Klein, D. F., Gittelman, R., Quitkin, F. and Rifkin, A. (1980), *Diagnosis and Drug Treatment of Psychiatric Disorders: Adults and Children*, 2nd edn, Baltimore.
Klerman, G. L. (1980), 'Overview of affective disorders', in H. I. Kaplan *et al.* (eds), *Comprehensive Textbook of Psychiatry III*, Baltimore.
Kovacs, M. and Beck, A. T. (1978), 'Maladaptive cognitive structures in depression', *American Journal of Psychiatry*, 135.
Vogel, G. W., Vogel, F., McAbee, R. S. and Thurmond, A. J. (1980), 'Improvement of depression by REM sleep deprivation: new findings and a theory', *Archives of General Psychiatry*, 37.
Weissman, M. M., Myers, J. K. and Thompson, W. D. (1981), 'Depression and its treatment in a US urban community – 1975–1976', *Archives of General Psychiatry*, 38.

Depth Perception

A classical problem in visual perception is understanding how an observer can perceive the world as extended in three dimensions from information registered on the two-dimensional retinas of the eyes. Unlike horizontal and vertical extensions in the world which are represented by proportional retinal extents, information or cues regarding the dimension of distance are coded indirectly in the visual system. There are two kinds of distance cues. One kind, called egocentric cues, provides information as to the distance of objects from the observer. The other, termed exocentric cues, indicates the depth between objects. Two instances of egocentric cues to distance involve motor adjustments of the eyes. In one of these (the cue of vergence), the two eyes turn in opposite directions in order to position the image of the object being viewed on the most sensitive portion of each retina (the fovea). In the other (the accommodative cue), the curvature of the lens of the eye is adjusted in order to focus clearly the image on the retina. These oculomotor cues are ineffective for objects beyond about three metres from the observer. A possible egocentric cue that by definition is learned and can apply to both near and distant objects is the known size of familiar objects. In general, exocentric cues are more precise than egocentric cues and help to extend the perception of distance to far distances from the observer. Among the exocentric cues that have been identified is the cue of binocular disparity, which is a consequence of the two eyes being laterally separated in the head and thus receiving slightly different views of scenes extended in depth (Ogle, 1962). Another exocentric cue occurs between different successive views of the world as the head is moved laterally, and is called relative motion parallax (Hochberg, 1972). Although the contribution and limitations of these and other sources of distance information have been examined in many studies, less is known about how the different cues are put together to help determine the perception of a unified visual world.

Walter C. Gogel
University of California, Santa Barbara

References

Hochberg, J. (1972), 'Perception II. Space and movement', in J. W. Kling and L. A. Riggs (eds), *Woodworth and Schlosberg's Experimental Psychology*, 3rd edn, New York.

Ogle, K. N. (1962), 'Spatial localization through binocular vision', in H. Davson (ed.), *The Eye*, vol. 4, *Visual Optics and the Optical Space Sense*, New York.

See also: *sensation and perception; vision.*

Developmental Psychology

Developmental psychology studies growth and change in psychological processes from before birth, through childhood, adolescence and adulthood, to old age. In its nineteenth-century origins it was strongly influenced by evolutionary theory, which saw childhood as a phase in which the transition from 'animal' to 'human' nature could be studied *in vivo*, rather than through fossils. The growth of the discipline was also stimulated by the notion – itself a bone of contention among developmentalists – that the conditions of early development strongly influence adult potential, and therefore contain the key to many social problems. As an applied science, it mainly addresses itself to practical interventions and social policy concerning the care and education of children, and has considerable overlap with experimental and clinical psychology, psychiatry, and the study of personality.

To a large extent the theoretical ideas of developmental psychology have been borrowed or adapted from other branches of psychology, and much research on development has accordingly been merely an application of whatever approaches were currently dominant in the rest of psychology. Psychoanalytic principles, for example, informed the pre-war work of Anna Freud, Melanie Klein and others on the stages of emotional development and the role of fantasy and play, and the influential post-war work of John Bowlby on attachment and the need for security. In turn, psychoanalysis came to be overshadowed by the behaviourist 'social learning' approach, which sought to explain development in terms of external contingencies, invoking general laws of learning rather than stage-related 'inner processes'.

Another major theme of developmental psychology – the development of intelligence – has been largely divorced from the study of emotional growth, and reflects social concern with sorting and grading individuals and maximizing their cognitive potential. Intellectual development has been studied from both quantitative and qualitative angles. The main instrument of quantitative study has been the IQ test, and a veritable industry has grown up around the refinement of such tests and the question of whether performance on them reflects innate endowment or environmental influences. Indeed, the construction of norms of all kinds has been a major activity of developmental psychology, through which it helps to propagate social values and regulate individual conduct.

It is in the qualitative study of cognitive development that most of developmental psychology's original contributions to the rest of psychology are to be found. Within mainstream American and British psychology, the behaviourist emphasis on studying observable stimuli and responses discouraged interest in mental processes for several decades, but a major breach in this position was made in 1959 by Chomsky, who demonstrated that the child's ability to learn language could not possibly be explained on stimulus-response principles. With mental activities once again accepted as a proper object of study, Piaget's 'cognitive-developmental' approach to the child's active structuring of the world – developed several decades earlier – was widely adopted, along with his more sensitive and detailed methods of observation. The particular theories of both Chomsky and Piaget have been heavily criticized, but their emphasis on the distinctively human activities of language and thought – to which behaviourism could not do justice – helped to displace mechanistic and biologistic thinking from psychology.

Since the 1960s, the study of linguistic and cognitive development has become one of the most fertile areas of psychology. The renewed influence (after half a century) of the Russian psychologist Vygotsky, who saw cognitive structures as rooted in social interaction, reflects growing discontent with the study of development in a social vacuum, and gradual recognition of its cultural and historical variability.

David Ingleby
University of Utrecht, The Netherlands

Further Reading
Bee, H. (1981), *The Developing Child* (3rd edn), New York.
Bower, T. G. R. (1979), *Human Development*, San Francisco.

Sants, J. and Butcher, H. J. (eds) (1975), *Developmental Psychology: Selected Readings*, Harmondsworth.
See also: *Piaget; psychoanalysis*.

Dreams

Despite their power to bewilder, frighten or amuse us, dreams remain an area of human behaviour little understood and typically ignored in models of cognition. As the methods of introspection were replaced with more self-consciously objective methods in the social sciences of the 1930s and 1940s, dream studies dropped out of the scientific literature. Dreams were neither directly observable by an experimenter nor were subjects' dream reports reliable, being prey to the familiar problems of distortion due to delayed recall, if they were recalled at all. More often dreams are, of course, forgotten entirely, perhaps due to their prohibited character (Freud, 1955 [1900]). Altogether, these problems seemed to put them beyond the realm of science.

The discovery that dreams take place primarily during a distinctive electrophysiological state of sleep, Rapid Eye Movement (REM) sleep, which can be identified by objective criteria, led to a rebirth of interest in this phenomenon. When REM sleep episodes were timed for their duration and subjects woken to make reports before major editing or forgetting could take place, it was determined that subjects accurately matched the length of time they judged the dream narrative to be ongoing to the length of REM sleep that preceded the awakening. This close correlation of REM sleep and dream experience was the basis of the first series of reports describing the nature of dreaming: that it is a regular nightly, rather than occasional, phenomenon, and a high-frequency activity within each sleep period occurring at predictable intervals of approximately every 60 to 90 minutes in all humans throughout the life span. REM sleep episodes and the dreams that accompany them lengthen progressively across the night, with the first episode being shortest, of approximately 10–12 minutes duration, and the second and third episodes increasing to 15 to 20 minutes. Dreams at the end of the night may last as long as 45 minutes, although these may be experienced as several distinct stories due to momentary arousals interrupting sleep as the night ends. Dream reports can be retrieved from normal subjects on 50 per cent of the occasions when an awakening is made prior to the end of the first REM period. This rate of retrieval is increasd to about 99 per cent when awakenings are made from the last REM period of the night. This increase in ability to recall appears to be related to an intensification across the night in the vividness of dream imagery, colours and emotions. The dream story itself in the last REM period is farthest from reality, containing more bizarre elements, and it is these properties, coupled with the increased likelihood of spontaneous arousals allowing waking review to take place, that heighten the chance of recall of the last dream. The distinctive properties of this dream also contribute to the reputation of dreams being 'crazy'. Reports from earlier dreams of the night, being more realistic, are often mistaken for waking thoughts.

Systematic content analysis studies have established that there are within-subject differences between dreams collected from home versus laboratory sleep periods, with home dreams being on the whole more affect-laden. This calls into question the representativeness of laboratory-collected dreams, particularly when subjects have not been adapted to the laboratory and the collections are carried out only for a limited period. More often, between-group comparisons are being made. Here clear differences have been reported between the home-recalled dreams of males and females, old and young, rich and poor, and between those of different ethnic groups living in the same geographical area. These differences reflect the waking sex-role characteristics, personality traits, and sociocultural values and concerns of these groups. These findings raise the question of whether dreams make some unique contribution to the total psychic economy, or merely reflect, in their distinctive imagistic, condensed language and more primitive logic, the same mental content available during wakefulness by direct observation or interviewing techniques.

The question of uniqueness of dream data and function may well be answered differently for home and laboratory retrieved dreams. Home dreams are so highly selected, whether from dream diaries or those recalled in response to questionnaires, that they yield culturally common material much like the study of common myths. In the laboratory, where the data base includes all of the dreams of a night in sequence and where experimental controls can be instituted to ensure uniform collection, the yield is more individual and varied. Despite this, the question of dream function has continued to be an area of controversy over the past thirty years of modern sleep research. It has been approached empirically through studies of the effects of dream deprivation with little progress. Neither awakenings at REM onset to abort dreams nor nights of drug-induced REM sleep deprivation have been followed by reliable deficits in waking behaviour or the appearance of dream-like waking hallucinations.

It is possible that these studies have not been carried out long enough or that the dependent measures have not been appropriately designed. Other studies have proceeded by manipulating the pre-sleep state to heighten a specific drive, such as thirst or sex, or to introduce a problem requiring completion such as a memory task and testing for the effects on dream content or subsequent waking behaviour. Again, effects have been small and rarely replicable. The laboratory setting and experimenter effects have been implicated in masking the very phenomenon the studies were designed to reveal, being more powerful stimuli than the experimental manipulation itself (Cartwright and Kaszniak, 1978).

Seldom have theoretical models of dream function been tested. These have varied widely in the psychological processes implicated. Learning and memory have been prominent, as in the Hughlings Jackson (1932) view that sleep serves to sweep away unnecessary memories and connections from the day. This was recently revised by Crick and Mitchison (1983) and stated as a theory that dream sleep is a period of reversed learning. However, the opposite view that dreaming has an information-handling, memory-consolidating function (Hennevin and Leconte, 1971) is also common. Other writers stress an affective function. Greenberg and Pearlman (1974) and Dewan (1970) hold that during dreaming, reprogramming of emotional experiences occurs, integrating new experiences and updating existing programmes. The modern psychoanalytically oriented view is an adaptation of Freud's conception of dreams as safe ways for unconscious drive discharge to take place (Fisher, 1965; French and Fromm, 1964). Beyond the issue of what psychological process is involved is the further problem posed by those who deny that studies of dream content can make any headway without taking into account their latent as well as their manifest content. This requires obtaining waking associations to each dream to plumb their function fully. Such a design would produce confounding effects on subsequent dreams.

Despite the theoretical morass and methodological problems rife in this field, systematic headway in understanding dreams has been made. One such advance came from a ground-breaking longitudinal collection of home and laboratory dreams of boys and girls by Foulkes (1982). These were analysed to explore the age- and sex-related changes in dream structure and content in terms of the cognitive and other aspects of the developmental stages of these children. Another advance came in the area of methodology with the development of standardized content analysis systems (Foulkes, 1978) and rating scales (Winget and Kramer, 1979). Another recent improvement in design combines the advantages of the methods of the laboratory with the reality of a field study by predicting dream-content differences in the laboratory-retrieved dreams among groups of persons differing in response to a major affect-inducing life event.

The study of dreams is ready to move beyond the descriptive. Many facts have been amassed about this distinctive mental activity without any clear understanding of its basic nature. How is a dream put together into a dramatic format without the contribution of any voluntary intent of the dreamer? How are the new perceptions formed that often express in such highly economical terms a coming together of old memories and current waking experiences? Do dreams have effects despite the fact that they are forgotten? What do these processes tell us about how the mind works? Dreams are a difficult challenge. They deserve our best response.

Rosalind D. Cartwright
Rush-Presbyterian-St Luke's Medical Center, Chicago

References

Cartwright, R. and Kaszniak, A. (1978), 'The social psychology of dream reporting', in A. Arkin *et al.* (eds), *The Mind in Sleep*, Hillsdale, N.J.

Crick, F. and Mitchison, G. (1983), 'The function of dream sleep', *Nature*, 304.

Dewan, E. (1970), 'The programming "P" hypotheses for REM sleep', in E. Hartmann (ed.), *Sleep and Dreaming*, Boston.

Fisher, C. (1965), 'Psychoanalytic implications of recent research on sleep and dreaming. II. Implications of psychoanalytic theory', *Journal of American Psychoanalytical Association*, 13.

Foulkes, D. (1978), *A Grammar of Dreams*, New York.

Foulkes, D. (1982), *Children's Dreams*, New York.

French, T. and Fromm, E. (1964), *Dream Interpretation: A New Approach*, New York.

Freud, S. (1955 [1900]), *The Interpretation of Dreams*, ed. J. Strachey, New York.

Greenberg, R. and Pearlman, C. (1974), 'Cutting the REM nerve: an approach to the adaptive role of REM sleep', *Perspectives in Biology and Medicine*.

Hennevin, E. and Leconte, P. (1971), 'La fonction du sommeil paradoxal: faits et hypotheses', *L'Ann. Psychologique*, 2.

Jackson, J. H. (1932), *Selected Writings of John Hughlings Jackson*, ed. J. Taylor, London.

Winget, C. and Kramer, M. (1979), *Dimensions of Dreams*, Gainesville.

Further Reading

Cartwright, R. (1977), *Night Life: Explorations in Dreaming*, Englewood Cliffs, N.J.

Cohen, D. (1979), *Sleep and Dreaming*, New York.
Fishbein, W. (1981), *Sleep, Dreams and Memory*, New York.
See also: *fantasy; sleep.*

Drugs
See Drug Use, Psychopharmacology.

Drug Use
The ingestion of mind-altering substances is very nearly a human universal; in practically every society, a sizeable proportion of its members take at least one drug for psychoactive purposes (Weil, 1972). This has been true for a significant stretch of history. Fermentation was one of the earliest of discoveries, predating the fashioning of metal; humans have been ingesting alcoholic beverages for some 10,000 years. Several dozen plants contain chemicals that influence the workings of the mind, and have been smoked, chewed or sniffed by members of societies all over the world. These plants include coca leaves, the opium poppy, marijuana, the psilocybin mushroom, the peyote cactus, quat leaves, nutmeg, tobacco, coffee beans, tea leaves, and the cocoa bean. During the past century or more, hundreds of thousands of psychoactive chemicals have been discovered, isolated or synthesized by scientists or physicians. Thousands have been marketed for medicinal purposes. According to the journal, *Pharmacy Times*, approximately 1.5 billion medical prescriptions for drugs are written each year in the United States alone. Although most of these drugs are not psychoactive, roughly one out of six of these prescriptions is written for a substance that significantly alters the workings of the human mind. Drug-taking is one of the more widespread of human activities.

Most of the time that psychoactive chemicals are ingested, they are used 'in a culturally approved manner' (Edgerton, 1976), with little or no negative impact on the user or on society. However, in a significant minority of cases, drugs are taken in a culturally unacceptable or disapproved fashion: a condemned drug is taken instead of an approved one, it is taken too frequently or under the wrong circumstances, for the wrong reasons, or with undesirable consequences. With the establishment of the modern nation-state and, along with it, the elaboration of an explicit legal code, certain actions came to be deemed illegal or criminal. The use, possession or sale of certain kinds of drugs, taking drugs in certain contexts, or the ingestion of drugs for disapproved motives, have been regarded as crimes in nearly all countries, punished with a fine or imprisonment of the offender. The catch-all term 'abuse' is commonly used to refer to somewhat different types of drug use: (1) any use of an illegal drug for non-medical purposes, or (2) any use of a drug, legal or illegal, to the point where it becomes a threat to the user's physical or mental well-being, or interferes with major life goals or functioning, such as educational or occupational achievement, or marriage. 'Misuse' is the term that is commonly used to refer to the inappropriate use of a legal prescription drug for medical purposes.

It must be emphasized that drug use is not a unitary phenomenon. There are, to begin with, different types of drugs, classified according to their action. Drugs are commonly categorized on the basis of their impact on the central nervous system (the CNS) – the brain and spinal cord. Some drugs speed up signals passing through the CNS; they are called *stimulants* and include cocaine, the amphetamines, caffeine, and nicotine. Other drugs retard signals passing through the CNS, and are called *depressants*. Depressants include *narcotics* (such as opium, heroin, and morphine), which dull the sensation of pain, *sedatives* (such as alcohol, the barbiturates, and mathaqualone) and 'minor' *tranquillizers* (such as Valium), which reduce anxiety, and 'major' tranquillizers or *antipsychotics*, which inhibit the manifestation of symptoms of psychosis, especially schizophrenia. Hallucinogens (such as LSD) and marijuana do not fit neatly into this stimulant-depressant continuum.

Psychoactive drugs, even of the same type, are taken for a variety of reasons: to attain religious or mystical ecstasy, to suppress fatigue, hunger, or anxiety, to enhance hedonism and pleasure, to heal the body or the mind, to facilitate socializing or interpersonal intimacy, to follow the dictates of a particular group or subculture, and to establish an identity as a certain kind of person. A drug's psychoactive properties may be central to the user's motive for taking it, or incidental to it; the intoxication may be experienced for intrinsic reasons (that is, the drug is taken by the user to get 'high') or the drug taken for instrumental purposes (that is, to attain a specific goal, such as alleviating pain). Of the many varieties of drug use, perhaps the three most common and important are: (1) legal recreational use, (2) illegal recreational use, and (3) legal medical use. Each of these modes of use will attract strikingly different users and will have strikingly different consequences. Even the same drug will be used by a different set of individuals for entirely different purposes with different effects. It is a fallacy to assume that the pharmacological properties of a drug dictate the consequences following its use; factors such as the motives for its use, the social context in which use is embedded, social norms surrounding use, methods of use, and so on, all play a major role in a drug's impact on the individual and on society. It is misleading, therefore, to assume that the use of even the same drug in different cultural settings will result in the same effects, consequences or impact. In parts of India, for example, holy men (*sadhus*) smoke cannabis to quell their appetite for food and sex; in the West, the same drug is successfully used to enhance precisely the same appetites.

(1) *Legal recreational use* refers to the attempt to alter one's consciousness by ingesting a psychoactive substance whose possession is not against the law. For the most part, in Western nations, this refers mainly to alcohol consumption. When the term 'drug' is used to apply to substances consumed outside a medical context, it usually connotes those whose use is illegal and/or strongly condemned and disvalued. It rarely refers to substances such as alcohol. Although not generally perceived or regarded as a drug, alcohol qualifies for the term in a pharmacological and a physiological sense: not only is it psychoactive, and widely used for this reason, but it can produce a physical dependence, or 'addiction', in heavy, long-term, chronic users, and it causes or is associated with a wide range of medical maladies. Many estimates place the proportion of alcoholics at roughly one drinker in ten, and argue that

alcoholism is the West's most serious drug problem. In short, alcohol is 'a drug by any other name' (Fort, 1973).

(2) Of all types of drug use, *illegal recreational use* attracts the most public attention and interest. In the two decades following the early 1960s, Western Europe and North America experienced an unprecedented rise in the recreational use of illegal psychoactive drugs. The most widely used of these drugs are marijuana and hashish, products of the plant *Cannabis sativa*. In most countries, there are as many episodes of cannabis use as episodes of the use of all other illegal drugs combined. And of all illegal drugs, cannabis is the one that users are most likely to continue using regularly, and least likely to abandon or use extremely episodically. Of all illegal drugs, marijuana is the one with the highest ratio of current to lifetime users. In one study, 52 per cent of all at least one-time marijuana users had taken this drug one or more times in the past month; for cocaine, this was 34 per cent, for the other stimulants, 19 per cent, for the hallucinogens, 18 per cent, and for the sedatives, 16 per cent (Fishburne *et al.*, 1980). Cannabis is the illegal drug that people most frequently 'stick with'. As with alcohol, the majority of users take the drug in a fairly moderate, controlled fashion. Approximately 10 per cent of all cannabis users become so involved with their drug of choice that it becomes an obsession or a psychological dependency, threatening their health and occupational or educational attainment. While the recreational use of more dangerous drugs, such as heroin, cocaine, and barbiturates, is considerably less than for cannabis, the potential for abuse of these substances is far greater. It is estimated that there are as many as half a million heroin addicts in the United States alone (Goode, 1984).

(3) The *medical use* of psychoactive chemicals in the Western world has undergone dramatic changes over the past century. Late in the nineteenth century, over-the-counter preparations containing psychoactive substances such as morphine and cocaine were freely available and were widely used to treat or cure medical ailments. Legal controls on what these nostrums contained were practically non-existent. When authorities became aware of widespread abuses of these drugs, dispensing

them became tightly controlled, and medical prescriptions became necessary to obtain them. In the United States, the number of prescriptions written for psychoactive drugs rose steadily until the early 1970s when, again, misuse and abuse of these substances was publicized. Since that time, there has been a steep decline in the number of psychoactive drug doses dispensed by physicians. For instance, in the United States in 1975, 61.3 million prescriptions were written for Valium, that nation's number one prescription drug; in 1980, this figure had dropped to 33.6 million (Rosenblatt, 1982). The number of prescriptions written for morphine in 1981 was half the number for 1976. Benzedrine, a once popular stimulant, was prescribed one-sixth as often in 1981 as in 1976 (Goode, 1984). There has been a dramatic downward trend in the use of psychoactive prescription drugs between the 1970s and the 1980s; the trend continues unabated. With some of these drugs, such as the barbiturates, this cut-back has translated into a decline in illegal recreational or 'street' usage; with other drugs, such as methaqualone and amphetamine, this has not taken place.

In contrast, the treatment of psychotic disorders, mainly schizophrenia, with the use of anti-psychotic drugs such as Thorazine, has been increasing dramatically since their discovery in the 1950s. The impact of the medical use of anti-psychotic drugs, also called 'major' tranquillizers, can be measured by the dramatic decline in the number of resident patients in mental hospitals. Between 1945 and 1955, in the United States, there was a yearly average increase of 13,000 patients residing in state mental hospitals; in the latter year, the total was just under 560,000. Between 1954 and 1955, psychoactive agents were introduced as treatment for psychosis. Because of the success of this modality in controlling the symptoms of schizophrenia, patients who were previously confined in hospitals were released as outpatients. By 1978, the number of resident state mental hospital patients in the United States had plumetted to under 150,000 (Ray, 1983). The average length of hospitalization dropped from six months in 1955 to 26 days in 1976. The decline in the number of mental patients in hospi-

tals can be traced directly to the use of anti-psychotic or pheno-
thiazine drugs, the 'major' tranquillizers.

Erich Goode
State University of New York at Stony Brook

References

Edgerton, R. B. (1976), *Deviance: A Cross-Cultural Perspective*,
   Menlo Park, Calif.
Fishburne, P. M. *et al.* (1980), *National Survey on Drug Abuse:
   Main Findings, 1979*, Rockville, Maryland.
Fort, J. (1973), *Alcohol: Our Biggest Drug Problem*, New York.
Goode, E. (1984), *Drugs in American Society*, 2nd edn, New
   York.
Ray, O. (1983), *Drugs, Society, and Human Behavior*, 3rd edn, St
   Louis.
Rosenblatt, J. (1982), 'Prescription-drug abuse', *Editorial
   Research Reports*, 1.
Weil, A. (1972), *The Natural Mind: A New Way of Looking at
   Drugs and the Higher Consciousness*, Boston.

Further Reading

Abel, E. L. (1982), *Marihuana: The First Twelve Thousand Years*,
   New York.
Grinspoon, L. and Bakalar, J. B. (1979), *Psychedelic Drugs
   Reconsidered*, New York.
Judson, H. F. (1974), *Heroin Addiction in Britain*, New York.
Young, J. (1971), *The Drugtakers: The Social Meaning of Drug
   Use*, London.
See also: *psychopharmacology*.

DSM III

DSM III is the third edition of the American Psychiatric Association's *Diagnostic and Statistical Manual of Mental Disorders*,
published in 1980. It is a guide for diagnosis of mental illnesses,
whether for clinical, administrative or legal purposes.

Historically, classification systems for mental disorders are
relatively recent. In 1863, Kahlbaum proposed the first classifi-

cation system based on observation rather than theory. In 1892, Kraepelin published such a classification, that separated for the first time those serious illnesses with a deteriorating course (such as, dementia praecox) from those that might be serious and episodic, but did not result in progressive dysfunction (for example, cyclic insanity). These conditions, now better understood, are referred to respectively as schizophrenia and manic-depressive disorder. In the United States, the first complete nomenclature, *The Standard Classified Nomenclature of Disease*, was printed in 1933. In 1952, the American Psychiatric Association issued the first DSM, and in 1968, the second. Both of these manuals used the traditional trichotomization of mental disorders: psychosis, neurosis and personality disorders.

DSM III makes a further attempt to specify and to clarify mental disorders, to avoid any implication of aetiology (for example, neuroses stemming from unconscious conflict) by using a 'descriptive approach', and to delimit sharply some diagnoses (such as schizophrenia) while moving toward a spectrum concept for others (for example, manic-depressive illness, now called affective disorders). While it is not explicitly stated, the fact that affective disorders and anxiety states can now be treated much more effectively, while schizophrenia remains more problematic, leads to exclusionary criteria favouring the spectrum approach to these more treatable illnesses.

DSM III defines five axes: (1) those illnesses previously considered neurotic or psychotic; (2) only the personality disorders – so that one may diagnose both a non-personality disorder (such as schizophrenia) and personality disorder (for example, schizoid); (3) physical disorders, some of which might previously have been considered 'psychosomatic'; (4) indicating the severity of the pre-illness stressors; and (5) the highest level of recent functioning. Since Axes 1 and 2 contain all the mental disorders, they will be the focus of further discussion.

DSM III begins with conditions that usually start in childhood, including mental retardation, and attention deficit, conduct, anxiety, eating, stereotyped movement (such as tics), and pervasive developmental disorders (for example, infantile autism). Next, the manual lists the organic mental disorders, whether acute (deliria) or chronic (dementias), and whether of unknown (primary degenerative dementia) or known (for example, alcohol or other abused substances) cause. Substance abuse itself is diagnosed separately. The schizophrenic disorders are divided into disorganized, catatonic, paranoid and undifferentiated types. Paranoid disorders, as well as several other psychotic conditions (such as, schizophreniform, brief reactive, and schizo-affective), are listed separately. The affective disorders group contains those illnesses which are major (previously considered manic-depressive), other (previously neurotic or characterological), and atypical (such as present with hypersomnia rather than insomnia). The anxiety disorders emcompass phobias (with or without panic attacks), anxiety states (including obsessive-compulsive disorders) and post-traumatic stress disorders. An entirely new concept, that of somatoform disorders, incorporates somatization, conversion, psychogenic pain and hypochondriacal disorders. Then there are the dissociative (amnesia, fugue, and so on) and psychosexual disorders – the latter divided into paraphilias (for example, transvestism, voyeurism, sadism) and dysfunctions (for example, inhibited orgasm). Finally there are separate categories for factitious, impulse control and adjustment disorders. As mentioned previously, the personality disorders are all classified in Axis 2 and include paranoid, schizoid, schizotypal, histrionic, narcissistic, antisocial, borderline, avoidant, dependent, compulsive, passive-aggressive, and mixed personality disorders.

John A. Talbott
Cornell University Medical College
The Payne Whitney Psychiatric Clinic
The New York Hospital

References
American Psychiatric Association (APA) (1952), *Diagnostic and Statistical Manual of Mental Disorders*, 1st edn, Washington, DC.

APA (1968), *Diagnostic and Statistical Manual of Mental Disorders*, 2nd edn, Washington, DC.

APA (1980), *Diagnostic and Statistical Manual of Mental Disorders*, 3rd edn, Washington, DC.

Commonwealth Fund (1933), *The Standard Classified Nomenclature of Disease*, New York.

Kahlbaum, K. L. (1973 [1862]), *Catatonia*, Baltimore.

Kraepelin, E. (1921 [1892]), *Manic Depressive Insanity and Paranoia*, Edinburgh.

See also: *mental disorders*.

Dyslexia

The general meaning of dyslexia is an impairment of the ability to read. Such impairments can arise in either of two ways: (1) There are cases of people who learned to read normally and reached a normal level of skill in reading, and who subsequently suffered some form of damage to the brain, a consequence of which was a reduction or even loss of their reading ability. This is often referred to as acquired dyslexia. (2) There are cases of people who fail to learn to read adequately in the first place and who never reach a normal level of skill in reading. The condition from which they suffer is known as developmental dyslexia. (An alternative terminology is to use the words *alexia* for acquired dyslexia, and *dyslexia* for development dyslexia.) These are two rather different conditions.

A parallel term is dysgraphia, the general meaning of which is an impairment of the ability to spell (in writing or aloud). This too can be an acquired or a developmental disorder, so that acquired and developmental dysgraphia are distinguished. The terms agraphia and dysgraphia are sometimes used to express this distinction.

A child's intelligence is strongly related to the likelihood that an adequate level of reading will be attained. Therefore there will be children whose reading ability is less than would be expected for their age but is what would be expected for their level of intelligence. In contrast, however, there are also children who are of normal intelligence but who read less well than would be expected for their age and intelligence. The first kind of dyslexia might be thought of as a non-specific concomitant of below-normal intelligence, whilst the second kind is specific to reading and associated abilities, since other intellectual abilities are at a normal level. It has been argued by Rutter and Yule (1975) that this distinction is important. Hence they proposed the term *reading backwardness* to refer to a condition in which poor reading is accompanied by similarly poor performance in other, unrelated, intellectual spheres, and the term *specific reading retardation* to refer to a condition in which only reading and closely related abilities are impaired.

Current progress in understanding the nature of acquired and developmental dyslexia and dysgraphia is being achieved largely through taking seriously the obvious fact that neither reading nor spelling is an indivisible mental activity: each relies on the correct functioning of a considerable number of independent cognitive subsystems. It follows that impairment of any one of the various cognitive subsystems involved in reading will produce some form of dyslexia. The particular form of dyslexia which will be seen will depend upon the particular cognitive subsystem which is imperfect. Theories about which cognitive subsystems actually underlie reading and spelling thus permit one to offer interpretations of the different sets of symptoms manifest in different varieties of dyslexia and dysgraphia.

Max Coltheart
Birkbeck College, University of London

Reference
Rutter, M. and Yule, W. (1975), 'The concept of specific reading retardation', *Journal of Child Psychology and Psychiatry*, 16.

Further Reading
Coltheart, M. (1982), 'The psycholinguistic analysis of acquired dyslexias', *Philosophical Transactions of the Royal Society*, B298.
Ellis, A. W. (1984), *Reading, Writing and Dyslexia*, London.

Jorm, A. F. (1983), *The Psychology of Reading and Spelling Disabilities*, London.

Eastern Psychology

Eastern psychology is the widely used, though rather unfortunate, label for a rapidly growing field of study that is concerned to translate the insights and techniques of various spiritual and mystical traditions into the languages and mechanisms of contemporary psychology. These traditions are to be found in Europe (mystical Christianity) and the Middle East (Hasidism and Sufism) as well as in India (Buddhism), China (Taoism) and Japan (Zen). And the geographical distinction becomes even more inappropriate as increasing numbers of practitioners from these 'schools' come to settle and to teach in Western Europe and America.

Spiritual traditions are best seen neither as systems of belief nor as codes of conduct, but as practical psychologies and psychotherapies of considerable depth, sophistication and subtlety. Their goal is not to inform but to transform the serious student. Man lives, they all agree, under an almost universal misapprehension – that there is such a thing as an individual Self, and that we all 'have' one, or 'are' one. While to most people it is second nature that 'I' exist as something *separate* from other things, *persisting* through space and time, and at least partially *autonomous* in what 'I' choose and think and do, nevertheless this creation of a boundary is an error. Or rather it is an error if we take it as referring to a 'real' discontinuity in nature rather than as a convention that exists only within thought and speech. Contour lines convey useful information about mountains, but we should not fear lest we trip over them as we climb, nor do we expect Everest to ascend in neat hundred metre steps. The illusion of the Self is of the same sort, and it leads to the same kinds of bizarre actions and expectations – which we do not see as strange only because everybody else is under the same spell. 'The (Self) is an imaginary, false belief which has no corresponding reality . . . It is the source of all the troubles in the world from personal conflicts to wars between nations' (Rahula, 1967). This is what Buddha, Lao

Tsu, Rinzai, Jesus, Muhammad and all other disillusioned masters have taught.

Where Eastern psychology goes beyond much of humanistic psychology and psychotherapy, therefore, is that it focuses on what is seen as the *root* of all misery, rather than on its many forms; and its goal is not improvement but insight. Liberation and integration occur not as a result of the effort and intention to change, but simply and automatically through inspecting clearly what is the case and what is not. When one observes closely the conjurer's sleight-of-hand, the magic is dispelled. This unbiased wide-eyed scrutiny of the details of life is *meditation*.

Eastern psychology's fascination lies in its bringing together of the theoretical and the experimental with the experiential. Conceptual advances are being made. Empirical research about the physical and neurophysiological effects of meditation is accumulating. And at the same time the only real proof of the pudding is in the eating: the student is his or her own subject, and what could be of greater interest to me than my self?

Guy Claxton
Chelsea College
University of London

Reference
Rahula, W. (1967), *What the Buddha Taught*, Bedford.

Further Reading
Claxton, G. L. (Swami Anand Ageha) (1981), *Wholly Human: Western and Eastern Visions of the Self and its Perfection*, London.
Wilber, K. (1977), *The Spectrum of Consciousness*, Wheaton, Ill.

Educational Psychology
Educational psychology covers two related, but distinguishable, fields. One is a branch of academic psychology that seeks to understand the processes of teaching and learning. The other is a profession – specifically that which is concerned to diagnose

and to treat those handicaps and lacks that impede or impair a person's ability to learn. To aid this distinction the academics tend to refer to themselves as 'psychologists of education' while the professionals are more generally known as 'educational psychologists'.

In practice both the descriptions given above are too general. Academic educational psychology has focused almost exclusively on specific *contexts* of teaching and learning, and specific *types of knowledge* that are acquired. The contexts are formal institutions of education – schools, colleges and universities. The types of knowledge are predominantly conceptual, symbolic, verbal and rational.

These overemphases arise because psychologists have been as guilty as anyone of confusing 'schooling' with 'education', and thereby assuming that what is important in school reflects what is important psychologically. The best example of this is the fact that there is still no integrative framework for viewing human learning. There are many *cognitive* theories (e.g. Smith, 1975) but they neither contain, nor are readily coupled to, ways of construing feeling, need, intuition, physical skill, social demeanour or personality. Yet, while intellect forms the *de jure* matter of schools, these other domains are central parts of its *de facto* curriculum, at least for the young people.

This links to a second underlying assumption of the psychology of education, namely that because teachers are important in schools they are important in learning. Many people would agree with Ausubel (1968) that it is the teachers's prime task to 'ascertain what the learner knows and teach him accordingly'. But this demand has unsettled generations of student teachers, for it is clearly impossible to keep tabs on the shifting states of knowledge and readiness of twenty or thirty other people. The best way to ascertain what the learner already knows is to feed him and let him spit out what he doesn't want. But teachers acquire from psychologists a lack of trust in the learner's ability to chew and to choose, and from the examin ation boards the assumption that the menu has been so well designed that to wish to leave some on the plate is a symptom of either ill-health or sacrilege. In general, psychologists of education are beginning to suspect that teaching is neither necessary nor sufficient to produce learning, and that it can have many unintended, unacknowledged, conflicting and counterproductive effects.

The relationship of the 'psychology of education' to 'educational psychology' is similar to that of physiology to medicine: the former generates knowledge which the latter adapts and uses to remedy disabilities of learning (though, like medicine, educational psychology generates and conducts its own applied research as well). In practice, educational psychologists concern themselves mostly with the problem of school-age children, although their statutory responsibility in England and Wales is for the 2 to 19-year-old range. Most educational psychologists in the UK are employed by local Education Authorities, and work within the School Psychological Service. They may also have responsibilities within Child Guidance Clinics.

The work in academic psychology on which educational psychologists can draw is extensive. They tend, however, to make use of any or all of three main areas: (1) psychometrics, from which come the specialist tests, diagnostic tools and measuring instruments which are the stock-in-trade of many educational psychologists; (2) psychotherapy, which provides methods of treatment, particularly for emotional and neurotic problems, that are based on empathic conversation (though play and fantasy may be used as well) with the child and/or his family; (3) behaviourism or 'learning theory', which has generated the principles and techniques of behaviour modification. There is sometimes acrimony between those who favour one or the other of these approaches to behavioural and learning problems. The testers are said to use their tests in mechanical and insensitive ways. The behaviourists, it is claimed, degrade and dehumanize their clients by treating them simply as faulty machines to be fixed. And those of a therapeutic or humanistic persuasion are accused of being romantic and ineffective. These criticisms have some force when levelled – in less crude terms – at *abuses* of the methods: they are not valid comments on the methods as such.

Trained educational psychologists help to ensure that the best possible decisions are made in respect to children who are having trouble at school. To this end they will spend time talking with, and perhaps administering tests to, the child in question; consulting with teachers, parents and other professionals (education welfare officers, social workers, remedial teachers, child psychiatrists and psychotherapists); finding out what suitable provisions (special schools, tutorial centres, residential homes) are available, and writing detailed reports and recommendations. This latter activity is an increasingly prominent and time-consuming part of the work, In addition to this, educational psychologists may work directly with parents or teachers to help them set up and monitor programmes of training or other conditions that will be helpful to the child. And they act too in an advisory and consultative capacity to schools, local authorities and other interested parties. Senior members of the profession will also be involved in formulating policy on how to deal with the various types of child in need of special educational help. Whether children with such 'special education needs' (Warnock, 1978) are best helped within normal schools, or whether they do better in specially designed schools, is such an issue, the preferred solution to which alternates from generation to generation.

The educational psychologist's clients fall into three main groups – the physically handicapped (those with serious impairments to vision, hearing or co-ordination, for example); the mentally handicapped (those with learning or other predominantly intellectual problems that have some clearly identifiable and usually irremedial physical basis); and those whose problems are seen as primarily emotional or social. Some of the latter children are labelled 'maladjusted' or as having 'behavioural problems', though the questions of to whom the behaviour is a problem, and whether it is healthy for a particular young person to adjust to a school system that may be damaging his dignity and denying him a sense of worth or purpose, are sometimes not explored as fully as they might be (Hargreaves, 1982). It is currently thought to be an advance to dispense with labels for different kinds of client, and to categorize instead the types of educational provision that they are deemed to require.

Guy Claxton
Chelsea College, University of London

References
Ausubel, D. (1968), *The Psychology of Meaningful Verbal Learning*, New York.
Hargreaves, D. H. (1982), *The Challenge for the Comprehensive School*, London.
Smith, F. (1975), *Comprehension and Learning*, New York.
Warnock, M. (1978), *Special Educational Needs*, London.

Further Reading
Chazan, M., Moore, T., Williams, P., Wright, J. and Walker, M. (1974), *The Practice of Educational Psychology*, London.
See also: *learning*.

Electroconvulsive Therapy

Electroconvulsive therapy (ECT) is essentially the induction of a cerebral seizure by application of an electrical stimulus to the scalp. The convulsive procedure was introduced after clinical observations suggested sudden improvement in psychiatric patients after spontaneous convulsions. The use of electricty to induce seizures was first introduced by two Italian psychiatrists, Cerletti and Bini, in 1938. Today the use of muscle relaxants almost entirely avoids the actual physical convulsion, which was similar to an epileptic seizure. The physiological reaction in the brain, however, which is like that associated with an epileptic seizure, is unaffected by the relaxing drugs, and is the essential therapeutic event in the treatment. The usual therapeutic course involves a total of eight to twelve treatments administered at the rate of two or three per week.

From the outset, clinical improvement was noted when the treatment was administered to patients with severe depressive illness or psychosis. Because of dramatic clinical improvement following the use of ECT in some patients, and with new control over adverse side-effects such as fractures and dislocations, some psychiatrists tended to use ECT for conditions other than depression. However, although ECT is occasionally of benefit to patients with other conditions, its continued use is in the main justified by the positive response of depressed patients for whom other treatments may be less effective; it has also led to improvement in catatonic states and in other cases of schizophrenia.

One of the concerns about ECT regards possible loss of memory. Memory loss following ECT varies, Some patients return to intellectually demanding jobs with no sense of impairment. Others complain of problems with memory. When both electrodes are placed over the non-dominant hemisphere, memory complaints are fewer. Almost all memory difficulties disappear over days or weeks, although occasionally memories of the treatment period itself may be persistently lost.

It has been postulated that the efficacy of ECT as an anti-depressant results from the increased release and distribution of hypothalamic peptides in the brain. Understanding the therapeutic effect of ECT in this and other conditions will require further investigation.

Fred H. Frankel
Harvard University
Beth Israel Hospital, Boston

Further Reading
American Psychiatric Association Task Force on
    Electroconvulsive Therapy (1978), *Report no. 14*. APA,
    Washington, D.C.
See also: *biological psychiatry; depressive disorders*.

Emotion

William James wrote that he would 'as lief read verbal descriptions of the shapes of the rocks on a New Hampshire farm' as toil again through the classic works on emotion, which lacked a 'central point of view, a deductive or generative principle'. Since then, many theories of emotion have been advanced, but none has succeeded in gaining widespread acceptance. Indeed, one hundred years after James's famous essay in *Mind* (1884), 'What is an emotion?', we are hardly better placed than James to answer the question he posed – a situation which is partly attributable to the neglect of emotion by psychologists during the behaviourist era. Recently, however, there has been a notable resurgence of interest from psychologists and other social scientists in the study of emotion. Most theories of emotion adopt a biological or psychological level of analysis, although more emphasis is also given nowadays to social and cultural factors.

The issues that preoccupy modern emotion theory are remarkably similar to those that arose from James's (1884) theory of emotion and its subsequent rebuttal by Cannon. Briefly, James advocated what has come to be called a *peripheral* theory of emotion, in which he argued that the perception of an arousing stimulus causes changes in peripheral organs such as the viscera (heart, lungs, stomach, and so on) and the voluntary muscles, and that emotion is quite simply the perception of these bodily changes. To use James's own example, it is not that we run because we are afraid; rather, we are afraid because we run. This view clearly implies that there should be as many discrete patterns of physiological activity accompanying emotion as there are discernible emotional states. Cannon (1927) published what was widely regarded as a devastating critique of James's theory, although later research has shown that some, if not all, of Cannon's objections were ill-founded.

The essence of Cannon's critique was that the visceral changes that occur during emotion are too non-specific to serve as the basis for differentiated emotional experience. This point led later researchers to abandon the search for an explanation of emotion couched exclusively in terms of bodily changes, and to consider more carefully the role played by cognitive factors – the individual's interpretation of external and internal events. Two cognitive theories of emotion have attracted some attention. The more complex theory is the one proposed by Lazarus and his associates (Lazarus *et al.*, 1970), basic to which is the notion that emotion is based on the individual's *appraisal* of his circumstances. Thus the appraisal of a stimulus as 'threatening' instigates various responses (cognitive, expressive and instrumental) which together comprise the experience of fear. One limitation of Lazarus's theory is that it was developed with specific reference to the understanding of stress, and it is by no means clear how easily it generalizes to other emotions.

The other influential cognitive theory of emotion is Schachter's (1964) two-factor theory. One of Cannon's objections to James's theory was that the artificial induction (by adrenaline injection) of bodily changes characteristic of emotion does not result in emotional experience. Schachter reasoned that this is because the individual knows the bodily changes to be the product of the injection, rather than an emotional stimulus. Therefore, emotion is the joint product of *two* factors, namely a general state of physiological arousal, and the cognition that this arousal is caused by an emotional stimulus. The arousal creates the conditions necessary for *any* emotion to be experienced, while the cognition determines which emotion is actually experienced. Thus the same physiological arousal could, in principle, be experienced as any of a variety of emotions, depending on cognitive factors. Although this theory has an appealing elegance and simplicity, there is little evidence to support it (Manstead and Wagner, 1981).

Whereas Schachter treats bodily changes accompanying emotion as undifferentiated arousal, recent research findings support the Jamesian notion that discrete patterns of physiological change accompany emotion. For example, Ekman, Levenson and Friesen (1983) found that flexing the facial muscles into emotional expressions has effects on measures such as heart rate and skin temperature, and that anger and fear expressions have different effects from those produced by happiness, surprise and disgust. It would therefore seem that the facial musculature is intimately related to the autonomic nervous system, which controls functions such as heart rate. It seems likely that future research on bodily changes in emotion will take emotion theory away from Schachter's view that cognitive factors are solely responsible for differentiating emotional experience into qualitatively distinct states such as anger and joy, and towards the type of view advocated by theorists such as Izard (1971), who argues that (for some emotions, at least) there are discrete, innate patterns of neural, facial-postural, and motor activity, awareness of which generates the subjective experience of emotion.

Apart from work aimed at elucidating the roles played by cognitive and physiological processes in the generation of emotion, there are two other notable lines of research on emotion. One is concerned with facial expression. More specifically, some investigators have examined whether the way in which emotion is expressed in the face is the same across diverse cultures (Ekman, 1982), while others have studied individual differences, both in facial expressiveness during emotional experience and in the ability to recognize from facial expressions what emotions others are experiencing (Rosenthal, 1979). A second line of research, much of it conducted by sociologists, is concerned with what is referred to as the 'socialization of the emotions'. Here the focus is on how social and cultural factors influence 'feeling rules' (Hochschild, 1979), that is, rules concerning how to express emotions, when to express emotions, how emotions are managed, how emotions are labelled, and how emotions are interpreted (Lewis and Michalson, 1982).

A. S. R. Manstead
University of Manchester

References

Cannon, W. B. (1927), 'The James-Lange theory of emotions: a critical examination and an alternative theory', *American Journal of Psychology*, 39.

Ekman, P. (1982), *Emotion in the Human Face* (2nd edn), New York.

Ekman, P., Levenson, R. W. and Friesen, W. V. (1983), 'Autonomic nervous system activity distinguishes among emotions', *Science*, 221.

Hochschild, A. R. (1979), 'Emotion work, feeling rules, and social structure', *American Journal of Sociology*, 85.

Izard, C. E. (1971), *The Face of Emotion*, New York.

Lazarus, R. S., Averill, J. R. and Opton, E. M. (1970),

'Toward a cognitive theory of emotion', in M. B. Arnold (ed.), *Feelings and Emotions*, New York.

Lewis, M. and Michalson, L. (1982), 'The socialization of emotions', in T. Field (ed.), *Emotion and Early Interaction*, Hillsdale, N.J.

Manstead, A. S. R. and Wagner, H. L. (1981), 'Arousal, cognition and emotion: an appraisal of two-factor theory', *Current Psychological Reviews*, 1.

Rosenthal, R. (1979), *Skill in Nonverbal Communication: Individual Differences*, Boston.

Schachter, S. (1964), 'The interaction of cognitive and physiological determinants of emotional state', in L. Berkowitz (ed.), *Advances in Experimental Social Psychology* (vol. 1), New York.

Further Reading

Izard, C. E. (1977), *Human Emotions*, New York.
Mandler, G. (1975), *Mind and Emotion*, New York.

See also: *activation and arousal; aggression and anger; empathy and sympathy.*

Empathy and Sympathy

Empathy has been conceived as being a cognitive process or an emotional-cognitive one. The former conception relates primarily to an individual's intellectual understanding of another's ideation and feelings, and has led to studies of the accuracy of predicting another's responses to questionnaire items and of other adjustments about others. These studies have been fraught with methodological difficulties.

The emotional-cognitive conception has focused on a person's perceiving – veridically or not – that another is experiencing an emotional state and, as a consequence, experiencing the same type of emotion. The degree of similarity of the two emotional states is in some dispute. Furthermore, the other's state can be inferred from the situation, from direct observation, or from other information. This conception does not include the trivial case in which the other's emotional state is a precursor of an affect causing experience for the 'empathizer'.

Emotional-cognitive empathy has been found to be an outcome definitionally required of 'taking the role of the other', although it may also be based on learned associations between one's own and other's experiences. Emotional-cognitive empathy has been found to be related to helping the other person, when such help appears to be a means of reducing negative affect in the other; and it also appears to be related to moral behaviour. However, recent research has suggested that if the empathizer is motivated only to free himself from the empathized negative emotion, then he may do so by escaping the situation as well as by helping the other, whichever is less costly and more effective. In fact, if the empathized negative emotion is very strong, the individual may flee from the other person.

On the other hand, if the empathizer also has a positive attitude toward the other and is motivated to help him, then his empathy becomes a form of sympathy. Sympathy may be viewed as a state in which a person is concerned about another's welfare. Whether or not empathy is a necessary correlate of sympathy is undetermined as yet, since a person may sympathize with another even when the latter is not experiencing any relevant emotion.

Ezra Stotland
University of Washington

Further Reading

Hoffman, M. L. (1977), 'Empathy, its development and prosocial implications', in C. B. Keasey (ed.), *Nebraska Symposium on Motivation: 1977 Social Cognitive Development*, Lincoln.

Stotland, E., Mathews, K., Hansson, R., Richardson, B. and Sherman, S. (1978), *Fantasy, Empathy and Help*, Beverly Hills.

Stotland, E., Sherman, S. and Shaver, K. G. (1971), *Empathy and Birth Order: Some Experimental Explorations*, Lincoln.

See also: *emotion*.

Employment and Unemployment: Social Psychological Aspects

Employment as the dominant institution through which people earn their living is largely the result of the Industrial Revolution. Since then social scientists of all kinds have thought about its impact on individuals and society. Their powerful ideas influenced the climate of thought about industrialism long before social psychology came of age. Karl Marx and Max Weber had proposed conflicting ideas on work motivation: alienation versus the Protestant work ethic. Frederick Taylor (curiously acclaimed by Lenin) concentrated on productivity through changes in work organization. Few social psychologists based their work explicitly on these forerunners, but when they began systematic study they adopted their themes: work motivation and productivity.

A considerable number of early studies were based on a combination of both themes and searched for ways to improve morale in the expectation that increase in productivity would follow. The results of these efforts are ambiguous. On the positive side, an enormous amount has been learned about how to improve morale: job enrichment and enlargement, flexible working hours, group organization, participation in decision making, profit-sharing and co-operative organization have all been demonstrated as capable of strengthening morale, even though less effectively for workers in the most routinized jobs. The expectation that productivity would increase correspondingly, however, was not universally fulfilled: it happened in some cases, not in others, and in a few instances improved morale occurred even with lowered productivity. The reasons for these inconclusive results have so far not been identified (see Klein, 1976, for a full discussion).

Recently it has become recognized that productivity is more a function of technology, less of morale. Continuing studies of morale and motivation are undertaken in the belief that improvement in these matters is a legitimate goal in its own right, even if it does not increase productivity.

The current wave of mass unemployment in Western societies has induced many social psychologists to switch from their concern with these issues to the study of the psychological impact of unemployment. For the second time in this century the tragic opportunity has arisen to elucidate the taken-for-granted meaning of employment by the systematic study of its absence.

During the Great Depression of the 1930s the psychological impact of unemployment was documented in over 100 studies (summarized in Eisenberg and Lazarsfeld, 1938). They showed the suffering of the unemployed through abject poverty and lack of work; they were often without public support and depended on charity. Many felt depressed and bored, time had lost its meaning, voluntary activities that previously could be accommodated after a long working day were abandoned, self-respect was undermined, people felt thrown on the scrap-heap. Of course there were individual differences, but the general picture was one of resignation or deeply felt frustration.

Was this response due more to living in extreme poverty or more to the absence of employment? A comparison with the impact of unemployment in the 1980s, when economic deprivation is as a rule relative and not absolute, suggests the answer: the current response to unemployment shows many similarities to those in the 1930s. The majority of unemployed suffer from depressive moods, boredom and loss of time orientation, feel socially useless and abandoned by the larger community.

This similarity, notwithstanding the enormous social changes that have occurred since the 1930s, suggests that the meaning of employment has remained relatively constant. Like every other institution, employment has not only conscious, manifest purposes but also latent consequences that inevitably enforce, for better or worse, experiences within certain categories on those who participate in it. These enforced categories of experience (more fully discussed in Jahoda, 1982) are: a specific organization of time, an enlarged horizon through contact with others, a demonstration of the need for collective effort, and an assignment of social identity and regular activity.

The frustrations of the unemployed (also of many housewives whose children have left home and of many retired people) suggest that some experiences within these general categories are needed to make sense of one's daily life, and that the majority of those who were used to the social support provided by the organization of employment in meeting these needs feel deprived when this support is withdrawn. In the 1980s, as was also the case in the 1930s, those few unemployed who manage out of their own initiative and against the norms of society to meet these needs in voluntary work do not suffer psychologically, even if they do economically, when they lose their jobs. But it is unrealistic to expect that most of the unemployed – consisting of unskilled workers and young people without any work experience – could manage.

Social psychological thought and research thus support the notion that people need work beyond economic considerations, though not necessarily under conditions of employment, to make sense of their daily lives. For the foreseeable future, economic necessity will, however, continue to make employment the central institution through which most people satisfy their often unrecognized psychological needs as well as their aspirations for a high material standard of living. The identification of the five basic needs helps not only to understand why the unemployed suffer, but also provides a concrete agenda for the humanization of employment. While all employment is psychologically preferable to unemployment, there exist some employment conditions where the time experience, the quality of the social contact, the collective purpose, the social identity and the actual activity are deeply unsatisfactory. There is great scope for future research-based changes in all these areas.

Marie Jahoda
Science Policy Research Unit, University of Sussex

References

Eisenberg, P. and Lazarsfeld, P. F. (1938), 'The psychological effects of unemployment', *Psychological Bulletin*, 35.

Jahoda, M. (1982), *Employment and Unemployment*, Cambridge.

Klein, L. (1976), *New Forms of Work Organisation*, Cambridge.

Environmental Psychology

Canter and Craik (1981) define environmental psychology as: 'That area of psychology which brings into conjuction and analyses the transactions and interrelationships of human experiences and actions with pertinent aspects of the socio-physical surroundings.' This approach emphasizes that although the 'environment' of environmental psychology is usually regarded as essentially physical (typically the designed architectural environment or the natural environment), it is always treated as part of the socio-physical matrix. The field of environmental psychology emerged from the collaboration of perceptually oriented psychologists and design decision makers, but it now overlaps considerably with many aspects of social psychology, especially the developments in situational theory (Canter, 1985).

In Europe the initial impetus for environmental studies came from the practical problems produced by the devastation of World War II. The need to build quickly on a vast scale for unidentified individuals and large groups led to user require-ment studies and surveys, which tried to establish recurring patterns and preferences to be considered in design. In the 1960s these studies extended to the evaluation of existing build-ings, social scientists being called upon to provide 'feedback' about psychological successes and failures. It was paralleled in the design professions by an examination of the nature of the design process. This examination gave rise to the consideration of various forms of systematic design which clearly required as a basis some scientific underpinnings concerned with the ways in which the built environment influenced behaviour.

In North America, pressures from the design professions, whilst present, have not been so strong. The consideration of psychological implications of environmental design has grown out of developing interests (and the search for social relevance) of university-based psychologists. In general, the pioneering environmental psychologists such as Ittelson et al. (1974) have emphasized the need to consider perceptual problems on an environmental scale, given the advances in perceptual psychology, and social psychologists such as Sommer (1983) have seen the need to take into account the physical setting.

Measurement techniques in environmental psychology have concentrated on standardized questionnaire procedures on the one hand and detailed observations of actions *in situ* on the other. The relative efficacy of these two forms of measurement was debated in the late 1960s, but the emerging consensus is that both are necessary for a full account of action and experience in relation to the physical environment.

Research design has taken many forms, with the laboratory experiment being dominant only in studies dealing with heat, light and sound. Questionnaires and observational studies of users of existing facilities have attempted to highlight the strengths and defects of the particular environment under study, and findings are consequently difficult to generalize. More novel field experiment techniques have been developed which appear to offer the possibility of both minimizing interference with the environment under study while at the same time testing hypotheses and providing results of general applicability. A further method is to represent the environment in some form and then to modify these representations in order to produce environments which differ in controlled ways.

Most of the laboratory research following in the footsteps of classical psychophysics has explored the human correlates of design variables such as temperature, noise level and luminance, although also increasingly considered are issues such as air pollution and other hazards and environmental risks. In general, two separate sets of psychological variables have been examined, the effects upon task performance and the relationship to comfort or satisfaction. These studies have been fruitful in establishing meaningful relationships and providing information for design decision makers.

The relationship between satisfaction and performance has been found to be quite complex (Canter, 1983). Another growing area of investigation considers the consequences for general health and well-being of a combination of environmental features (Evans, 1983).

From the variety of studies of institutional environments, a number of themes have emerged: (1) It is essential to examine the institution and its setting over time in order to reveal the effects of the physical surroundings. (2) The institutional administration is a crucial influence in modifying the interaction between environment and behaviour. It follows from these two points that the way in which a person makes use of, or is affected by, his physical surroundings relates to a marked degree to his role in the organization.

Within the theoretical approaches underlying all the research two distinct trends have emerged. One set of researchers draws its impetus from the formulations of the ecological psychologists and learning theorists. They assign a deterministic role to the environment, which influences behaviour. They are concerned with detailed descriptions based upon observations of ongoing behaviour and with describing the physical environment as one aspect of the general ecological system (Kaminski, 1983).

The alternative trend has its roots in cognitive and phenomenological psychology. These studies attempt to understand the ways in which people experience and understand their environments, relating these processes to the built forms involved. The emphasis here is on the interactions which occur between people and places (Canter, 1977). Increasingly, however, these two approaches complement one another, and a variety of hybrid theories are emerging which will contribute both to the development of academic psychology and to real world decision making.

David Canter
University of Surrey

References

Canter, D. (1977), *The Psychology of Place*, London.

Canter, D. (1983), 'The physical context of work' in D. J. Oborne and M. M. Ginsburg (eds), *The Physical Environment at Work*, Chichester.

Canter, D. (1985), 'Putting situations in their place', in A. Furham (ed.), *Social Behavior in Context*, New York.

Canter, D. and Craik, K. H. (1981), 'Environmental psychology', *Journal of Environmental Psychology*, 1.

Evans, G. W. (ed.) (1983), *Environmental Stress*, London.

Ittelson, W. H., Proshansky, H. M., Rivlin, L. G. and Winkel, G. H. (1974), *An Introduction to Environmental Psychology*, New York.

Kaminski, G. (1983), 'The enigma of ecological psychology', *Journal of Environmental Psychology*, 3.

Sommer, R. (1983), *Social Design*, Englewood Cliffs, N.J.

Existential Psychology

Existential psychology developed in Europe between World Wars I and II and gradually spread to America in the 1950s. The seeds of existentialism were found in the writings of Kierkegaard, the Danish philosopher, but the principal founders of existential philosophy were two Germans, Heidegger and Jaspers. In France its leading protagonists were Marcel, Sartre and Merleau-Ponty.

Existential psychology did not claim to be a new branch of psychology, nor even a new theory. It viewed itself as a new orientation, essentially idiographic, as opposed to the nomothetic tendencies of other forms of psychology, such as behaviourism.

The general characteristics of existential psychology are as follows:

(1) It is not a school, but a *movement* which focuses its inquiry on the individual person as being-in-the-world.

(2) Several basic tenets underlie this movement: (a) every man is unique in his inner life, perceptions and evaluations of the world, and in his reactions to it; (b) man as a person cannot be understood in terms of functions of elements within him. He cannot be explained in terms of physics, chemistry, or neurophysiology; (c) psychology, if patterned after physics, cannot fully understand human nature; (d) neither the behaviouristic nor psychoanalytic approach is totally satisfactory.

(3) As a *human* psychology, it attempts to complement, not to replace or suppress, other existing orientations in psychology.

(4) It attempts to develop a comprehensive concept of man

and an understanding of man in his total existential reality. It concerns itself with the person's consciousness, feelings, moods, and experiences relating to his individual existence in the world and among other humans. Its ultimate goal is to discover the basic force in human life that would provide a key to understanding human nature in its entirety.

(5) Its themes are person-to-person relationships, freedom and responsibility, individual scales of values, the meaning of life, suffering, anxiety, and death.

(6) Its principal method is phenomenological, including *intuiting* (or intense concentration on the phenomena of consciousness), *analysing* (or focusing on aspects of consciousness and how they relate to each other), and *describing* (or rendering an intelligible account to others). Existential psychology seeks to grasp the essence of whatever appears in consciousness and to describe what is perceived, imagined or felt.

(7) Its contributions have been primarily to personality theory, psychotherapy, and counselling.

In Europe one of the leading existential psychologists, Ludwig Binswanger, developed *Daseinsanalyse* (existential analysis). This method seeks to describe an individual's relationship with the world (*Umwelt*), with his fellow-men (*Mitwelt*) and with himself (*Eigenwelt*) in order to help the person become his own authentic self.

Two important American existential psychologists are Carl Rogers and Rollo May. Stressing the developmental aspect of *becoming*, Rogers seeks to help the person achieve greater self-actualization. Like Rogers, May has been concerned with existential psychotherapy. He emphasizes understanding the basic nature of man and insists that through existential psychology man will be able to understand the characteristics that make him human.

Existential psychology has been criticized by behaviourists and rigorous experimentalists for its lack of verifiable data, subjectivism and strong attachment to philosophy.

Virginia Staudt Sexton
St John's University, New York

Further Reading
Binswanger, L. (1963), *Being-in-the-World: Selected Papers by Ludwig Binswanger*, New York.
May, R. (1969), *Existential Psychology*, 2nd edn, New York.
Misiak, H. and Sexton, V. S. (1973), *Phenomenological, Existential and Humanistic Psychologies: A Historical Survey*, New York.
Rogers, C. (1961), *On Becoming A Person*, Boston.
See also: *Rogers*.

Eysenck, Hans J. (1916–)

A voluntary expatriate from Germany in 1933, Eysenck studied at University College London, and thus in the psychometric tradition of Galton, Spearman and Burt; he was later to extend the methodology of the study of intellectual ability to the study of human personality, and so to create one of the major schools of personality theory. The war forced him into the clinical field, and he was eventually to found the first university-based course in clinical psychology, a profession in Britain that owes much to his early initiative and scientific approach. He is quite unusual in his literary output, being the author or joint author of well over 50 books and 600 journal articles: many of the layman's modern concepts of psychology as a scientific discipline owe much to his popular writings. He has been at the centre of the longstanding debate concerning the role of genetic factors in determining individual differences in intellectual ability, with its strong overtones of political controversy, and he appears to enjoy controversy. Although reputed to be a hard-nosed scientist, and having been a leading figure in the critical onslaught against the vagaries of psychoanalytic theory, Eysenck has shown a surprising fondness for treating seriously such fringe topics as astrology and psychic research. Retiring from the chair of psychology at the age of 67 in 1983, he is still a man of remarkable intellectual and physical vigour, and in terms of citations in learned journals, he proves to be quite the most influential of living British psychologists.

H. B. Gibson
Cambridge

Further Reading

Broadbent, D. E. (1981), 'Introduction', in R. Lynn (ed.),
Dimensions of Personality: Papers in Honour of H. J. Eysenck,
Oxford.

Eysenck, H. J. (1979), 'Autobiographical sketch', in G.
Lindzey (ed.), *A History of Psychology in Autobiography*, vol.
VII, San Francisco.

Gibson, H. B. (1981), *Hans Eysenck: The Man and His Work*,
London.

Family Therapy

Family therapy is both a theory of family functioning and a
treatment technique for troubled couples or families. The theory
maintains that the family is a functioning and cohesive system
with rules or patterns, which it maintains when faced with
stress. Thus, the family system is different from and greater
than the sum of its parts and must be observed as a whole in
action. Malfunctioning or pathological family systems often lead
to individual symptomatology.

To understand and change the family, the therapist requires
certain information, including details about its culture, ethnicity
and socioeconomic status, the facts about each member, and
the family's history and life-cycle phase. Each family has its
own traditions, marital contracts, myths, secrets and loyalties
to the past. Each individual in the family has his own dynamics,
expectations, hopes and life-experiences. Direct observations
are necessary in order to assess the roles, coalitions, hierarchies
and alliances between members, the communicational patterns
and their clarity, the patterns of rewards and punishments, and
the distribution of power. Finally, the experimental and ethical
aspects must be ascertained. This last step involves assessing
the empathic experience of the family from the perspective of
each member, learning whether they have been treated fairly
and justly and what debts and credits they have *vis-à-vis* other
family members.

The family therapist uses these observations to form a therapeutic alliance and meets with the appropriate family members
to design appropriate interventions in order to change family

functioning. In maximally distressed families, interventions should initially be aimed at preventing physical harm to members, strengthening the parental-marital coalition, appropriately controlling the children, and promoting suitable distance between over-involved pairs. Other goals include encouraging clear and open communication, exploring mistaken attributions made of members, particularly as these are related to the past, and rebalancing the family towards fairness and justice.

Techniques commonly employed include: (1) The explorations of projective identification, where disowned aspects of the self are attributed to others, who are both related to as though the attribution was correct, and are often pressured to act in accordance with it. (2) The assignment of tasks to the family with the purpose of altering behavioural reinforcements, interrupting malfunctioning aspects of the family system, particularly when the family resists change, and providing a new and novel experience. (3) Helping the family to find ways of redressing past injustices and finding new and fairer ways of functioning.

Family therapy is considered more effective than individual treatment when the problems involve a dysfunctional marriage, and at least as effective in the treatment of disturbed children and adolescents – particularly if the problems are neurotic or psychosomatic. Psycho-educational work with families has recently been found valuable in preventing relapse in schizophrenia. The family is educated about the disease, its course and treatment, and is helped to attend to and comment on the patient's behaviour rather than to criticize thoughts and feelings. Finally, meetings with the families of individual psychotherapy patients have been found to be a useful adjunct to the treatment of adults in marital difficulties.

Henry Grunebaum
Harvard University

Further Reading

Grunebaum, H. and Glick, I. (1983), 'The basics of family treatment', in L. Grinspoon (ed.), *Psychiatry Update: The American Psychiatric Association Annual Review*, vol. II.

McFarlane, W. R., Beels, C. C. and Rosenheck, S. (1983), 'New developments in the family treatment of the psychotic disorders', in L. Grinspoon (ed.), *Psychiatry Update: The American Psychiatric Association Annual Review*, vol. II.

Fantasy

Fantasy is a form of human thought characterized by a freedom from the thinker's ordinary concerns about evaluating such activity in terms of its relevance to specific problem solutions, or about responding to objects or tasks in the immediate environment. Modern psychological investigators generally use 'fantasy' as an alternative to the term 'daydreaming'. Fantasy reflects a shift of one's attention away from an immediate task set for oneself, mental or physical, towards the sometimes almost effortless unfolding of a sequence of images or interior monologues typified by a mixture of playful consideration of often improbable or at least 'as if' occurrences (Singer, 1981), and story-like projections in which the thinker or others may serve as protagonists. Fantasies are more often thought sequences involving interpersonal transactions, but they may also take the form of juxtapositions of unlikely or unexperienced natural events, as in the case of scientists or engineers using 'thought experiments' – such as imagining the consequences of men flying faster than the speed of light, or of 'big bangs' which initiate the structures and dynamics that characterize our solar system or galaxy.

Fantasy thought or daydreaming has often been regarded as primitive, regressive or as a distraction or escape from directed, logical problem-solving thought (except when it is turned into the socially-approved product of a work of literature). Recent systematic research suggests that it may essentially be a normal feature of human cognition and that, properly employed, it can serve a variety of adaptive functions, from self-entertainment in dull situations to the effective use of mental rehearsal for later social interaction or even athletic performances (Richardson, 1969; Singer, 1981). Fantasy thought is often also used loosely in connection with terms like mental or imagination imagery. The human imagery capacity, which involves the private reduplication in some roughly analogous form of objects or persons in one's environment, is certainly a common feature of fantasy and daydreaming. The latter processes may be viewed as ongoing or continuous, in William James's phrase 'a stream of thought' in which sequences of images, for example, sights, sounds and tastes, are linked along with interior self-conversations.

Psychological Research on Fantasy and Daydreaming

Our knowledge of fantasy processes rests largely on personal experience and introspection or on the verbal reports of other persons, as well as on the observations of children's play and their often unlimited verbalizations during make-believe play (Piaget, 1962; Singer, 1973). There is some research evidence of various physiological processes that accompany fantasy or daydream-like thought. But we cannot as yet infer private fantasy activity in other persons solely from such physiological processes, and must therefore depend ultimately on written or verbalized reports or, at least, on the same pre-agreed-upon signal from the research participants that such fantasy thought is under way. Important advances have occurred, however, in the elaboration of a number of methods for studying patterns of fantasy and the behavioural correlates of such activity from verbal reports.

Projective Techniques in Personality Assessment

Clinical methods such as the Rorschach inkblots or the Thematic Apperception Test have been employed to infer characteristic fantasy activities for individuals or groups of subjects. Persons who respond to Rorschach inkblots by reporting associations involving human figures or persons in action (M responses) have been shown in various studies to be more prone to imaginative or creative thought on other measures, as well as more likely to be more planning, controlled, deliberate and restrained in overt action. The extensive studies of stories told to the ambiguous pictures of the Thematic Apperception Test indicate that recurrent themes of achievement, power-striving or affiliation in a respondent's verbalized fantasies are predictive of diverse behavioural activities such as entrepreneurial endeavours, alcohol abuse or marital relationships (McClelland, 1966).

Questionnaire Methods

Direct questions of people about the forms and content of their daydreams and fantasies in the form of psychometrically sophisticated questionnaires have yielded evidence that daydreaming and various aspects of fantasy are common phenomena. Normative data for a wide variety of persons from various age and social-class cohorts have been emerging, although cross-national data from non-English-speaking countries remain sparse. Factor analyses of questionnaires for large numbers of respondents repeatedly identify three general clusters of self-reported inner activity: (1) Positive-constructive daydreaming, which involves acceptance and enjoyment of fantasy and constructive use of one's imagery; (2) Guilty-dysphoric fantasies; (3) Poor attentional control with little elaboration of fleeting, often fearful, fantasies (Segal, Huba and Singer, 1980). Only the third of these patterns has been consistently linked to measures of anxiety or emotional disturbance. Behavioural or psychometric correlates of questionnaire reports of fantasy suggest some congruent validity for such self-report measures.

Laboratory Studies Using Signal Detection

By training individuals to an agreed-upon definition of task-irrelevant thought and imagery, it is possible to study the occurrence of fantasy activities – by having them signal periodically while they are engaged in a variety of continuous absorbing mental or perceptual tasks such as auditory or visual signal detection watches. Such procedures make it possible to estimate the conditions conducive or detrimental to the occurrence of spontaneous fantasy or daydreaming, the extent to which such activities occur concurrently with (parallel processing) or during interruptions in signal detections (sequential processing) and so on (Antrobus, Singer, Goldstein and Fortgang, 1970). Data indicate that some fantasy activity is a regular feature of almost all circumstances in which attention is chiefly being paid to processing external stimulation. Content reports suggest that such daydreaming often involves (playful or fearful) attention to and elaboration of recurrent unfulfilled intentions or 'current concerns', as well as wishful or aesthetic elaborations of recent experiences or anticipated social encounters.

Thought-Sampling

Although psychoanalysts and other clinicians have long relied heavily on fantasies reported during psychotherapy sessions, recent approaches have used continuous talking or intermittent report methods throughout several days (using randomly-gener-ated portable electronic 'beepers' to alert participants to report on thoughts) in order to obtain more reliable samples of 'natu-ral-occurring' fantasy. Such methods further demonstrate the extent to which fantasy is a recurring feature of normal human thought and may reflect a major way in which humans orient themselves toward a variety of potential futures and keep track of previously established intentions or goals (Klinger, Barta, and Maxeiner, 1981).

Psychophysiological Measurement

Fantasy or daydream-like thought has been found in various studies to be associated with reduced ocular motility in the waking state, or to leftward eye-shifting preceding reflection (presumably reflecting greater right brain hemispheric involve-ment). Imagery involving events that evoke different emotions have been found to yield differential blood pressure patterns or brainwave activity.

Psychotherapeutic Uses of Fantasy

A wide variety of behaviour modification and psychotherapeutic or stress reduction procedures rely on our human capacity for producing fantasies. These range from the transference and dream interpretation procedures of psychoanalytically-derived therapies through the guided imagery approaches increasingly prevalent in Germany and France. Behavioural techniques such as covert modelling, covert aversive conditioning or symbolic elaboration all can be shown to rely on the client's capacity to generate vivid or detailed daydreams (Singer and Pope, 1978; Singer, 1973). Research findings in these spheres further point to the value of regarding our capacity to travel mentally to potential futures, or to take an 'as if' stance in our thought, as an inherently adaptive feature of our evolutionary development, even with the misuse we may often make of 'the vanity of human wishes'.

Jerome L. Singer
Yale University

References

Antrobus, J. S., Singer, J. L., Goldstein, S. and Fortgang, M. (1970), 'Mindwandering and cognitive structure', *Transactions of the New York Academy of Science*, Series II, 32.

Klinger, E., Barta, S. and Maxeiner, M. (1981), 'Current concerns: assessing therapeutically relevant motivation', in P. Kendall and S. Hollon (eds), *Assessment Strategies for Cognitive-Behavioral Interventions*, New York.

McLelland, D. (1966), 'Longitudinal trends in the relation of thought to action', *Journal of Consulting Psychology*, 30.

Piaget, J. (1962), *Play, Dreams and Imitation in Childhood*, New York.

Richardson, A. (1969), *Mental Imagery*, New York.

Schwartz, G., Weinberger, D. and Singer, J. L. (1981), 'Cardiovascular differentiation of happiness, sadness, anger and fear, following imagery and exercise', *Psychosomatic Medicine*, 43.

Segal, B., Huba, G. J. and Singer, J. L. (1980), *Drugs, Daydreaming and Personality: A Study of College Youth*, Hillsdale, N.J.

Singer, J. L. (1973), *The Child's World of Make-Believe*, New York.

Singer, J. L. (1981), *Daydreaming and Fantasy*, London.
Singer, J. L. and Pope, K. S. (1978), *The Power of Human Imagination*, New York.
See also: *dreams; projective methods; thinking – cognitive organization and processes.*

Free Association

The requirement for free association is often referred to as the fundamental rule of psychoanalysis. The patient in psychoanalytic treatment attempts to express in words all thoughts, feelings, wishes, sensations, images, and memories without reservation, as they spontaneously occur. Originally, Sigmund Freud introduced free association to assist in the abreaction of traumatic experiences. Later it served him especially well in deciphering the language and grammar of dreams and in describing the vicissitudes of human passion, emotion, and motivation. Gradually, as psychoanalysis progressed, free association became the vehicle for elucidation of unconscious conflicts and of the history of their formation in the life of the individual.

Free association replaced hypnosis in Freud's early investigative and psychotherapeutic work in the 1890s. The approach was consonant with his general conviction about the determinism of mental life and the importance of unconscous influences. It served and continues to serve as the principal method of psychoanalysis and of psychoanalytic psychotherapy. The word 'free' in this term indicates relative freedom from *conscious* determination. Unconscious determinants, both those that seek expression and those that oppose it (resistance), can be inferred from the many varieties of sequence, content and form of the free associations. The analyst's interventions, based on a grasp of conscious and unconscious determinants, aim at expansion of the patient's *freedom* of association mainly through clarification and interpretation, with a concomitant development of the patient's insight. The analyst is guided by his own associations and by the requirement of maintaining a nonjudgemental attitude characterized by personal anonymity, neutrality and abstinence.

Free association can be seen to promote continuity in mental functioning – the continuity, for example, of thought, feeling, memory, styles of loving, and sense of self. Discontinuities in these functions and corresponding restrictions in the freedom of association are characteristic of the psychopathology which may be expected to respond favourably to psychoanalytic treatment. In a narrower sense, free association aims to make conscious what is unconscious, to revive lost experience, to expand what is condensed, to express the components of inner conflict, and to put thought and feeling, as much as possible, into words. Although not all of mental life can be put into words, emphasis on the intimate connection between language, reason, consciousness, and the capacity for decision and resolution has been an explicit feature of the psychoanalytic method from the beginning. The considerable variety of perspectives and theoretical formulations with which psychoanalysts perform their work can regularly be shown to relate to these features of the free association method.

Anton O. Kris
Boston Psychoanalytic Institute

Further Reading
Kris, A. O. (1982), *Free Association: Method and Process*, New Haven.
See also: *psychoanalysis; unconscious*.

Freud, Anna (1895–1982)

The youngest of Sigmund Freud's six children, Anna Freud was born in Vienna in 1895. As the only one of his children to follow her father's profession, she referred to psychoanalysis as a sibling. She was for many years her father's caretaker and confidante, and she promulgated his theories during the generation after his death. Her own work focused on child analysis and adolescence.

Beginning her career as a teacher of young children, Anna Freud presented her first paper to the Vienna Psychoanalytic Society in 1922 and joined the Society soon after. One of her first and most important works was *The Ego and the Mechanisms of Defense* (1936). In it she stressed that for psychoanalytic understanding of ego development, the defences are as important as the instincts. This insight was a major contribution not only to psychoanalytic theory, but to psychoanalytic therapy as well. She also focused on adolescence as a crucial period of ego and super-ego transformation.

Among her other notable publications are two monographs derived from her wartime experience: *Infants Without Families* (1943) and *War and Children* (1943). These studies marked the beginning of detailed and systematic psychoanalytic observation of children and its relation to the reconstruction of childhood in the psychoanalysis of adults. *Normality and Pathology in Childhood: Assessment in Development* (1965) brought a new, developmental direction to the so-called psychoanalytic metapsychology. *Beyond the Best Interests of the Child* (1973), written with collaborators from the Yale School of Law, was an attempt to apply psychoanalytic theories to legal policy affecting children.

Anna Freud escaped with her father to London following the Nazi occupation of Austria in 1938. There, in order to advance the study and treatment of children, she established a nursery school which evolved into the Hampstead Child Therapy Course and Clinic. Anna Freud died in London in 1982.

Leo Rangell
University of California, Los Angeles
University of California, San Francisco

Further Reading
Freud, A. (1936), *The Ego and the Mechanisms of Defense*, New York.
Freud, A. (1965), *Normality and Pathology in Childhood*, New York.
See also: *Freud, Sigmund.*

Freud, Sigmund (1856–1939)

Ernest Jones, the foremost biographer of Freud, comments that Freud gave the world an incomplete theory of mind, but a new vista on man (Jones, 1953–57). The insights Freud arrived at and shared with the world changed and developed as he expanded his knowledge and understanding of himself, pursued his clinical work with patients, and broadened his interest in the world of science and letters. The perilous times in which he lived had a profound impact on his personal and professional life.

Freud was born on 6 May 1856, in Schlossergasse, Moravia, a small town in what is now Czechoslovakia (Freud, 1959 [1925]). His parents were Jewish, and though he was an agnostic he always maintained his identity as a Jew. The family moved to Vienna when Freud was four, and he lived there until 1938 when he and his family fled the Nazis to London (Hampstead). He died a year later, on 23 September 1939.

Although the family was not well off, no pressure was put on Sigmund, the oldest child, to seek a career that would be economically advantageous. Stimulated by Darwin's theories, he saw new hopes for understanding human nature. An essay by Goethe, 'On Nature', read at a popular lecture, sparked his interest in becoming a natural scientist and strengthened his desire to go to medical school. Freud's interests in social sciences, human interactions, developmental processes and ancient history were already evident during his childhood and youth; they were later to give richness to the discipline he founded: psychoanalysis.

At the university, he experienced serious disappointments. Yet the fact that his Jewishness made him an outsider seemed to strengthen his independence of mind. In Ernst Brücke's physiological laboratory, where he *was* allowed to work, he found role models he could respect, not only Brücke himself but his assistants, Sigmund Exner and Ernst Fleischl von Marxow. Brücke asked him to work on the histology of the nervous system, which he did before undertaking his own independent research. In 1882, when he had been at the laboratory for six years, Brücke strongly advised him, in view of his 'bad financial position', to abandon his research and theoretical career for a clinical one.

Freud entered the General Hospital in Vienna, where he

pursued his neurohistological interests at the Institute of Cerebral Anatomy, published several short papers, and was encouraged by Professor Theodore Meynert to devote himself to the study of the anatomy of the brain.

In 1882 Freud's friend Josef Breuer told him about his work with a patient suffering from hysterical symptoms. After putting the patient into deep hypnosis, Breuer had asked her to tell him what was on her mind. In her awakened state she could not repeat what she had revealed under hypnosis. The major contribution of the case of Anna O. (whose real name was Bertha Pappenheim) was the discovery of a technique that was a precursor to psychoanalystic treatment – free association.

In 1885 Freud won a travelling grant and went to Paris, where he became a student at the Saltpêtrière of the eminent neurologist, Jean-Martin Charcot. Freud's interest in Breuer's work had made him eager to find out more about Charcot's studies on hysteria. Charcot demonstrated quite convincingly the genuineness of hysterical phenomena and their conformity to laws, the frequent occurrence of hysteria in men (contrary to current theories), the production of hysterical paralyses and contractures by hypnosis, and the finding that artificially induced states showed features similar to those of spontaneous attacks that were initiated traumatically. Freud determined to study neuroses in greater depth. Before returning to Vienna, he spent a few weeks in Berlin in order to gain more knowledge of childhood disorders. During the next few years he published several monographs on unilateral and bilateral cerebral palsies in children.

In 1886 he settled in Vienna as a physician, married Martha Bernays, to whom he had been engaged for several years, and became known as a specialist in nervous diseases. He reported to the Vienna Society of Medicine on his work with Charcot, an account which the medical society did not receive with favour. Some of his critics doubted that there could be hysteria in males. In response to their scepticism he found a male with a classical hysterical hemianesthesia, demonstrated it before the medical society, and was applauded – but ultimately ignored.

Once again he was an outsider. He was excluded from the laboratory of cerebral anatomy, had no place to deliver his lectures, withdrew from academic life, and ceased to attend meetings of the professional societies.

Freud's therapeutic armamentarium was limited. He could use electrotherapy or hypnotism. Since it became known that the positive effects of electrotherapy were in fact the effects of suggestion, Freud turned his sole attention to hypnosis. With this shift he thus became more firmly committed to psychological rather than organic treatment. He had observed in Paris how hypnotism could produce symptoms similar to hysteria and could then remove them again. In 1889 he went to Nancy where he observed the technique developed by Liébeault and Bernheim which used suggestion, with or without hypnosis, for therapeutic purposes. As he wrote in his autobiographical study (1925), '[I] received the profoundest impression of the possibility that there could be powerful mental processes which nevertheless remained hidden from the consciousness of men.' This was one of the first statements presaging Freud's monumental discovery of the unconscious.

In the early 1890s, Freud attempted to persuade Breuer to renew his interest in the problems of hysteria and to share with the world the discoveries he had made in the case of Anna O. *Studien über Hysterie* (1895) (*Studies on Hysteria*) was the result – a collaborative effort in which Breuer and Freud presented their ideas on the origin and treatment of hysterical symptoms. Freud described the unconscious in detail and introduced two key concepts: that a symptom arises through the restraining of a conflictful affect, and that it results from the transformation of a quantum of energy which, instead of being used in other ways, was converted into the symptom. Breuer described the way in which the technique he used with Anna O. allowed for the cathartic discharge of feelings (abreaction) with symptom relief. Although subsequent clinical research has questioned the universality of the effectiveness of this technique, it was *Studies on Hysteria* that introduced psychoanalysis to the world.

Breuer ultimately left the field of psychological treatment, but Freud, undeterred by the unfavourable reception given to the *Studies* by the experts of the day, pursued his studies of patients. He discovered that what was strangulated in neurosis was not just any kind of emotional experience but those that were primarily sexual in nature. Freud then began to study the so-called neurasthenics as well as the hysterics. As a consequence of these investigations, he believed at that time that the neuroses, without exception, resulted from disturbances in sexual function.

Freud's study of Breuer's patient, Anna O., led to the discovery of the concept of 'transference', a key to clinical and applied psychoanalysis. In a patient's relationship with his analyst, Freud thought, the patient re-experiences the early emotional relations that he had with his parents. It is the analysis of this transference that becomes the most fruitful instrument of analytical treatment. As a result of his discovery of transference, Freud abandoned hypnotism and began to use other procedures that evolved into the technique used in psychoanalysis today. The patient lies on a couch with the analyst sitting behind. The patient associates freely, and the analyst listens for patterns of transference, linkages, feelings, dreams, and other products of the associative process.

Once he had abandoned the use of hypnosis, Freud came to understand that there were forces which he called resistances which kept certain patterns, linkages, and connections from awareness. An impulse barred from access to consciousness was in fact retained and pushed into the unconscious (that is, repressed), from which it was capable of re-emerging when the counterforces were weakened or the repressed impulses strengthened. Freud considered repression a mechanism of defence, comparable to the flight mechanism used to avoid external conflict. In order to keep the debarred impulse repressed in the unconscious, the mental apparatus had to deploy 'energy'. The amount of energy available for other nonconflicted activities was thereby depleted, and as a result symptoms appeared. The theory of repression became the cornerstone of the newer understanding of the neuroses, which in turn affected the task of therapy.

Freud's early 'topographic model' of the mind separated the

unconscious into the preconscious and the unconscious proper. The topographic model was later to evolve into the 'structural model' of the mind, which consisted of the id, the ego, and the ego ideal or super-ego.

As Freud investigated his patients' lives, he was struck by the significance of events that had seemingly occurred during the first years of childhood. The impressions of that early period of life, though buried in the unconscious, still played a significant role in the individual's personality and vulnerability to later emotional disturbance. Freud's assertion that sexuality is present from the beginning of life and has a subsequent course of development was a pivotal concept of psychoanalysis and one that evoked a good deal of controversy.

At the time of this discovery, Freud believed that experiences of sexual seduction in childhood were universally the basis of neurosis. The evidence for this was derived from his clinical work. Subsequently, however, he came to realize that the seductions had not actually taken place but were fantasies. That such wishful fantasies were of even greater importance than actual external reality, however, was one of Freud's most significant discoveries.

Freud's ideas of infantile and childhood sexuality became the basis of his developmental theory of sexual progression. Initially, he believed that sexuality is connected with what he called 'component instincts', i.e., instincts which are connected with erotogenic zones of the body but which have an independent wish for pleasure. These are usually connected with the vital biological activities necessary for survival. For example, oral activities involve sucking and feeding as well as oral pleasures; anal activities involve excretion as well as anal pleasures; and genital pleasures are related to reproduction and conception. Freud called the energy of sexual instincts libido. In the course of psychosexual development, fixations of libido may occur at various points which may be returned to when later threats force a withdrawal to an earlier level. Freud called this process 'regression'. Freud also noted in *An Autobiographical Study* (1925) that, 'The point of fixation is what determines the *choice of neurosis*, that is, the form in which the subsequent illness makes its appearance.'

The first object of libidinal gratification and fulfilment is the mother. Her breasts serve as the source of oral pleasure, and she takes on the significance of the external source from which later confidence, self-esteem, and self-regulation are derived. This relationship with the mother plays a pivotal role in a developmental stage that Freud named the Oedipus complex, after the famous Greek tragic hero. Using the male child as an illustration, and reducing this developmental stage to a simple formulation that did not take into account variations, complexities and consequences, Freud noted that boys focus their sexual wishes upon their mothers and become hostile to and rivalrous with their fathers. The incestuous object choice and its feared and fantasied consequences of genital damage and retaliation give rise to a stage of latency during which the conscience (super-ego) becomes evident through feelings of morality, shame and disgust. At puberty, the earlier conflicts, including the Oedipus complex, may become reanimated. Although Freud's discoveries of the sexuality of children were made from the psychoanalyses of adults, direct observation of children as well as the analyses of children and adolescents have confirmed, extended, detailed and modified his ideas.

Freud also made a major contribution to the study of dreams – their meaning and their use in the therapeutic situation. In one of his major works, *Die Traumdeutung* (1900) (*The Interpretation of Dreams*, 1913), Freud described his researches on dreams, dream work and formation, symbolism, and his wish-fulfilment theory of the function of dreams.

In *Zur Psychopathologie de Alltagslebens* (1904) (*The Psychopathology of Everyday Life*), Freud turned his attention to slips and lapses of memory. Such symptomatic acts, so common in everyday life, he believed, have meaning, can be explained and interpreted, and indicate the presence of conflicting impulses and intentions. The study of dreams and of symptomatic acts has applicability to both pathological situations and normal healthy mental functioning.

For ten years after he and Breuer parted (1895–96 through

1906–7) Freud worked in isolation, rejected by the German-Austrian establishment. In 1900–1902, however, Bleuler and Jung, working at the Burghölzli, a large hospital near Zurich, became interested in psychoanalysis and began to extend the application of Freudian theories beyond the confines of upper-middle-class Vienna.

In 1909, Freud, Jung, and Sandor Ferenczi, a member of Freud's circle in Vienna, gave lectures at Clark University in Worcester, Massachusetts. James J. Putnam, a neurologist at Harvard, and William James were among those present. The trip was a success, and marked the beginning of international recognition. In 1910 the International Psycho-Analytic Association was founded, an organization that still exists. Several journals, institutes, and societies were organized in Vienna, Berlin, Moscow, New York, Zurich, and London.

Although many of the earlier pioneers remained loyal to Freud and to psychoanalysis, some of his followers ultimately left him to found their own movements (for example, Adler, Jung, Reich, Rank, and Stekel).

Freud's research continued at an intense pace, but gradually his students and colleagues took over increasingly from him. In 1923 he became ill with a malignancy of the jaw which was to give him pain and anguish for the rest of his life. His contributions to our understanding of art and artists, literature and writers, jokes, the psychology of religion, anthropology, myths and fairy tales, rituals, the emotional aspects of group psychology, philosophy, education, child care and rearing, and the question of educating nonphysicians to be psychoanalysts were some of the by-products of his lifelong struggle to penetrate the science of the mind.

Freud was a brilliant and a learned man, a researcher, clinician, theoretician, and writer. Psychoanalysis allowed us to understand what previously was seen as irrational human behaviour from a new perspective. His contributions to psychiatry, psychology, sociology, and biology are monumental. The science of psychoanalysis has moved on since Freud's time, correcting some of his errors and expanding into areas that he did not develop. One can only do so much in a lifetime, and

Freud gave us so much that it will many lifetimes before we have fully understood him.

George H. Pollock
Institute for Psychoanalysis, Chicago

References
Freud, S. (1953–74), *Standard Edition of the Complete Psychological Works of Sigmund Freud*, 24 vols, ed. J. Strachey, London.
Included are: Vol. XX: *An Autobiographical Study, Inhibitions, Symptoms, Anxiety, Lay Analysis and Other Works* (1925–6).
Vol. II: *Studies on Hysteria* (1893–5) (with J. Breuer).
Vol. IV and V: *The Interpretation of Dreams* (I) and (II) (1900–1).
Vol. VI: *The Psychopathology of Everyday Life* (1901).
Jones, E. (1953–7), *The Life and Work of Sigmund Freud*, 3 vols, London.

Further Reading
Schur, M. (1972), *Freud: Living and Dying*, London.
Sulloway, F. J. (1979), *Freud: Biologist of the Mind*, New York.
Wollheim, R. (1971), *Sigmund Freud*, London.
See also: *psychoanalysis*.

Genetic Aspects of Mental Illness

Differences in the prevalence of mental illnesses may be partly explained by genetic factors (breeding effects and higher consanguinity rates), or by differences in ethnic backgrounds. However, environmental factors may also be implicated, while some divergences could be a result of sampling errors.

Affective Disorders

One may conclude from the more reliable lifetime-risk studies that at least 1 per cent of the population suffers from manic-depressive illness. If one were to include milder forms of bipolar illness and unipolar illness, where a considerable number of subjects are being treated as outpatients, the general prevalence may well be as high as 10 per cent. Most studies have reported an appreciable difference between the sexes in the distribution of manic-depressive illness. The sex ratio generally accepted is two females to one male. The interpretation of this excess of females is still controversial. It is conceivable that for cultural reasons, women are more likely to be hospitalized for manic-depressive illness than men. If this were true, one would expect to find the same phenomenon for schizophrenia, and this is yet to be proved. Another possible explanation is the fact that male suicides outnumber female suicides by a ratio of about 2 to 1. Finally, one could also invoke the hypothesis of sex-limited factors, for example, hormonal fluctuations or sex-linked genetic factors which increase the expressivity of manic-depressive illness in females predisposed to this disorder (Mendlewicz and Fleiss, 1974).

The twin method allows comparison of concordance rates for a trait between sets of monozygotic (MZ) and dizygotic (DZ) twins. Both types of twins share a similar environment, but whereas monozygotic twins behave genetically as identical individuals, dizygotic twins share only half of their genes and thus behave as siblings. Most twin studies show that the concordance rate for manic-depressive illness in MZ twins is significantly higher than the concordance rate for the disease in DZ twins (Zerbin-Rüdin, 1969). This observation is taken as evidence in favour of a genetic factor in manic-depressive illness.

Price reviewed the twin studies literature in order to locate pairs of identical twins, reared separately since early childhood, where at least one had been diagnosed as having an affective disorder (Price, 1968). Price was able to find twelve such pairs of MZ twins. Among these pairs, eight were concordant for the disease, an observation suggesting that the predisposition to manic-depressive illness will usually express itself regardless of the early environment.

The complex interaction between hereditary and environmental factors underlying the aetiology of manic-depressive illness cannot be elucidated by the twin method, nor can it tell us anything about the type of genetic mechanisms that may be involved in the transmission of manic-depressive illness.

Most of the early studies on manic-depressive illness have

shown that this illness tends to be familial (Kallmann, 1954). The lifetime risk for the disease in relatives of manic-depressive probands is significantly higher than the risk in the general population.

Most of the early family studies were influenced by Kraepelin's classification. As a result, the investigators included among their subjects patients suffering from mania and depression (bipolar) and patients presenting depression only (unipolar) without distinguishing between these. Thus, the samples investigated in the various studies are relatively heterogeneous. Leonhard (1959) was one of the first investigators to make a clinical distinction between bipolar and unipolar forms of affective disorders on genetic grounds. This genetic distinction between unipolar and bipolar illness has recently been confirmed in the United States (Winokur et al., 1969).

When correction has been made for age, diagnoses, and statistical procedures, the morbidity risks for manic-depressive illness in different types of first-degree relatives (parents, siblings, children) are similar. This observation is consistent with a dominant mode of transmission for this disease. Mendlewicz and Fleiss (1974) were able to demonstrate close linkage between bipolar illness and both deutan and protan colour blindness in seventeen pedigrees, suggesting that an X-linked dominant factor is involved in the transmission of the manic-depressive phenotype in at least some families. The linkage studies conducted so far on manic-depressive illness are of great value, since they are able to discriminate between sex-linked and sex-influenced types of inheritance, and they provide an estimate of the significance of the results. They all point to the presence of an X-linked dominant factor in the transmission of manic-depressive illness. This methodological approach has great potential and should be extended to the study of other psychiatric conditions, such as schizophrenia, using other genetic markers.

A recent study of adoption showing more psychopathology of the affective spectrum in biological parents of manic-depressive adoptees as compared to their adoptive parents is further evidence in favour of the genetic hypothesis of affective illness (Mendlewicz and Rainer, 1977).

Schizophrenia

Family risk studies, twin surveys, the model of adoption, and longitudinal investigations of high-risk children have been used successively to approach the numerous problems at issue in the area of schizophrenia. These special problems are (1) diagnosis; (2) the separation, at least conceptually, of heredity and environment; (3) the forms of inheritance; and (4) the developmental expression of genetic predisposition.

Despite the absence of hard data on the heritability of schizophrenia, the genetic-oriented approach has been valuble in that it has facilitated the distinction between schizophrenia and other psychotic illnesses, particularly manic-depressive psychosis, and the correlation of schizophrenia with such syndromes as involutional psychosis. The schizophrenic spectrum is a group of disorders exhibited, for example, by the biological children of schizophrenics reared in adoptive homes (Rosenthal and Kety, 1968). It encompasses various disorders, including schizophrenia itself and borderline states, schizoid disorders, and inadequate personality.

Roberts (1963) believes that 'genetic advice on mental disease must be left to psychiatrists. Some of those interviewed, and the histories they give, need psychiatric appraisal. What is even more important is the difficulty to anyone not a psychiatrist of interpreting and assessing psychiatric reports.' A second contribution of psychiatry to genetic counselling concerns ways of presenting material and discussing it with persons who need help. Marriage choice, family planning, child rearing, adoption, and foster care are all questions that fall under the wider sphere of genetic counselling.

Empirically, risks run from about 40 per cent for the children of two schizophrenic parents, to about 15 per cent in children of one schizophrenic parent. Risks of 100 per cent in the former case (theoretical recessive) or 50 per cent in the latter (theoretical dominant) have not been observed. Since most people do not consider risks below 10 per cent to be serious, the clearest indication for a warning of caution is in the case of dual matings; with one parent affected, the empirical risk for the offspring is low, though not negligible. It is necessary in such cases to help the family to consider also the possible effect of having a child on the course of illness in the disabled parent, and, second, the effect of a possibly disrupted home on the development of the child regardless of genetic considerations. In all cases, the psychiatrically trained genetic counsellor will have the opportunity to utilize all of his diagnostic abilities, psychological understanding, clinical experience, and biological sophistication in dealing with the many family problems presented by schizophrenia. This multidisciplinary approach can best be utilized in longitudinal studies of high-risk children.

Julien Mendlewicz
University Clinics of Brussels
Department of Psychiatry
Erasme Hospital

References

Kallmann, F. J. (1954), 'Genetic principles in manic-depressive psychoses', in P. Hoch and J. Zubin (eds), *Depression*, New York.

Leonhard, K. (1959), *Aufteilung der Endogenen Psychosen*, Berlin.

Mendlewicz, J. and Fleiss, J. L. (1974), 'Linkage studies with X-chromosome markers in bipolar (manic-depressive) and unipolar (depressive) illness', *Biological Psychiatry*, 9.

Mendlewicz, J. and Rainer, (1977), 'Adoption study supporting genetic transmission in manic depressive illness', *Nature*, 268.

Price, J. (1968), 'The genetics of depressive behaviour', in A. Coppen and A. Walk (eds), *Recent Developments in Affective Disorders, British Journal of Psychiatry*, Special Publication, no. 2.

Roberts, J. A. F. (1963), *An Introduction to Medical Genetics*, London.

Rosenthal, D. and Kety, S. (eds) (1968), *Transmission of Schizophrenia*, Oxford.

Winokur, G., Clayton, P. J. and Reich, T. (1969), *Manic-Depressive Illness*, St Louis.

Zerbin-Rüdin, E. (1969), 'Zur Genetik der depressiven Erkrankungen', in H. Hippius and H. Selbach (eds), *Das Depressive Syndrome*, Munich.

See also: *biological psychiatry; genetics and behaviour.*

Genetics and Behaviour

In the late nineteenth century, Sir Francis Galton collected information on accomplishments, physical traits and occupational status of members of families and began the correlational approach to behaviour genetics. In agreement with the prevailing sentiment of the British establishment, the finding that these characters aggregated in families was used as a biological justification for the social class structure of the time and even for the predominance of the British Empire. Kamin (1974) points out that similar reasoning by American psychologists responsible for the administration of intelligence tests to immigrants to the United States led to Congressional passage of the Immigration Act of 1924 which restricted immigration to the US from southern and eastern Europe. Thus over the past hundred years the issues involved in the relationship between genetics and behaviour have had serious political ramifications.

R. A. Fisher's 1918 paper reconciled particulate Mendelian transmission genetics with the continuously varying phenotypes that interested the biometricians. This paper led to the variance-analysis approach to familial data on continuously varying traits, in particular, behavioural characters. The idea is that overall phenotypic variance, P, can be partitioned into contributions due to variation in gene action, G, those due to environmental variation, E, and interactions between genes and environment. Later, animal breeders termed the ratio of G to P the 'heritability' of the trait. The sense in which animal breeders used heritability was as an index of amenability to selective breeding. Of course, this is inappropriate in the context of human behaviour, and in this context it unfortunately developed the connotation of an index of biological determination and refractivity to environmental intervention.

The use of heritability in situations where experimental controls are lacking has been criticized by geneticists, who prefer to think in terms of the 'norm of reaction'. The norm of reaction for a given genotype is the graph of the phenotype against the environment. It emphasizes the dependence of gene action on the particular environment; a genotype that performs better than another in one environment may do worse in a second. An example is the human genetic disease phenylketo-nuria, PKU, in which sufferers accumulate toxic concentrations of phenylalanine resulting in extreme mental retardation. Under a diet that restricts intake of phenylalanine from birth, normal mental function occurs. The norm of reaction approach informs us that even if the heritability of IQ were 100 per cent, this would say nothing about its potential for environmental manipulation.

Fisher's approach to the genetics of continuous variation produces expected values for correlations between relatives of all degrees which can then be compared to observed correlations and heritability estimated. In principle the most powerful data of this kind uses adoptions and, in particular, identical twins reared apart. Such twins are extremely difficult to find and unfortunately the largest sample, that published by Burt in his analysis of the heritability of IQ, has since been shown to be fraudulent. The remaining samples of this kind normally suffer from nonrandomness in the adoption procedure. Nevertheless, until about 1970 the estimates obtained using data that included Burt's produced the widely accepted statistic that genes accounted for about 80 per cent of variation in IQ.

In the past ten years Wright's (1934) method of path analysis has become the predominant one for estimating heritability. In 1974 this method produced an estimate of genetic heritability of 67 per cent. The latest path-analytic treatments make allowances for assortative mating and for the transmission of environments within families, that is, cultural transmission. The most recent estimates by Rice et al. (1980) and Rao et al. (1982) suggest that genetic and cultural transmission each account for about one-third of the variance in IQ. As with Fisher's variance analysis, the path-analysis approach is based on linear models of determination and has been criticized for that reason. Among the other criticisms are that most adoptions are not random, that the increase in mean IQ of adoptive children over that of their biological parents is ignored, and that the estimates of genetic and cultural heritability depend on how the environment is defined and its transmission modelled.

It has frequently been claimed that a high heritability of a trait within a group makes it more likely that average differences between groups, for example, races, are genetic. This is false since heritability is strictly a within-group measure strongly dependent on the range of environments in which it is measured.

In studies of the distribution of human behaviours within families, where the data base is not as large as that used for IQ and where the trait in question is a clinically defined disorder, the twin method and the method of adoptions have been widely used. In the twin method the fraction of identical (monozygous or MZ) twin pairs in which both members are affected is compared to that in fraternal (dizygous or DZ) twin pairs. A significant margin in favour of the former is taken as evidence of genetic aetiology. Numerous studies of these concordance rates for criminality, neuroses, homosexuality, drinking habits, affective disorders such as manic depression, and schizophrenia have generally shown greater agreement among MZ than DZ twins. In these studies the twins are usually not reared apart and the role of special environmental influences, especially on MZ twins, cannot be discounted. Other problems such as the mode of ascertainment of the proband, heterogeneity in syndrome definition and variation among the concordance rates in different studies also raise doubts about the efficacy of the twin method.

In the adoption method, the incidence of a trait in the adoptive relatives of an affected adoptee is compared with that in the biological relatives. If the latter is higher than the former the inference is usually drawn that there is some genetic aetiology to the disease. Adoption studies of behavioural disorders from among those mentioned above have generally produced higher agreements between biological than between adoptive relatives.

Again the interpretation of a genetic basis for the behavioural abnormality must be viewed with circumspection since truly random adoption is extremely rare and frequently adoption occurs relatively late in childhood. In none of the behavioural disorders mentioned above has any biochemically distinguishable genetic variant been identified, although research directed at the role of variation in properties of catecholamine and indole metabolism still continues.

The evolution of social behaviour has provided something of a puzzle to natural historians since Darwin. This field of study was subsumed under ethology and behavioural ecology, and until recently was relatively immune to the developments in evolutionary population genetics by Fisher, Wright (1934) and Haldane (1932; 1955). 1975 saw the publication of E. O. Wilson's book *Sociobiology* in which he not only stressed that social behaviours were similar across the animal kingdom from termites to humans, but also claimed that these behaviours were genetically determined. Ethology and much of behavioural ecology were then subsumed under a new name, 'sociobiology'.

J. B. S. Haldane had speculated in 1932 as to how alarm calls in birds might have evolved genetically but concluded that a simple genetic basis for the evolution of self-sacrifice might only apply to the social insects. In 1955 he foreshadowed sociobiology by asking for how many cousins should one's self-sacrifice be equivalent to that for a brother. These speculations were formalized in 1964 by Hamilton, who modelled the evolution of a single gene one allele of which conferred 'altruistic' behaviour on its carrier. Altruism here means that the fitness of the altruistic individuals is reduced by their performance of a behaviour which increases the fitness of others in the population. Hamilton arrived at conditions on the degree of relatedness between the donor and recipient of the behaviour that would enable 'altruistic' genotypes to increase in the population. The condition is usually stated in the form $\beta r > \gamma$ where β and γ measure the gain in fitness to recipients and loss in fitness to donors and r is a coefficient of relatedness. Hamilton noted that in the haplodiploid insects like the hymenoptera his measure of relatedness between sisters is higher than for any other relationship. Since the above inequality is then easier to satisfy than in species where both sexes are diploid, this could explain on a simple genetic basis the evolution in the social hymenoptera of the social caste system with sterile workers. This theory of the evolution of the kin-directed behaviours is now called 'kin selection'.

Hamilton's theoretical analysis was made using a mathematical approximation that allows the allele frequency of the 'altruistic' variant, the 'altruistic gene' frequency, to play the central role. With this approximation the mathematics gives the impression that it is possible to add fitness contributions from all relatives affected by the altruism to produce the 'inclusive fitness' of the allele. It has recently been shown that inclusive fitness is an unnecessary concept and that the theory of kin selection can be developed in terms of classical population genetic models with frequency-dependent Darwinian fitness differences. Hamilton's formulation contains many assumptions, but when these are removed his theory remains qualitatively true: the closer is the degree of the relatedness between the donor and recipient of an individually disadvantageous behaviour (controlled by a single gene), the easier it is for that behaviour to evolve.

In *Sociobiology*, E. O. Wilson extrapolated from Hamilton's theory to posit that the evolution of social behaviour throughout the animal kingdom including *Homo sapiens* has followed these rules of kin selection. Of course this position ignores the general criticism that none of the social behaviours discussed have been shown to have a genetic basis and are certainly not under simple genetic control. Although many behavioural ecologists took Wilson's position in the years immediately following the publication of his book, the difficulty of empirical measurement of relatedness, and fitness gains and losses, as well as technical criticism by population geneticists, have had a moderating effect. Kinship still plays a central role in behavioural ecology, but the explanatory limitations of the simple kin selection theory are now more widely appreciated.

In *Homo sapiens* the position of sociobiology is to minimize the role of learning and cultural transmission of social behaviours. In particular, the human sociobiologists have taken the position that such phenomena as aggression, incest taboos, sex-differentiated behaviours, sexual preferences, conformity and spite have largely genetic antecedents. There is clear political danger in acceptance of this assertion that such human behaviours have a genetic basis. We have the precedent of the politics of IQ based on erroneous inferences drawn from data of dubious quality. Sociobiology adopts a position of pan selectionism in which the terms adaptive and genetic are interchangeable. Cultural transmission, under which the properties of evolution are obviously different from those under genetic transmission, is ignored. Clearly sociobiology tried to claim too much: 'Sooner or later, political science, law, economics, psychology, psychiatry and anthropology will all be branches of sociobiology' (Trivers in *Time*, 1 August 1977). Fortunately, we are all biologists enough to tell the tail from the dog.

Marcus W. Feldman
Stanford University

References

Fisher, R. A. (1918), 'The correlation between relatives on the supposition of Mendelian inheritance', *Transactions of the Royal Society*, 52.

Haldane, J. B. S. (1932), *The Causes of Evolution*, New York.

Haldane, J. B. S. (1955), 'Population genetics', *New Biology*, 18.

Hamilton, W. D. (1964), 'The genetical evolution of social behaviour, I and II', *Journal of Theoretical Biology*, 7.

Kamin, L. (1974), *The Science and Politics of IQ*, Hillsdale, N.J.

Rao, D. C., Morton, N. E., Lalouel, J. M. and Lew, R. (1982), 'Path analysis under generalized assortative mating, II, American IQ', *Genetical Research Cambridge*, 39.

Rice, J., Cloninger, C. R. and Reich, T. (1980), 'The analysis of behavioural traits in the presence of cultural transmission and assortative mating: application to IQ and SES', *Behavior Genetics*, 10.

Wilson, E. O. (1975), *Sociobiology*, Cambridge, Mass.

Wright, S. (1934), 'The method of path coefficients', *Annual of Mathematical Statistics*, 5.

Further Reading
Cavalli-Sforza, L. L. and Feldman, M. W. (1978), 'Darwinian selection and altruism', *Theoretical Population Biology*, 14.
Cavalli-Sforza, L. L. and Feldman, M. W. (1981), *Cultural Transmission and Evolution*, Princeton.
Feldman, M. W. and Lewontin, R. C. (1975), 'The heritability hangup', *Science*, 190.
See also: *intelligence*.

Gestalt Therapy

Gestalt therapy is a particular approach to psychological growth and change rooted in psychoanalysis and existentialism. It was developed in the 1940s by Laura and Fritz Perls, trained psychoanalysts who had worked with Kurt Goldstein (developer of the holistic organismic approach) and with Karen Horney and Wilhelm Reich. Gestalt therapy and Gestalt perceptual theory are not directly related but do share a few similar ideas, such as the whole being greater than the parts and the notion of a constantly shifting figureground relationship (our awareness of the world is always shifting, so that one aspect will become important at one moment and then move into the background as another replaces it).

The goal of Gestalt therapy is to make someone responsible for his own life. It resembles Eastern approaches to growth, for example, Theravada Buddhism and insight meditation. The therapist begins by concentrating on what a person is attending to at that moment: by focusing on the present it is possible to articulate better the rules and assumptions that govern a person's life. The therapy emphasizes not so much change *per se* but an awareness of what choices the person is making. With awareness comes freedom, and with freedom responsibility.

A second common theme in Gestalt therapy is behavioural integration. People are assumed to have both tacit rules and inconsistent sets of behaviours, ideas and feelings. A person may express one idea intellectually and, at the same time, just the opposite idea with his body – facial expression, muscle tension and so on. (The man who says, 'I am not mad at my wife' in a loud voice while beating on the table would be an example of this situation.) The aim in therapy would be to integrate these modes of expression. The therapist might merely draw his patient's attention to his voice and pounding fist, or he might use the technique of getting the patient to exaggerate his movements or tone of voice. There are, in fact, no required techniques in Gestalt therapy, although in the past Perls did utilize certain specific modes of therapy. The therapist is more or less free to use any process that will help to increase awareness.

Many of the people who came to Perls for therapy were not sensitive to bodily sensations and compensated through overintellectualizing. To Perls, bodily and emotional expressions were positive, natural processes, not to be feared or kept under control, and the techniques he used were directed at eliciting these processes. Many critics treated his views as anti-intellectual – which they were to the extent that Perls regarded overintellectualizing as a barrier to full self-awareness.

Three other notions inform Gestalt therapy: (1) The patient knows all he needs to know for change to occur – he just does not know that he knows it. The therapist must try to increase awareness and through therapy help the patient to see, feel, function and relate better. (2) Life and change take place in the present. From this derives the Gestalt focus on 'what is going on now', and the emphasis on how one feels, thinks and what one does right now. This is not to deny the capacity to remember or be influenced by the past, but the effects of the past are in the present. Therefore important past events will be manifested now, at this moment, in therapy. (3) Everything is personal. Whatever a person says or does expresses his own consciousness and internal processes; in everything he does, he is talking about himself. This leads to the various techniques used by Gestalt therapists to elicit from the patient his statements concerning others and the world, and to help him to see them as part of his own psyche.

The therapy examines, brings forth, and explores ways in

which people stop themselves from functioning properly. The techniques of Gestalt borrow from Freud (for example, free association) and Jung (for example, active imagination), but these are carried a step further by stressing the patient's active participation – motor, emotional, intellectual and spiritual – in the course of therapy.

William Ray
Pennsylvania State University

Further Reading
Perls, F. (1972), *Gestalt Therapy Verbatim*, New York.
See also: *Eastern psychology; existential psychology; Horney; Reich.*

Group Dynamics

'Group Dynamics' was originally the term used, from the 1930s to the early 1950s, the characterize the study of changes in group life by Kurt Lewin and his followers (Lewin, 1943). Gradually, however, the term lost its restricted reference and came to be more or less synonymous with 'the study of small groups'. It is in this broader, second, sense that it will be used here.

A small group consists of from three to about three dozen persons, every one of whom can recognize and react to every other as a distinct individual, and the members are likely to manifest sustained interaction, perception of group membership, shared group goals, affective relations, and norms internal to the group which may be organized around a set of roles. These are amongst the most commonly invoked criteria of groups.

According to Hare (1976), by end of the first decade of this century about twenty social scientific articles on small groups had appeared, and many of the subsequent concerns of small-group research had been identified. Triplett (1898) posed questions and conducted experiments investigating the effect of the group on individual performance. Within the next half-dozen years, Cooley had written about the importance of the primary group, Simmel had discussed some of the consequences of group size, Taylor, the apostle of 'scientific management' techniques, had started to examine pressures on individuals to conform to group norms regarding productivity, and Terman (1904) had studied group leaders and leadership. From about 1920 onwards the rate at which relevant publications appeared started to increase. The 1930s saw the appearance of three classic lines of research: the work of Lewin *et al.* on different styles of leadership, parts of the programme of research at the Western Electric Company's Hawthorn plant, together with the beginnings of Mayo's misleading popularization of its findings (see Rose, 1975), and reports by Moreno and others of socio-metric techniques designed to represent choices, preferences or patterns of affect in a group.

By the late 1930s, the developing study of group processes, in the United States at any rate, was seen as part of the defence of conventional democratic practices in the face of authoritarian threats, and these hopes and expectations continued through the 1940s to the heyday of small-group research, the 1950s and early 1960s. During that period Bales produced his category system for the relatively detailed description of group interaction processes, the sensitivity or experiential group appeared on the scene (Hartman, 1979) and those not preoccupied with experiential groups increasingly studied laboratory experimental ones. From the mid-1950s onwards, Hare calculated that about 200 articles or books on groups were appearing each year. The quantity of work has not abated, but the sense of excitement and enthusiasm has. Mainly via laboratory experiments, a variety of delimited issues, often refinements of earlier topics, have provided successive foci for attention, including co-operation and competition, aspects of group cohesion, leadership styles, social influence processes including minority influences, group decision making and group polarization, personal space and density, and interpersonal attraction. Increasing methodological sophistication has been claimed and the absence of major theoretical advances bemoaned (Zander, 1979; McGrath and Kravitz, 1982).

Let us examine some of the field's achievements in the four

major areas of (1) group structure; (2) leadership; (3) processes; and (4) products, before turning to a brief critique.

(1) Various aspects of the structure of groups have been studied. Of these the most common have been the affective or liking structures, communication networks, power relations and role structures. Rather less attention has been paid to the inter-relations of conceptually distinguishable types of group structures.

(2) Hierarchically organized structures may suggest the existence of leaders, and from Terman (1904) onwards considerable effort was invested in attempts to specify recurring personality and social correlates of individuals who were leaders, but with only limited success. After a brief flirtation with the opposite strategy of attempting to relate the emergence of leaders to features of specific situations, in recent decades the emphasis has been on increasingly sophisticated attempts to understand leadership, which may or may not be concentrated in a particular individual leader. Leadership functions, roles and styles have all been examined in some detail (for example, Fiedler, 1967).

(3) A major part of the study of group processes has been concerned with social influence processes. Classic laboratory studies by Sherif and Asch demonstrated the powerful impact on group members of internal groups norms and led to a continuing emphasis on conformity within groups. More recent work from Europe, however, has shown that conformity need not always be on the part of a minority towards a majority (Moscovici, 1976) and that a group consensus or decision need not represent a mere averaging of individuals' views (Fraser and Foster, 1984).

(4) From Triplett onwards, the outcomes or effectiveness of groups has been a major issue. It has become conventional to distinguish two sets of criteria of group effectiveness. (a) Criteria such as quantity, quality, economy and speed measure success on the extrinsic task and can be regarded as assessing a group's productivity. (b) Measures of interpersonal pleasure, socio-emotional effectiveness and group stability are assessments of group satisfaction. While productivity and satisfaction are often

assumed to go together, there have been many empirical demonstrations that they need not, so that a strong relationship between productivity and satisfaction is better seen as an ideal to aim at rather than a fact of life. Attempts to specify the determinants of group effectiveness are virtual summaries of research on group dynamics (see Hare, 1976).

Initially the study of group dynamics was held to offer answers to a number of democracy's problems (Zander, 1979), but the group dynamics movement's most tangible legacy was the spawning of, first, group-centred training groups and then individual-centred existential groups. This move from a concern with the world's problems to the soothing of personal anxieties is perhaps symptomatic of the failure, as yet, of the study of groups to fulfil its potential (Steiner, 1974). All too often narrow questions have been studied by increasingly restricted methods, leading, at best, to mini-theories which have failed to sustain interest in the issues. Some of the reasons for this reflect North American experimental social psychology more generally. But the nature of the 'groups' studied, particularly in recent decades, must be a prime contributing factor. In practice, the study of small groups has not been primarily concerned with families, friends, committees, and the multitude of naturalistic groups that mediate between individuals and the societies they live in. Instead it has examined small collectivities of student strangers meeting for no more than an hour at a time; it is possible that a majority of 'groups' studied have manifested few, if any, of the defining properties of actual groups. In an analogy with 'nonsense syllables', Fraser and Foster (1984) have dubbed them 'nonsense groups', and if group dynamics is to regain its position as a major field in the social sciences, the rediscovery of real social groups would appear to be a necessity.

Colin Fraser
University of Cambridge

References
Fiedler, F. E. (1967), *A Theory of Leadership Effectiveness*, New York.

Fraser, C. and Foster, D. (1984), 'Social groups, nonsense groups and group polarization', in H. Tajfel (ed.), *The Social Dimension: European Developments in Social Psychology*, vol. II, Cambridge.

Hare, A. P. (1976), *Handbook of Small Group Research*, 2nd edn, New York.

Hartman, J. J. (1979), 'Small group methods of personal change', *Annual Review of Psychology*, 30.

Lewin, K. (1948), *Resolving Social Conflicts: Selected Papers on Group Dynamics*, New York.

McGrath, J. E. and Kravitz, D. A. (1982), 'Group research', *Annual Review of Psychology*, 33.

Moscovici, S. (1976), *Social Influence and Social Change*, London.

Rose, M. (1975), *Industrial Behaviour: Theoretical Development since Taylor*, London.

Terman, L. M. (1904), 'A preliminary study of the psychology and pedagogy of leadership', *Pedagogical Seminary*, 11.

Triplett, N. (1898), 'The dynamogenic factors in pacemaking and competition', *American Journal of Psychology*, 9.

Zander, A. (1979), 'The psychology of group processes', *Annual Review of Psychology*, 30.

Further Reading

Steiner, I. D. (1974), 'Whatever happened to the group in social psychology?', *Journal of Experimental Social Psychology*, 10.

See also: *conformity; group therapy; social psychology.*

Group Therapy

Group therapy implies a group of people who, in an optimal environment with a leader or leaders skilled in psychodynamics, interact for the purpose of conflict resolution and social maturation. For such a process to occur, regularly scheduled meetings over an extended period of time are usually regarded as essential. This is the stand taken by most group psychotherapists whose basic training includes an extensive knowledge of Freudian psychodynamics and/or object relations theory.

As with any relatively new discipline, universal standards of training and practice have not yet been formulated, but most agree that a mix of didactic and experiential experiences is essential. Until we understand the details of group process more fully, it is inevitable that psychoanalytic theory remains the basis of didactic training and, also, that some form of exposure to actual group process is part of a group therapist's 'apprenticeship' (Roman and Porter, 1978).

Intellectual understanding of group phenomena is not enough, and the therapist must, among other things, be able to empathize with his clients' anxieties and gauge their stress tolerance if he is to help them grow. At the same time he must be acutely aware of his own subjective responses to the clients; it is here that a personal psychoanalytic training is often considered to be invaluable.

Perhaps the most intriguing part of group therapy is the way it forces one to recognize nuances of interpersonal behaviour that are usually missed (for a detailed discussion of therapy, see Yalom, 1970). In fact, it amounts to a depth perspective where the spoken word is no longer the pre-eminent aspect of communication but only a part. A subtle process is at work in the group where members begin to identify themselves with the group and place increasing trust in it. This build-up of trust is partly the result of the group's performance in assuming responsibility for its members and partly due to other more intangible factors, for example, man's need for a family or social support system. Little is as yet understood about intuition but it is linked with philosophy and religion in many cultures. Further research in this area is needed if we are to understand better the nature of evolution and change which are an integral part of group process. At a more tangible level we know that the wisdom of the group can amount to more than the total inputs of the individuals concerned – this synergism is part of a creative process and links group therapy with education and growth.

A training in group therapy can be invaluable in many areas of ordinary life where interpersonal conflict is seldom turned into a learning or growth experience. This is particularly true in our educational system where teachers lacking skills in group dynamics, tend to rely on punishment to redress deviant behaviour and thus lose an invaluable opportunity for learning at a formative age. Similar skills would seem to be called for in all walks of life, from arbitration in trade disputes, prison reform, or consumer advocacy to holistic issues world-wide.

Maxwell Jones
Nova Scotia

References
Roman, M. and Porter, K. (1978), 'Combining experiential and didactic aspects in a new group therapy training approach', *International Journal of Group Psychotherapy*, 28.
Yalom, D. (1970), *The Theory and Practice of Group Psychotherapy*, New York.
See also: *group dynamics; therapeutic community.*

Horney, Karen (1885–1952)

Born in Germany in 1885, Karen Horney trained as a Freudian psychoanalyst and was the first important 'feminist' critic of Freud's biological and mechanistic theories. Freud, as has often been noted, created a male-oriented psychology which stressed the psychological consequences of anatomical differences. Horney rejected his notion of penis envy as crucial to female psychology and emphasized instead the role of social and cultural factors in producing in women a lack of self-confidence and an overemphasis on the love relationship. Although her own theoretical ideas were not coherent or fully worked out, her psychological insights, her interpretations and her criticisms of Freud are none the less brilliant. Abandoning Freud's ego, id, and super-ego; she replaced them with a theory of the true and the false self. Central to her work is the idea that because of basic anxieties and insecurities, the person begins to develop strategies to cope with feelings of isolation and helplessness. A particular strategy can become characteristic, causing the person to develop and present a false or neurotic self to others. The goal of Horney's therapy was to help the patient to recognize his true self and to foster its growth.

Horney constructed a typology of the styles of the false self: the expansive, the perfectionist, and others. Her descriptions of these types are intriguing portraits filled with 'aperçus'. Horney anticipated many of the ideas in contemporary psychology: Laing's theory of the divided self, notions of self-actualization and authenticity, the emphasis on the division between the public and the private self, and the focus on self-esteem.

Like many other European psychoanalysts, Horney emigrated to the United States when Hitler came to power. She eventually developed her own 'school' of psychoanalysis in New York. More optimistic about human nature than Freud, Horney believed that neurotic conflict could be avoided and was not an inevitable consequence of civilization. Horney told her women patients who wanted to be good mothers and homemakers to lead lives more like men, counselling that modern women invest too much of themselves in love and thus leave themselves too vulnerable to rejection and loss of self-esteem. A generation of women has taken Karen Horney's advice.

Alan A. Stone
Harvard University

Further Reading
Horney, K. (1937), *The Neurotic Personality of Our Time*, New York.
Horney, K. (1939), *New Ways in Psychoanalysis*, New York.

Hull, Clark L. (1884–1952)

An American neobehavioural psychologist whose influence within psychology was most profound during the 1940s and 1950s, Clark L. Hull was himself influenced by Darwin's theory of evolution, Pavlov's concept of delayed or trace-conditioned reflexes, and Thorndike's law of effect. Hull firmly believed that psychology is a true natural science concerned with the 'determination of the quantitative laws of behaviour and their deductive systematization', and set out during his years at Yale University (1929–52) to develop a comprehensive general theory of behaviour constructed of variables linked systematically to experimentally derived data. An extensive study of rote learning led to the publication in 1940 of a monograph entitled *Mathematico-Deductive Theory of Rote Learning*. This work served as a prelude to a more general behaviour system first detailed in *Principles of Behavior* (1943) and later, with modifications, in *A Behavior System*, published posthumously in 1952. The system was based on the assumption that most response sequences leading to the reduction of bodily tension associated with need reduction are learned or reinforced. Hull proposed that the tendency for an organism to make a particular response when a stimulus is presented is a multiplicative function of habit strength (reflecting the number of previous reinforcements) and drive (based on bodily needs), minus certain inhibitory tendencies (associated with previous conditioning trials). These, along with other factors such as stimulus intensity and momentary behavioural oscillation, were seen as variables relating to response acquisition in the context of reinforced trials. Through careful experimentation, much of it with laboratory rats in mazes, Hull sought to quantify the functional relationships among these variables. While he failed to construct a comprehensive behaviour system, his theory led to important studies in the areas of motivation and conflict, frustration and aggression, manifest anxiety, social learning theory, and biofeedback. Early in his career Hull also made contributions in the areas of concept formation, hypnosis and aptitude testing. In the late 1930s and early 1940s, he conducted seminars to explore the congruencies between psychoanalytic and behavioural theories. These seminars did much to bring Freudian ideas to the attention of experimental psychologists.

Albert R. Gilgen
University of Northern Iowa

Further Reading
Hilgard, E. R. and Bower, G. H. (1975), *Theories of Learning*, New York.
See also: *behaviourism*.

Hypnosis

Hypnosis is an altered state of mind, usually accompanied by some or all the following:

(1) Increases in the intensity of focal concentration as compared with peripheral awareness.
(2) Changes in perception, memory and temporal orientation
(3) Alternations in the sense of control over voluntary motor functions
(4) Dissociation of certain parts of experience from the remainder.
(5) Intensification of interpersonal relatedness, with an increase in receptivity and suspension of critical judgement.

Individuals capable of experiencing some or all of these changes associated with a shift into the hypnotic-trance state may learn to employ them as tools in facilitating therapeutic change. This applies especially to people with disorders which involve the psychosomatic interface.

Hypnosis is not sleep but rather a shift in attention which can occur in a matter of seconds, either with guidance or spontaneously. Highly hypnotizable individuals are more prone to intensely absorbing and self-altering experiences, for example when reading novels or watching good films. All hypnosis is really self-hypnosis. Under guided conditions, a hypnotizable individual allows a therapist or other person to structure his own shift in attention. However, not everyone can be hypnotized. Recent research using a variety of standardized scales indicates that hypnotizability is highest toward the end of the first decade of life, and declines slowly through adulthood and more rapidly late in life. Approximately two-thirds of the adult population is at least somewhat hypnotizable, and about five per cent are extremely hypnotizable. Among psychiatric patients, this capacity for hypnotic experience has been shown to be higher in certain disorders such as hysterical dissociations, and lower in others such as schizophrenia. In general, the capacity to experience hypnosis is consistent with good mental health and normal brain function. Neurophysiological studies of hypnotized subjects indicate brain electrical activity consistent with resting alertness and some special involvement of the right cerebral hemisphere.

Hypnosis has been used successfully as an adjunctive tool in the treatment of a variety of psychiatric and medical conditions, including the control of pain; anxiety and phobias; habits, especially smoking; and in the treatment of traumatic neurosis. When used in treatment, the hypnotic state provides a receptive and attentive condition in which the patient concentrates on a primary treatment strategy designed to promote greater mastery over the symptom. Some individuals with hysterical fugue states and multiple-personality syndrome are treated with hypnosis because their high hypnotizability becomes a vehicle for the expression of symptoms. Hysterical amnesias can be uncovered, and shifts between different personality states can be facilitated with the goal of teaching the patient greater control over these transitions in states of mind.

All psychotherapies are composed of interpersonal and intrapsyphic components which facilitate change. Hypnotic trance mobilizes focused concentration, demonstrates the ability to change both psychological and somatic experience, and intensifies receptivity to input from others. This makes the hypnotic state a natural tool for use in psychotherapy and a fascinating psychobiological phenomenon.

David Spiegel
Stanford University

Further Reading

Hilgard, E. R. and Hilgard, J. R. (1975), *Hypnosis in the Relief of Pain*, Los Altos, California.
Spiegel, H. and Spiegel, D. (1978), *Trance and Treatment: Clinical Uses of Hypnosis*, New York.

Hysteria

Known to Hippocrates, hysteria is one of the very earliest psychiatric entities to be recognized. Yet the passage of time has produced more confusion than clarity and more diversity than unanimity as to its meaning.

For the ancients, hysteria was the result of the extravagant wanderings of the uterus (*hysteron* being Greek for womb) which, having broken loose from its moorings, was thought to career about the innards causing various stoppages, effluxions and diverse symptoms of disorder. Latent in this rather mythical formulation are two central ideas, still noteworthy in modern conceptualizations: (1) the tendency of the disorder to be more prevalent in women than men; and (2) the possibility of a multi-symptom clinical picture. Although the multiplicity of symptoms brought the disorder within the compass of medicine, the problem was poorly understood, highly resistant to the nonspecific treatments of former times, and complicated by the sexist perspective in which it was considered.

Sigmund Freud's work led to a major breakthrough. His careful analyses of these patients, long considered to be untreatable or malingering, revealed the underlying unconscious residues of past emotional conflicts, usually sexual, that led to the puzzling clinical picture. Hysterics, Freud discovered, suffered from reminiscences.

Since that time, other conflictual issues, such as aggression, have been found to gain expression in hysterical symptoms. To understand hysteria one must grasp a closely related concept, the idea of conversion: the tendency for intrapsychic conflict to express itself through 'conversion' into somatic symptomatology. These symptoms usually involve the voluntary nervous system and its organs, sturctures and actions. In addition, the symptom usually contains within itself, in symbolic fashion, both of the elements of the unconscious conflict. An example might be a person who has an unconscious sexual conflict about masturbation and whose symptom is paralysis of the right forearm which keeps the arm from movement. The conversion symptoms – here, paralysis – afflicts the organ that would express the impulse (the arm) and prevents the feared action (masturbation): both impulse and prohibition are thus captured in the symptom.

Unfortunately for conceptual clarity, the term hysteria is used in several different ways today:

(1) Internists and neurologists commonly use the designation

to refer to a multiplicity of non-organically based disorders, including conversion, psychosomatic illness, somatopsychic illness and simple malingering.

(2) Dynamic psychiatrists and psychoanalysts, in contrast, designate by hysteria those neurotic conflicts that stem from the Oedipal stage of development. This conceptualization implies primarily sexual conflicts and a tendency to see nonsexual issues in sexual terms (and therefore to deny or avoid them). A common concurrent finding is the tendency to have relationships that are triangular in configuration, or to experience existing relationships as if they were triangular.

(3) Descriptive psychiatrists may use the term to refer to dramatizing, histrionic and seductive patients, mostly women, who tend to somatize their emotional difficulties; such clinicians may speak of an hysterical personality rather than of hysterical conflicts.

The latest diagnostic and statistical manual of the American Psychiatric Association (DSM-III) deals with this dilemma by eliminating the term entirely. Instead, the historically accrued elements of hysteria are dispersed under a number of headings including somatoform disorders, conversion disorders, histrionic personality disorders, and dissociative disorders (the last relating to a tendency among patients with hysteria toward dissociative states, one dramatic but rare example of which is multiple personality).

Thomas G. Gutheil
Harvard University
Program in Law and Psychiatry
Boston

Further Reading

Breuer, J. and Freud S. (1947 [1895]), *Studies in Hysteria*, New York.

Chodoff, B. and Lyons, H. (1958), 'The hysterical personality and "hysterial" conversion', *American Journal of Psychiatry*, 114.

Marmor, J. (1956), 'Orality in the hysterical personality', *Journal of the American Psychoanalytic Association*, 1.
Veith, I. (1965), *Hysteria: The History of a Disease*, Chicago.

Industrial and Organizational Psychology

Industrial and organizational psychology (IO) is the application of psychological principles to commerce and industry. It is defined in terms of where and how it is practised rather than according to distinct principles or propositions. There are three clear areas within IO psychology: (1) personnel psychology, (2) industrial/social or industrial clinical psychology, and (3) human factors or engineering psychology.

(1) Personnel Psychology

Every organization has to make decisions about personnel selection, training, promotion, job transfer, lay-off, termination, compensation, and so on. In each case, the characteristics of both workers and jobs must be assessed. In job selection, for example, the personnel psychologist must be able to determine what are the demands of the job in question and which human abilities are required to meet these demands, and then find the most suitable candidate. Similarly, training (or retraining) requires knowledge of the job demands and the current skills levels of an employee. The personnel psychologist's task is to minimize the discrepancy between demands and skills levels. Other decisions, such as promotion or changes in amount of compensation, represent the same basic challenge for the personnel psychologist: to match the environmental characteristics with the individual's.

The personnel psychologist uses various tools, the two most common being job analysis and psychological aptitude testing. Job analysis helps to determine the most important and/or frequently occurring tasks in a particular job. It may involve surveys, observations, interviews, or combinations of these techniques, and data from current incumbents and supervisors are an important source of information. Psychological aptitude testing tries to identify the capacities amd limitations of the candidates in meeting the demands of the job in question. In the past, popular methods were short tests of intellectual ability, particularly verbal and arithmetic skills. Two of the most popular tests of this kind are the Wonderlic Personnel Test and the Otis Intelligence Test. More prominent in recent years are the special ability tests, such as the Bennett Mechanical Aptitude Tests, and Multi-ability test batteries, such as the Differential Aptitude Test Battery and the Flanagan Aptitude Classification Tests. Psychological testing implies a standardized sample of behaviour. The sample may be gathered by means of a standardized paper-and-pencil test with specific questions and limited alternative answers. Alternatively the sample might include broad questions and open-ended answers, with structure imposed by the respondent rather than by the test or test administrator. The sample could also include motor performance, interview behaviour, and even physiological measures, for example, colour vision tests of vulnerability to stress factors in the work environment.

(2) Industrial/Social or Industrial/Clinical Psychology

This area of IO concerns the reciprocal adjustment between the person and the environment, the emotional capacities of the individual and the environmental climate being the key factors under investigation. The individual worker is assessed on the following criteria: adjustment, motivation, satisfaction, level of performance, tendency to remain within the organization and absenteeism rates. The organizational characteristics which are looked at include, for example, efforts to facilitate a positive emotional climate, reward systems used, leadership styles, and the actual structure and operation of the organization. Most adjustment strategies involve real or imagined others – this is the province of industrial social psychology. The industrial/clinical aspect considers the employee's psychological well-being, and the fact that poor adjustment often creates stress and occasionally transient abnormal behaviour.

(3) Human Factors or Human Engineering Psychology

This area makes assumptions which are just the opposite to those of the personnel psychologist. The problem is still the same: accomplishing a match between the individual and the job. But the human factors psychologist assumes that the person is constant and the job is variable. He must arrange or design the environment in such a way that it is more compatible with the capacities and limitations of human operators. In order to effect a better match, the job must be changed, which usually involves modifications in operations or equipment according to the capacities of the operators. These capacities could be sensory (for example, visual acuity), or cognitive (for example, information processing time). The information input and output system is emphasized: display devices (digital read-out devices, gauges or dials, and so on) and control devices (such as knobs, levers, and switches) are examined and modified if found to have a negative effect on performance. The three areas of IO are seldom, if ever, independent of one another. They are all components of an interrelated system. Selection strategies will define the capacities and shortcomings of the operators. This will yield a range for equipment design and modification. Similarly available equipment will determine desirable capacities and characteristics of applicants. Finally, the interaction of worker characteristics, equipment and task design, and administrative practices will influence adjustment.

Frank J. Landy
Pennsylvania State University

Further Reading

Dunnette, M. D. (1976), *The Handbook of Industrial and Organizational Psychology*, New York.

Landy, F. J. (1985), *The Psychology of Work Behavior*, 3rd edn, Homewood, Ill.

See also: *aptitude tests; occupational psychology.*

Infancy and Infant Development

Infancy is variously defined from time to time and in different cultures, although technically it is the period from birth to the onset of walking or, put more poetically, the time of life prior to the emergence of independent behaviour. In humans, the onset of walking without support and the beginning of definable 'speech' appear almost simultaneously. Among the significant issues surrounding the nature of development from infancy onward have been: (1) The question of the relative influence of organic or biogenic factors, on the one hand, and environmental, psychogenic, or learned factors, on the other. (2) The role of early experience in the determination or control of later behaviour and development, a concern which includes questions about the durability of early influences, the reversibility of effects of infantile trauma, and the effects of educational interventions on the behavioural maturation of the young. (3) The ever-present reality of individual differences in psychological characteristics paralleling those like height, eye-colour, and hair texture in the biological realm. (4) The mechanisms and processes by which behaviour change and emotional development occur in the early months of life.

(1) This issue is sometimes known as the nature-nurture controversy. Many studies have sought to establish how much of our life destinies and our characteristics (like intelligence level) can be accounted for by genetic factors, and how much by environment. Both domains of influence are relevant and, in fact, affect one another. The assumption of a dichotomy, therefore, is misguided and, as Anastasi (1958) has suggested, developmentalists should be studying how genetics and the environment work their wonders instead of trying to assign numerical weights to represent the relative importance of congenital and experiential determinants.

(2) The role of early experience in the determination of later behaviour and development goes directly to the problem of the plasticity of the young. The assumption that there is a primacy effect of early experience – which is significantly more enduring and influential than the effects of the same experience later in life – has a long tradition and has strong supporters among both psychodynamic and behaviouristic theorists and researchers. The early-experience proposition derives some of its strength from neurobiological data, and from studies of lasting influences of severe deprivational conditions (nutritional and experiential). Both the psychodynamic and the behavioural

views allow, of course, for later alteration of patterns of behaviour acquired early; their derivative therapeutic intervention procedures require the further assumption that behaviour patterns acquired even under traumatic conditions must be alterable.

(3) The last concern, that of human individual differences in behaviour and development as in more strictly biological characteristics, has occupied much of the research time of developmental psychologists. The study of mental age in relation to chronological age, or the documentation of behaviour change as a function of age, has yielded the developmental quotient, similar to the IQ (a ratio of mental age and chronological age) by providing standards of capabilities at successive ages, including assessments of variability. Such norms have enabled refinements in the classification of infants with developmental aberrations or disabilities. An unfortunate consequence of the construction of behaviour norms from the examination of large numbers of infants, however, was the unwarranted tendency to assume that a developmental quotient was descriptive of an organic verity and, hence, a stable attribute of the infant. A decided constitutional bias inhered in labelling of an infant as developmentally delayed or behaviourally precocious.

(4) The last issue has occupied theorists the most, from Freud to Piaget to Erikson to Lewin to all others who would understand early development as gradual accommodation or adaptation of behavioural functioning, resulting from both biological and experiential inputs. This latter group includes, of course, those committed to an understanding of child behaviour in terms of learning theory principles and known processes by which new behaviours are acquired through social controls and incentives.

Often seemingly at odds but none the less fuelling one another's empirical defences, the developmentalists concentrating on learning processes include those whose orientation stems from Pavlov, and flows through Thorndike to John B. Watson. The group includes Hull, Spence, Spiker, Skinner, and Bijou, and insists upon the importance of learning processes, as in classical conditioning and operant learning, and the importance of reward events in the production of behaviour change and, thus, memory processes. An often unstated but ever-present presumption is that the promotion of pleasure and the thwarting of annoyance are critical incentives for the occurrence of psychological development.

Those who favour cognitive interpretations of development in the first year of life (emphasizing reorganizations of informational inputs as the hallmark of development) rely heavily, like the learning theorists, on explanations of behaviour change in terms of gradually accruing complexities of function. The capacity for object permanence, for example, is a talent of humans not present at birth but usually seen by eight months. It involves the manifest refusal to believe that something is 'gone' when it has disappeared. Appreciation of object permanence, an obvious prerequisite for attachment by infants to those who nurture them, requires the ability to perceive multiple continuous events, retain memory of the succession of at least some of these events, and express surprise when the prediction of subsequent events from the continuity of earlier events has been violated. It is not clear in such instances how this series of capacities unfolds, although it is plain that the process is both developmental and gradual, and that the eventual talent is dependent upon the earlier acquisition of subroutines. Observers of infants who are in the process of acquiring, or are first manifesting, object permanence behaviour are aware that positive affective expression almost invariably accompanies the infant's appreciation that the object has reappeared or been rediscovered. Little is known, however, of the psychobiological mechanisms inherent in the curiosity behaviour or hypothesis-formation underlying the search, or about the reward mechanisms inherent in the infant's ultimate satisfaction with the search and confirmation of the hypothesis. A fair appraisal of our present level of sophistication must acknowledge enormous gaps in our understanding of even such relatively simple mechanisms of behaviour change with increasing age in young children. Infant development specialists are far more expert in describing infantile behaviour and in noting correlated changes in behaviour with age than in explaining those behaviour changes.

All of the foregoing comments lead to an appreciation of infant behaviour in terms of principles espoused by Harriet L. Rheingold (1963): the infant is an active organism responsive to environmental stimulation, and is thus capable of learning. Moreover, infants are shaped by their environments, but they also control their shapers. This reciprocity between the developing child and the childrearing milieu has been cited by Sameroff and Chandler (1975) as requiring a 'transactional' model for an understanding, which, on the one hand, honours the complex interplay of constitutional and environmental factors, and on the other hand, acknowledges the *cumulative nature* of human experience and its lasting effects.

At birth the normal human infant is able to hear, see, smell, taste, and feel touch. Much of the baby's behaviour can be characterized in terms of approach and avoidance tendencies. The baby turns towards and prepares itself to receive substances, objects, and events that are pleasing, as in feeding, and avoids stimulation that is clearly unpleasant. Even the newborn child is capable of behavioural self-regulation, as is evident when something sweet is placed in its mouth. The same baby will resist 'smothering' with head shakes and hand swipes when, as often inadvertently happens, the head falls into a position, even at the breast, that causes or threatens blockage of the respiratory passages. Infants also manifest conflict behaviour, as when both approach and avoidance behaviours are simultaneously elicited. All of these rudimentary psychobiological processes, initially gifts of the species, are shaped by subsequent environmental events to dispose the child towards increasingly complex, 'socialized' behaviour.

Human infants double in weight in the first three months of life and triple in the first year. Behavioural gains during these periods are equally astonishing. Over this time, the infant undergoes numerous transitions, not the least important of which involves development from a largely subcortical status to a system of behavioural and social interaction requiring extensive cortical mediation, autonomic nervous system organization, and memory based upon learning. The very rapid growth of myelin tissue in the first year of life, along with the proliferating maturation of dendrites characteristic of this neuronal super-growth period, are doubtlessly responsible in part for the infant becoming capable so quickly of taking in such vast amounts of information, selecting salient stimulation, acquiring simple associations between events, and performing psychomotor acts necessary to enhance further development.

Lewis P. Lipsitt
Brown University

References

Anastasi, A. (1958), 'Heredity, environment, and the question "How" ', *Psychological Review*, 65.

Rheingold, H. L. (1963), *Maternal Behavior in Mammals*, New York.

Sameroff, A. J. and Chandler, M. J. (1975), 'Reproductive risk and the continuum of caretaking casualty', in F. D. Horowitz (ed.), *Review of Child Development Research*, Vol. 4, Chicago.

Further Reading

Bower, T. G. R. (1982), *Development in Infancy*, 2nd edn, San Francisco.

Bowlby, J. (1969), *Attachment and Loss* (vol. I), New York.

Field, T. M., Huston, A., Quay, H. C., Troll, L. and Finley, G. E. (eds) (1982), *Review of Human Development*, New York.

Garmezy, N. and Rutter, M. (eds) (1983), *Stress, Coping, and Development in Children*, New York.

Kagan, J., Kearsley, R. B. and Zelazo, P. R. (1978), *Infancy: Its Place in Human Development*, Cambridge, Mass.

Lipsitt, L. P. and Reese, H. W. (1979), *Child Development*, Glenview, Ill.

Stratton, P. (ed.) (1982), *Psychobiology of the Human Newborn*, Chichester.

See also: *attachment; Bowlby; conditioning; intelligence.*

Instinct

In common parlance instinct has a variety of meanings. For example, it can refer to an impulse to act in some way that is purposeful yet 'without foresight of the ends and without previous education in the performance' (James, 1890); to a propensity, aptitude, or intuition with which an individual appears to be born, or a species naturally endowed; to motives, compulsions, or driving energies instigating behaviour serving some vital functions. This multiple meaning seldom causes a problem in everyday conversation. However, a tendency to assume that evidence for one of the meanings entails the others as well has been a cause of confusion in scientific contexts.

Darwin

Most scientific uses of instinct derive from Darwin, He dodged the question of definition, in view of the fact that 'several distinct mental actions are commonly embraced by the term' (Darwin, 1859). He used the word to refer to impulses such as that which drives a bird to migrate, dispositions such as tenacity in a dog, feelings such as sympathy in a person, and in other senses. However he frequently argued as though 'instinct' stood for something that combined its several meanings into a single concept, licensing inference from one meaning to another. For example, when there was reason to think that some behaviour pattern was genetically inherited, he would assume its development to be independent of experience; and, conversely, he took opportunity for learning as a reason to doubt that he was dealing with an instinct, as though what is instinctive must be both hereditary and unlearned. But the relationship between hereditary transmission and ontogenetic development admits of all sorts of combination between the inborn and the acquired. To take one of Darwin's examples, there is no contradiction between a bird's having an inborn migratory urge, and its having to learn the flypath to follow.

In *The Descent of Man* (1871) Darwin focused on instinct as the underlying source of feeling, wanting and willing. Construed thus as impulse to action, instinct manifests itself as behaviour directed towards a goal. However, if the only evidence for an instinct in this sense is the goal-directed behaviour that it is supposed to account for, the account will be uninformative. Unless there are independently identifiable correlates, such as physiological variables, the inventory of an animal's instincts will amount to an inventory of the goals towards which the animal's behaviour can be seen to be directed. However, observers can differ about what and how many kinds of goal govern an animal's behaviour; and it is an open question whether all the behaviour directed at a particular kind of goal is internally driven and controlled by a single and unitary motivational system. For Darwin these difficulties did not greatly affect his argument for psychological continuity between man and beast. They have been a bother to more recent theories of instinct, as those of Freud, McDougall, and 'classical' ethology, will illustrate.

Freud
Freud held several theories about instinct. In an early version he viewed the psyche as subject to biologically based instinctive drives for self-preservation and reproduction; later a single supply of psychic energy was envisaged as giving rise to and becoming dispersed between the psychic structures of the id, ego, and super-ego, with their rival imperatives of appetite, accommodation, and moral value; and finally this trio incorporated contending instincts of life (*eros*) and death (*thanatos*). For Freud the manifest goals of overt behaviour were false guides to the underlying instincts, since experience works through the ego to suppress or distort their natural expression, in accordance with social constraints. Only by the techniques of psychoanalysis, such as those using word associations and dream descriptions, can true inner dynamics of human action and preoccupation be revealed.

However, Freud made little attempt to get independent empirical validation of his findings. Also he wrote at times as though instinct were a kind of blind energy, at least analogous to the energy of physics, and at other times as though instinct were an intentional agent employing strategies in the pursuit of ends. Consequently, to some critics, psychoanalysis lacks sufficient empirical anchorage and conceptual consistency to count as science, its instinct theory having more the force of a myth than of a material account. Psychoanalysis itself has come to question the usefulness of its instinct theories. Without denying the existence of biologically grounded factors affecting behaviour and mental life, analysts such as Horney (1937) have emphasized the roles of society and culture in the development, differentiation, and dynamics of the psyche.

McDougall

In his *Introduction to Social Psychology* (1908) William McDougall defined an instinct as '. . . an inherited or innate psycho-physical disposition which determines its possessor to perceive, and to pay attention to, objects of a certain class, to experience an emotional excitement of a particular quality upon perceiving such an object, and to act in regard to it in a particular manner, or, at least, to experience an impulse to such action'.

He thought of the connections between the three aspects of instinct as neural, yet insisted that the system is psycho-physical, by which he meant that perception, emotion and impulse, as mentally manifested, are essential to and active in the instigation, control and direction of instinctive action.

Although McDougall, being an instinctivist, is often represented as ignoring effects of experience, he did allow that instincts are capable of modification through learning. But he held that such modification could occur only in the cognitive and conative divisions; the emotional centre was supposed to be immune. Accordingly he argued that identification of the distinct primary emotions is the way to discover what and how many instincts there are, and that this is a necessary prelimi-nary to understanding of the derived complexes and secondary drives patterning behaviour and mental life. He gave a list of the primary emotions and hence principal instincts in man, together with speculation about their probable adaptive signifi-cance and hence evolutionary basis.

The plausibility of this analysis led to a fashion for instinct in psychology and adjacent fields (for example Veblen, 1914;

Trotter, 1919). However, as the lists of instincts multiplied so did their variety. Different people parsed their emotions differently, and there was no agreed way of deciding between them. Also McDougall's conception of the psycho-physical nature of instincts led him to vacillate between accounts in terms of causes and effects and accounts in terms of intentions and actions; and his theory and speculation gave little purchase for empirical correlation or experimental test.

Behaviourist critics were provoked into mounting an 'anti-instinct revolt'. This was instigated by Dunlap (1919), who argued that McDougall's theory was scientifically vitiated to unobservable subjective purposiveness. Other attacks struck at the prominence given to innateness, contending that wherever evidence was available it supported the view that all behaviour, apart from the simplest reflexes, is shaped by experience. By and large the behaviourists got the better of the fight in their insistence on the priority of hard facts and the requirement of experimental testability. McDougall's theory has little following today (however, see Boden, 1972).

Ethology
Ethology's 'classical' phase covers the period begining with Lorenz's publications in the thirties (for example, Lorenz, 1937) and culminating with N. Tinbergen's (1951) *The Study of Instinct*. Lorenz began with animal behavioural characteristics that are like certain anatomical features in being correlated with taxonomic relatedness in their distribution and variation. This evidence of genetic basis implied for Lorenz the other instinctive attributes: such behaviour must also be independent of experience in its development, independent of peripheral stimulation in its motor patterning, and internally driven by endogenous sources of 'action specific energy', which also causes 'appetitive behaviour' leading to encounter with 'sign stimuli' necessary to 'release' the instinctive act, and to which the mechanism controlling the act is innately tuned (Lorenz, 1950). N. Tinbergen (1951) built the components of this conception into a more comprehensive theory in which each of the major functional classes of behaviour – feeding, reproduction, and so forth

– is organized hierarchically, the underlying machinery consisting of control centres receiving motivational energy from above and distributing it to others below, depending on the sequence of alternative releasing stimuli encountered through the associated appetitive behaviour. For Tinbergen, the whole of such a functional system constituted an instinct, and to it he connected his conceptions of sensory and motor mechanisms, behavioural evolution, development, function and social inter-action to make the classical ethological synthesis.

However, the next phase of ethology's history was given largely to criticism of the Lorenz-Tinbergen instinct theories. Both within and without ethology, critics pointed to lack of agreement between the quasi-hydraulic properties of the theory, and what was known about how nervous systems actually work; the inadequacy of unitary motivational theories in general and ethological instinct theories in particular to deal with the full complexity of behavioural fact (for example, Hinde, 1960); the fallacy of arguing from evidence of hereditary transmission to conclusions about individual development and motivational fixity (Lehrman, 1953, 1970). Tough-minded reaction to what was perceived as tender-minded speculation led to conceptual reform to meet empirical demands, and methodological refinement to bring experimental test to theoretical implications and quantitative rigour to behavioural analysis. Even Tinbergen (1963) emphasized the importance of distinguishing between different kinds of questions applying to behaviour. The general trend in later ethology has been division of 'the study of instinct' among the several distinct kinds of problem it encompasses. Indeed ethologists now rarely talk of 'instinct', except to reflect on past uses and abuses, and on the present ambiguity of the word.

The ambition to arrive at an overall theory of animal and human behaviour persists, as some of the claims of sociobiolog-ists demonstrate (see, for example, Wilson, 1975). A reconsti-tuted concept of instinct remains a likely possibility for incor-poration in any future synthesis. But unless history is to repeat itself yet again, anyone deploying such a concept would do well to heed the lesson of its forerunners: they thrived on blurred distinctions, but to their ultimate undoing.

C. G. Beer
Rutgers University

References

Boden, M. (1972), *Purposive Explanation in Psychology*, Cambridge, Mass.

Darwin, C. (1964 [1859]), *On the Origin of Species*, Cambridge, Mass.

Darwin, C. (1948 [1871]), *The Descent of Man*, New York.

Dunlap, K. (1919), 'Are there instincts?', *Journal of Abnormal Psychology*, 14.

Hinde, R. A. (1960), 'Energy models of motivation', *Symposia of the Society for Experimental Biology*, 14.

Horney, K. (1937), *The Neurotic Personality of Our Time*, New York.

James, W. (1890), *The Principles of Psychology*, New York.

Lehrman, D. S. (1953), 'A critique of Konrad Lorenz's theory of instinctive behaviour', *Quarterly Review of Biology*, 28.

Lehrman, D. S. (1979), 'Semantic and conceptual issues in the nature-nurture problem', in L. R. Aronson, E. Tobach, D. S. Lehrmann and J. S. Rosenblatt (eds), *Development and Evolution of Behavior*, San Francisco.

Lorenz, K. (1937), 'Über die Bildung des Instinktbegriffes', *Naturwissenschaften*, 25.

Lorenz, K. (1950), 'The comparative method in studying innate behaviour patterns', *Symposia of the Society for Experimental Biology*, 4.

McDougall, W. (1908), *An Introduction to Social Psychology*, London.

Tinbergen, N. (1951), *The Study of Instinct*, Oxford.

Tinbergen, N. (1963), 'On the aims and methods of ethology', *Zeitschrift für Tierpsychologie*, 20.

Trotter, W. (1919), *Instincts of the Herd in Peace and War*, New York.

Veblen, T. (1914), *The Instinct of Workmanship and the State of the Industrial Arts*, New York.

Wilson, E. O. (1975), *Sociobiology*, Cambridge, Mass.

Intelligence and Intelligence Testing

The testing of intelligence has a long history (for psychology) going back to the turn of the century when Binet in Paris attempted to select children who might profit from public education. Since that time the notion of intelligence has been the subject of considerable scrutiny, especially by Spearman in Great Britain in the 1930s, and of much and often bitter controversy.

The Meaning of Intelligence

Intelligence is defined as a general reasoning ability which can be used to solve a wide variety of problems. It is called general because it has been shown empirically that such an ability enters into a variety of tasks. In job selection, for example, the average correlation with occupational success and intelligence test scores is 0.3. This is a good indication of how general intelligence is, as an ability.

This general intelligence must be distinguished from other abilities such as verbal ability, numerical ability and perceptual speed. These are more specific abilities which, when combined with intelligence, can produce very different results. A journalist and engineer may have similar general intelligence but would differ on verbal and spatial ability. The illiterate scientist and innumerate arts student are well-known stereotypes illustrating the point.

Intelligence Tests

Most of our knowledge of intelligence has come about through the development and use of intelligence tests. In fact, intelligence is sometimes defined as that which intelligence tests measure. This is not as circular as it might appear, since what intelligence tests measure is known from studies of those who score highly and those who do not, and from studies of what can be predicted from intelligence test scores. Indeed the very notion of intelligence as a general ability comes about from investigations of intelligence tests and other scores. Well-known tests of intelligence are the Wechsler scales (for adults and children), the Stanford-Binet test and the recent British Intelligence Scale. These are tests to be used with individuals. Well-known group tests are Raven's Matrices and Cattell's Culture Fair test.

The IQ (intelligence quotient) is now a figure which makes any two scores immediately comparable. Scores at each age group are scaled such that the mean is 100 and the standard deviation is 15 in a normal distribution. Thus a score of 130 always means that the individual is two standard deviations beyond the norm, that is, in the top 2½ per cent of his age group.

Modern intelligence tests have been developed through the use of factor analysis, a statistical method that can separate out dimensions underlying the observed differences of scores on different tests. When this is applied to a large collection of measures, an intelligence factor (or, strictly, factors, as we shall see) emerges which can be shown to run through almost all tests. Factor loadings show to what extent a test is related to a factor. Thus a test of vocabulary loads about 0.6, that is, it is correlated 0.6 with intelligence. Such loadings, of course, give a clear indication of the nature of intelligence.

The results of the most modern and technically adequate factor analysis can be summarized as follows (for a full description see Cattell, 1971). Intelligence breaks down into two components.

(1)g_f *Fluid ability*: This is the basic reasoning ability which in Cattell's view is largely innate (but see below) and depends upon the neurological constitution of the brain. It is largely independent of learning and can be tested best by items which do not need knowledge for their solution. A typical fluid ability item is:

○ is to ◙ as ▽ is to . . . with a multiple choice of five drawings. An easy item (correct answer: ▽).

(2)g_c *Crystallized ability*: This is a fluid ability as it is evinced in a culture. In Cattell's view crystallized ability results from the investment of fluid ability in the skills valued by a culture. In Great Britain this involves the traditional academic disciplines, for example, physics, mathematics, classics or languages. In later life professional skills, as in law or medicine, may become the vehicles for crystallized ability. A typical Crystallized Ability Item is: Sampson Agonistes is to Comus as the Bacchae are to . . . . A difficult item (correct answer: The Cyclops).

Many social class differences in intelligence test scores and educational attainment are easily explicable in terms of these factors especially if we remember that many old-fashioned intelligence tests measure a mixture of these two factors. Thus in middle-class homes, where family values and cultural values are consonant, a child's fluid intelligence becomes invested in activities which the culture as a whole values (verbal ability, for example). Performance in education is thus close to the full ability, as measured by gf, of the child. In children from homes where educational skills are not similarly encouraged there may be a considerable disparity between ability and achievement. On intelligence tests where crystallized ability is measured, social class differences are greater than on tests where fluid ability is assessed.

Thus a summary view of intelligence based on the factor analysis of abilities is that it is made up of two components: one a general reasoning ability, largely innate, the other, the set of skills resulting from investing this ability in a particular way. These are the two most important abilities. Others are perceptual speed, visualization ability and speed of retrieval from memory, a factor which affects how fluent we are in our ideas and words.

We are now in a position to examine some crucial issues in the area of intelligence and intelligence testing, issues which have often aroused considerable emotion but have been dealt with from bases of ignorance and prejudice rather than knowledge.

The Heritability of Intelligence

Positions on this controversial question polarize unfortunately around political positions. Opponents of the hereditary hypothesis were heartened by the evidence now generally accepted, that Sir Cyril Burt had manufactured his twin data which supported this hypothesis. However, the fact is that there are other more persuasive data confirming this position – data coming from biometric analyses.

First, what is the hereditary hypothesis? It claims that the variance in measured intelligence in Great Britain and America is attributable about 70 percent to genetic factors, 30 percent to environmental. It is very important to note that this work refers to variance within a particular population. If the environment were identical for individuals, variation due to the environment would be nought. This means that figures cannot be transported from culture to culture or even from historical period to period. This variance refers to population variance; it does not state that 70 percent of the intelligence in an individual (whatever that means) is attributable to genetic factors. Finally, a crucial point is that interaction takes place with the environment; there is no claim that all variation is genetically determined.

These figures have been obtained from biometric analysis (brilliantly explicated by Cattell, 1982) which involve examining the relationship of intelligence test scores of individuals of differing degrees of consanguinity, thus allowing variance to be attributed to within-family and between-family effects, as well as enabling the investigator to decide whether, given the data, assortative mating, or other genetic mechanisms, can be implicated. Work deriving from this approach is difficult to impugn.

Racial Differences in Intelligence

This is an even more controversial issue with potentially devastating political implications. Some social scientists feel that this is a case where research should be stopped, as for example with certain branches of nuclear physics and genetic engineering.

Whether suppression of the truth or the search for it is ever justifiable is, of course, itself a moral dilemma.

The root of the problem lies in the inescapable fact that in America Blacks score lower on intelligence tests than any other group. Fascists and members of ultra right-wing movements have immediately interpreted this result as evidence of Black inferiority. Opponents of this view have sought the cause in a variety of factors: that the tests are biased against Blacks, because of the nature of their items: that Blacks are not motivated to do tests set by Whites; that the whole notion of testing is foreign to Black American culture; that the depressed conditions and poverty of Black families contributes to their low scores; that the prejudice against Blacks creates a low level of self-esteem so that they do not perform as well as they might; that verbal stimulation in the Black home is less than in that of Whites.

Jensen (1980) has investigated the whole problem in great detail and many of these arguments above are refuted by experimental evidence, especially the final point, for Blacks do comparatively worse on nonverbal than verbal tests. But to argue that this is innate or biologically determined goes far beyond the evidence. Motivational factors and attitudes are difficult to measure and may well play a part in depressing Black scores. What is clear, however, is that on intelligence tests American Blacks perform markedly less well than other racial or cultural groups, while these tests still predict individual success in professional, high-status occupations.

Importance of Intelligence

Intelligence as measured by tests is important because in complex technologically advanced societies it is a good predictor of academic and occupational success. That is why people attach great value to being intelligent. Cross-cultural studies of abilities in Africa, for example, have shown that the notion of intelligence is different from that in the West and is not there so highly regarded. Many skills in African societies may require quite different abilities. Thus as long as, in a society, it is evident that a variable contributes to success, that variable will be valued; and even though intelligence is but one of a plethora of personal attributes, there is, in the West, little hope that more reasoned attitudes to intelligence will prevail.

Two further points remain to be made. First, the fact that there is a considerable genetic component does not mean that the environment (family and education) do not affect intelligence test scores. It has clearly been shown that even with 80 percent genetic determination, environmental causes can produce variations of up to 30 points.

Finally, the rather abstract statistically defined concept of intelligence is now being intensively studied in cognitive experimental psychology in an attempt to describe precisely the nature of this reasoning ability. Sternberg's (1977) analyses of analogous reasoning are good examples of this genre – the blending of psychometric and experimental psychology.

Paul Kline
University of Exeter

References
Cattell, R. B. (1971), *Abilities: Their Structure, Growth and Action*, New York.
Cattell, R. B. (1982), *The Inheritance of Personality and Ability*, New York.
Jensen, A. R. (1980), *Bias in Mental Testing*, Glencoe, Ill.
Sternberg, R. J. (1977), *Intelligence, Information Processing and Analogical Reasoning: the Componential Analysis of Human Abilities*, Hillsdale, N.J.

Further Reading
Kline, P. (1979), *Psychometrics and Psychology*, London.
Resnick, R. B. (ed.) (1976), *The Nature of Intelligence*, Hillsdale, N.J.
Vernon, P. E. (1979), *Intelligence: Heredity and Environment*, San Francisco.

See also: *genetics and behaviour*.

James, William (1842–1910)

William James, eminent psychologist and philosopher, was born in New York City. He, his novelist brother Henry, and his sister were the main recipients of an unusually unsystematic education supervised by their father which consisted largely of European travels and private tutors. After an interval in which he studied painting, James enrolled in the Lawrence Scientific School at Harvard in 1861. In 1864 he entered Harvard Medical School and received the MD in 1869. His life was marked by periods of acute depression and psychosomatic illnesses which occasioned solitary trips to Europe for rest and treatment. These periods, however, produced two benefits: they gave James firsthand experience of abnormal psychological states concerning which he was later to be a pioneer investigator; and they provided opportunities for extensive reading of science and literature in French, German and English. His marriage in 1878 appears to have been an important factor in improving his health and focusing his concentration on teaching and writing. His academic life was centred at Harvard where he became an instructor in psychology in 1875 and taught anatomy and physiology. Subsequently he offered courses in philosophy until his retirement in 1907.

James's work in psychology and philosophy was interfused and is not completely separable. His greatest effort and achievement was *The Principles of Psychology* (1890) which, some ten years in writing, made him world-famous and is now regarded a classic in both fields of study. James stated his intention to establish psychology as a natural science. By this he meant that metaphysical questions would be avoided and, wherever possible, explanations in psychology should be based on experimental physiology and biology rather than on introspective procedures which had dominated philosophic psychology since Locke and Hume. In contrast to a widely prevailing conception of mind as composed of ideas, like atoms, ordered and compounded by association, James proposed that mentality is a 'stream of consciousness' including in it feelings and interests. For James, the mental is to be construed in evolutionary and teleological forms: mental activity is evidenced where there are selections of means to achieve future ends. Darwinian theory had an important influence on James's psychological and philosophical views. Ideas and theories are interpreted as instruments enabling us to adapt successfully to and partly transform reality according to our interests and purposes of action.

In an address of 1898, 'Philosophical Conceptions and Practical Results', James inaugurated the theory of pragmatism which soon became the major movement in American philosophy. He also drew attention to the neglected work of Charles S. Peirce whom he credited with having originated pragmatism. The main thesis is that the value and significance of concepts, their meaning and truth, is determined not by their origins but by their future practical consequences. An application of this view is found in 'The Will to Believe' (1896) and in James's Gifford Lectures (1901–2); 'The Varieties of Religious Experience'; it is argued explicitly in *Pragmatism* (1907) and *The Meaning of Truth* (1909). In his later writings and lectures, James refined and defended his metaphysical doctrines of the pluralistic character of reality, indeterminism, and 'radical empiricism' according to which the world is conceived as a growing continuous structure of experience.

H. S. Thayer
The City College of The City
University of New York

Further Reading

James, W. (1975–), *The Works of William James*, ed. F. Burkhardt and F. Bowers, Cambridge, Mass.

Perry, R. B. (1935), *The Thought and Character of William James*, 2 vols, Boston.

Jung, Carl Gustav (1875–1961)

Carl Gustav Jung was a Swiss psychiatrist whose theories form the basis of Analytical or Jungian psychology. Concepts that Jung introduced to psychology include: the stages of life with age-related tasks, psychological types with differing attitudes (extraversion-introversion) and functions, the collective unconscious, archetypes, individuation or transformation as an aim of analysis, feminine and masculine principles, and synchronicity (meaningful coincidence).

Jung's depth psychology considers spirituality important. It is considered especially suitable for people in the second half of life, who may be well adapted but plagued by a sense of the meaninglessness of life. His psychology is also of particular value in working with psychosis, since his insights into symbolic material help make delusions and hallucinations, as well as dreams, intelligible.

Jung was a prolific writer; his *Collected Works* (1953–79) contains eighteen volumes. His theories have also had a major impact on literature, history and anthropology.

Training centres in Jungian analysis exist in Europe and the United States. Certified analysts are members of local or regional Societies of Jungian Analysts and the International Association for Analytical Psychology.

Jung's life and his theories are intertwined, as he emphasized in his autobiography, *Memories, Dreams, Reflections*, (1961): 'My life is a story of self-realization of the unconscious. Everything in the unconscious seeks outward manifestation, and the personality too desires to evolve out of its unconscious conditions and to experience itself as a whole.'

Jung was born in 1875 in Kesswil, Switzerland. A sensitive child who played alone in his early years, he mulled over questions raised by his dreams and by observations of himself and others. As a student, he was powerfully drawn to science, especially zoology, paleontology, and geology. His other fascinations were comparative religion and the humanities, especially Graeco-Roman, Egyptian and prehistoric archaeology. These interests represented his inner dichotomy: 'What appealed to me in science were the concrete facts and their historical background, and in comparative religion the spiritual problems, into which philosophy also entered. In science I missed the factor of meaning; and in religion, that of empiricism.' Later in his psychology, he would attempt to bridge the distance between these two poles.

Jung's medical studies were at the Universities of Basel

(1895–1900) and Zurich (MD, 1902). At that time psychiatry was held in contempt, mental disease was considered hopeless, and both psychiatrists and patients were isolated in asylums. Jung had no interest in psychiatry, until he read the introduction to Krafft-Ebing's textbook. It had a galvanizing effect; 'My excitement was intense, for it had become clear to me, in a flash of illumination, that for me the only possible goal was psychiatry. Here alone the two currents of my interest could flow together and in a united stream dig their own bed. Here was the empirical field common to biological and spiritual facts, which I had everywhere sought and nowhere found. Here at last was the place where the collision of nature and spirit became a reality.' Jung became an assistant at the Burghölzli Mental Hospital in Zurich in 1902, which alienated him from his medical colleagues.

At Burghölzli, Jung concerned himself with the question: 'What actually takes place inside the mentally ill?' He developed the word association test, which provided insight into emotion-laden complexes, discovered that a patient's secret story is a key in treatment, and found that delusions are not 'senseless'. He became a lecturer in psychiatry at the University of Zurich, senior physician at the Psychiatric Clinic, and acquired a large private practice.

In 1903, Jung discovered the convergence of Freud's *The Interpretation of Dreams* with his own ideas. Jung had frequently encountered repressions in his experiments in word association. In 1907, he published *Über die Psychologie der Dementia Praecox* (*The Psychology of Dementia Praecox*, 1953) which led to a meeting with Freud. Jung considered Freud the first man of real importance he had encountered; Freud believed he had found in Jung his spiritual son and successor.

An idealized father-son relationship betwen Freud and Jung ended over theoretical differences. Jung could not agree with Freud that all neuroses are caused by sexual repression or sexual traumata. Freud considered Jung's interest in religion, philosophy and parapsychology as 'occultism'. The final personal and theoretical divergence concerned mother-son incest; Jung considered incest symbolically, in opposition to Freud's literal, sexual interpretation.

After the break with Freud in 1914, Jung was professionally alone. Then followed a four-year period of uncertainty that Jung called his 'confrontation with the unconscious'. In his private practice, he resolved not to bring any theoretical premises to bear upon his patient's dreams, instead asking them, 'What occurs to you in connection with that?' This method, which arose from theoretical disorientation, became the basis of the 'amplification' approach to dreams in analytical psychology.

This period was characterized by intense inner confusion and discovery for Jung. As he groped to understand himself, he became emotionally engaged in building a small villa out of stones and sticks at the lakeshore. Going about this project with the intensity of a participant in a rite released a stream of memories, fantasies and emotion. (This experience would later influence the development of sandplay therapy.)

Jung had vivid and frightening dreams, fantasies and visions, and feared that he was menaced by a psychosis. Despite his fear of losing command of himself, and motivated in part by 'the conviction that I could not expect of my patients something I did not dare to do myself', Jung committed himself to the 'dangerous enterprise' of plummeting down to the 'underground'. He kept a record of his fantasies and dreams, and painted and conversed with the figures populating his inner world. (This technique would lead to 'active imagination' as a therapy tool.) Jung's effort to understand and assimilate the meaning of his inner reality proved to be a germinal period for ideas that he would develop and write about for the rest of his life.

In 1918, the phase of Jung's intense journey inward ended, and a period of writing followed. The first major work, *Psychologische Typen*, was published in 1921 (*Psychological Types, Collected Works* vol. 6). In it, he introduced his concepts of introversion and extraversion as fundamental differences in attitude, and the four functions by which experience is assessed and perceived: thinking, feeling, intuition and sensation. Through this work, he came to understand why he, Freud and Adler could have such divergent theories about human nature.

He continued to write prolifically until his death in Zurich in 1961. Everything he wrote about began as an inquiry into a subject that was personally relevant. He sought empirical data, read widely and travelled considerably. Jung remains of continuing interest to students of religion, literary criticism and humanities. There has been some controversy about Jung's supposed racial theories of the collective unconscious and his alleged sympathies with ideologies of racial superiority.

Jean Shinoda Bolen
Training Analyst, C. G. Jung Institute, San Francisco

References
Jung, C. G. (1961), *Memories, Dreams, Reflections*, recorded and edited by A. Jaffe, New York.
Jung, C. G. (1953–79), *Collected Works of C. G. Jung*, 20 vols, eds, H. Read, M. Fordham and I. Adler, Princeton, N.J.

Further Reading
Jacobi, J. (1969), *The Psychology of C. J. Jung*, London.
Storr, A. (1973), *C. G. Jung*, London.
See also: *analytical psychology*.

Klein, Melanie (1882–1960)

Born to an intellectual Jewish Viennese family, Melanie Klein had intended to study medicine until an early engagement and marriage intervened. Then, in her thirties, when she was a housewife and mother of three, she discovered Freud's writing. Entering analysis with Ferenczi, she began an analytic career. Ferenczi encouraged her interest in analysing children, virtually an unknown procedure. In 1921, she accepted Abraham's invitation to continue her work in Berlin, and began publishing her observations on child development. After Abraham's death in 1925, she took up permanent residence in London, where she became doyenne of a distinct psychoanalytic school and the centre of a still active, and sometimes passionate, theoretical controversy.

Klein began her psychoanalytic career by developing a technical innovation – play therapy – which permitted the analysis of very young children. Klein came to believe that two broad formations successively organize the child's inner world: 'the paranoid-schizoid position' and the 'the depressive position'. While she ascribes them initially to the first and second half-year of life (an inference which has occasioned considerable criticism), Klein views these 'positions' as constellations of anxieties, defences, and object relations which are reactivated continually throughout development.

The paranoid-schizoid position is established before the achievement of object constancy. During this period, the real external mother contributes a number of quite separate figures to the child's inner world, via introjection of aspects of her in different situations. Thus there come to be 'good objects', introjected during gratifying experiences with the real mother, and eventually these images develop temporal continuity and merge. Moments of deprivation and pain are experienced by the infant as wilful persecution by his care-givers, so introjection during these states establishes sadistic, 'bad objects' in the inner world. The child's anxieties in this stage are that the persecutory objects will succeed in annihilating either the self or the good objects.

In normal development, this fantasy structure is gradually modified so that the various separate internal images of the real mother coalesce into a single object, with aspects both gratifying and frustrating, good and bad. But when the 'bad mother' begins to coalesce with the beloved mother in the child's internal psychic reality, the child comes to feel that his own (fantasized) attacks against the persecutor also damage the adored, essential good object. Guilt and mourning now develop. A new inner constellation, 'the depressive position', gradually emerges.

In addition to defensive regression ('splitting' of the internal object), the pain of the depressive position can also be temporarily assuaged through denial of the effects of one's own aggression (the 'manic defences'). But resolution of the depressive position depends on a different response: acceptance of responsibility, with attempts to repair the damaged objects. The cement for internal integration is the child's growing confidence in the reparative powers of his love.

While Klein's play therapy technique became universally accepted, her conclusions generated intense controversy and led to a schism within the psychoanalytic community. Most of the controversy concerns not the descriptive theory summarized above, but subsidiary issues – such as the timing of psychic phases in development, and the relative influence of constitutional versus environmental factors. Currently, as psychoanalysis struggles to conceptualize more primitive mental states, Klein's formulations are increasingly being integrated into the main body of analytic thought.

Alan S. Pollack
McLean Hospital, Belmont, Massachusetts
Harvard University

Further Reading

Klein, M. (1975), *Love, Guilt, and Reparation and Other Works 1921–1945*, New York.

Segal, H. (1964), *Introduction to the Work of Melanie Klein*, New York.

Lacan, Jacques (1901–83)

Jacques Lacan has been called the 'French Freud'. He was probably the most original and certainly the most controversial European psychoanalyst of the post-Second World War era. Lacan was a scathing critic of the 'American' developments in psychoanalysis which moved away from Freud's unconscious to what was called 'ego psychology'. In America, psychoanalytic therapy focused on forming an alliance with the healthy ego, interpreting pathological defences, and promoting the growth of conflict-free adaptation. Lacan entirely rejected this approach. There was, in his view, no conflict-free sphere: the 'ego' was hostile to the unconscious and the essential analytic process.

Analysis was an inquiry, not a cure. Lacan, in his characteristic play-on-words style, described American empirical research intended to make psychoanalysis an experimental science as 'ex-peri-mental' (that is, ex-mental and peri-mental). To Lacan, such research with animals left out the mental, because the mental has to do with language, meaning and signification.

Lacan regarded Freud's early and introspective works such as *The Interpretation of Dreams* (1913) as the essence of psychoanalysis. Lacan theorized that the unconscious is structured as a natural language; psychoanalysis, as a theory and as a therapy, was the discovery of this other language by recapturing associative chains of signification. An example of Lacan's theoretical emphasis on linguistics is his reinterpretation of the Oedipal complex. In greatly oversimplified terms, he believed it encompasses the child's movement from the order of images to the order of polysemic symbols. Lacan describes the infant's mental life as beginning in a mirror phase, like Narcissus by the stream seeing reflected images. When language and symbols are acquired, these images are mediated, their signification changes, and the infant becomes a divided subject. The unconscious is 'The Other' and the other language. The hydraulic and mechanistic theories of Freud are replaced in Lacan by a linguistic theory, for example, repression as metaphor formation.

Lacan's writing is arcane, convoluted, technical, poetic and difficult. Existentialist, neo-Hegelian and linguistic theories all influenced Lacan as much as did Freud. Lacan's later work became even more difficult as he emphasized the centrality of topology and mathematics to his theories.

Lacan became a central figure in French intellectual and radical thought, and was of particular interest to literary and social criticism in the West. Whatever Lacan's place may be in the history of modern thought, he was rejected by organized psychoanalysts because of his clinical methods. Most notable was his practice of dismissing patients after 5- or 10-minute sessions because, he said, they had nothing interesting to say or they were getting into a routine which silenced the unconscious. Lacan, in turn, attacked the psychoanalytic establishment which sought to 'authorize' those who would be analysts. Lacan claimed that analysis was a calling and the analyst must authorize himself.

Alan A. Stone
Harvard University

Further Reading

Bär, E. S. (1974), 'Understanding Lacan', in *Psychoanalysis of Contemporary Science*, vol. 3, New York.

Lacan, J. (1966), *Ecrits*, Paris. (English translation, *Ecrits*, London, 1977.)

Schneiderman, S. (1983), *Jacques Lacan: The Death of an Intellectual Hero*, Cambridge, Mass.

Laing, Ronald David (1927–)

The philosopher Kant wrote, 'The only general characteristic of Insanity is the loss of a sense of ideas that are common to all and its replacement with a sense for ideas peculiar to ourselves.' The question remains, however, how does one decide which *peculiar ideas* are delusions? R. D. Laing, born in Glasgow in 1927, began his career as a psychiatrist by attempting to make the *peculiar ideas* of schizophrenic patients (which he assumed were delusions) comprehensible. But in his subsequent work as a psychiatrist-philosopher he concluded that normality, 'the ideas that are common to all', is madness and, therefore, a psychiatry founded on such ideas was unable to declare any beliefs delusions.

Laing, his critics would say, went further than this epistemological relativism; he romanticized insanity and particularly schizophrenia. Madness became a breakthrough, a way of being in the world that rejects the 'pseudo-social' reality, the most awesome psychedelic trip.

Laing's early writings are both psychoanalytic and existential in character, as he attempted to portray the subjective experience of the schizophrenic. There are brilliant descriptions of the divided self unable to be a 'whole person with the other'. Perhaps most powerful are his descriptions of the family interactions out of which comes 'schizophrenic disorder'. It is the family that seems mad in Laing's description, and the patient's delusions and 'bizarre communication' are explained as a symbolic and visionary commentary on that family's madness (Laing and Esterson, 1964). His subsequent writings are less detailed, more prophetic in tone. The schizophrenic experience becomes a divination of the madness of society, not to be cured by drugs or to be interfered with by psychiatrists but perhaps to be learned from. As one of Laing's critics noted, 'Schizophrenia became a State of Grace.' Laing's writings were seized upon by the radical critics of psychiatry and by other radicals seeking liberation during the late 1960s and the 1970s. Laing's influence in psychiatry was short-lived. He turned to mysticism and poetry as his own liberation. In *The Politics of Experience* (1967) he wrote, 'True sanity entails in one way or another the dissolution of the normal ego, that false self competently adjusted to our alienated social reality: the emergence of the "inner" archetypal mediators of divine power, and through this death a rebirth, and the eventual re-establishment of a new king of ego-functioning, the ego now being the servant of the divine, no longer its betrayer.'

Alan A. Stone
Harvard University

References
Laing, R. D. (1967), *The Politics of Experience*, London.
Laing, R. D. and Esterson, A. A. (1964), *Sanity, Madness and the Family*, London.

Further Reading
Laing, R. D. (1959), *The Divided Self*, London.

Language Development

Learning a language is probably the stellar intellectual achievement across the species. It is robust. Children will learn a normal language right down to an IQ of around 50, before what they learn suffers appreciably. People try to teach children things about language in school, but the real bulk of language is learned in the preschool years, and is learned without anything resembling tutoring. We know now, for example, that parents do not reward children differentially on the basis of how well they put words together to make sentences, even though they may think they do. Nor do less correct sentences seem to communicate appreciably less well than accurate ones. Yet children inexorably learn the complexities of language – the arbitrary noun gender systems of Indo-European languages, the seventeen noun classifications of Bantu, the complex vocabulary of mental terms and modal verbs or particles that seem to be present in all languages.

In doing this, we now know, what they abstract is an underlying system of *rules*, rules for which the utterances they hear only provide examples. It is as though children induced physics from hanging around physics labs. We know they induce such rules partly because of the necessary nature of language, and partly because such rules show themselves in children's acquisition in utterances like *he feeled good*, or *where we should put this*? These show, respectively, application of a rule which happens not to cover all the terms it should (an irregularity), or overgeneralization of a rule from one context of use to another, slightly inappropriate one. Their learning of grammar – the sentence structure of language – is probably no more impressive than their ability to figure out word meanings, or to learn how to communicate to others. It can be estimated, for example, that the average child is learning nine new word meanings a day from the age of 2 to 6.

How do they do this? Chomsky (1980), whose linguistic work was the cause of the modern resurgence of language development work, argues that all these things – the complexity of language, the robustness of its learning, its relative ease of acquisition without tutoring or correction, the child's choice of some rules over others that should be justified by the same examples – all argue that the child approaches the problem with a rich, innately given biological programme for what languages can be like or are likely to be like. This position recently finds some empirical support in the work of Bickerton, who has studied creole languages, the languages that presumably children create out of the fragmentary and conflicting pidgins they are exposed to. Bickerton (1981) finds that these creoles have more in common than the pidgins the children built them from, and this argues they have strong ideas about what languages should be. On the other hand, many, perhaps a large majority in the field of normal acquisition, still think language is constructed by the child using what must be a very rich system of general intelligence. If this is so, the preschool child is far more intellectually powerful than has seemed so in the past, but this is turning out to be true in many areas besides language development.

Michael Maratsos
University of Minnesota

References
Bickerton, D. (1981), *Roots of Language*, Ann Arbor, Mich.
Chomsky, N. (1980), *Rules and Representations*, New York.

Further Reading
Maratsos, M. (1983), 'Some current issues in the study of the acquisition of grammar', in P. Mussen (ed.), *The Handbook of Child Psychology*, 4th edn, New York.
Brown, R. (1973), *A First Language: The Early Stages*, Cambridge, Mass.
Carey, S. (1982), 'Semantic acquisition: the state of the art', in E. Wanner and L. Gleitman (eds), *Language Acquisition: The State of the Art*, Cambridge, Mass.

Learning

For hundreds of years, learning meant the formation of associations, and was considered the means by which society transmitted its acquired cultural capital. Learning was the cliché which lay behind almost every explanation in the social sciences. Increasingly, however, the study of learning has been transformed into the study of the human mind. Nowadays when one speaks of learning one must speak of representations, of knowledge, of modularity, of innate and specific structures of mind. While the new view of learning is still mostly restricted to the cognitive sciences – the social sciences as a whole have not been affected – one would expect that it will ultimately have a powerful impact on the social sciences.

In philosophy and psychology, learning has traditionally been regarded as a potential solution to the problem of knowledge. How is it that a human being comes to have knowledge of the world? In this context, the study of learning has long been central to the study of the human mind. Empiricist philosophers, such as Locke and Hume, conceived of knowledge as a system of association of ideas. Hume invoked principles which explained how these associations were formed. For example, the principle of contiguity said that if two ideas occurred near each other in time, then it was likely that an association was formed between these ideas. In the latter part of the nineteenth century these principles became the focus of experimental study. With the behaviourist revolution in American psychology in the twentieth century, association theory was modified so that it no longer was ideas that were associated. Rather, a stimulus was associated with a response. But the basic underlying notions of association theory persisted: that human knowledge is to be represented as a system of associations and that these associations are learned.

The study of learning thus became the experimental study of the learning of associations. To make these associations experimentally testable, the learning of arbitrary associations was studied, for example, the associations between nonsense syllables, like *dax* and *gep*. From this emerged the famous learning curve, showing the probability of a person's forming an association as a function of the number of times the associated items were shown to him simultaneously. Not surprisingly, it was discovered that the more practice a person has on an association, the better he learns it.

Grand theoretical schemes developed to explain learning, for example, those of Hull. These envisioned learning as a unitary phenomenon. In essence, human and animal learning were conceived to be the same thing, though there might be a quantitative difference. And within a species what appeared to be different kinds of learning really were not. In short, the principles of learning remained unchanged across species and content of what was learned. A number of theoretical disputes arose over the precise character of these principles, but the different theories shared many underlying assumptions of breathtaking simplicity and elegance. These were that all learning was the same and that there were a few general principles of learning. The theory must have had simplicity and elegance, for what else could explain the fact that learning theory in this form lasted for so long? For the matter, plain and simple, was that learning theory did not work. If one actually considered real domains of human knowledge, it quickly became apparent that learning theory could not explain how that knowledge was acquired. The nonsense syllables of the laboratory, like the 'ideas' of the philosophers (or the 'quality spaces' of Quine), were abstractions which lost the essence of the problem.

The ideas which have replaced association theory are rich and interconnected. There is no way here even to hint at the extensive justification that has been developed for them. We will simply list some of the themes of the new study.

(1) Language and Innate Principles

Perhaps the major critique of the adequacy of association theory, as well as the most extensive development of an alternative theory for human learning, has come from the field of linguistics, namely from Chomsky (1965, 1975). Chomsky argues that the structure of language is such that there is no way that a human could learn language given any of the traditional notions of learning (call these 'learning theory'). Since every normal person masters a natural language, learning theory could not possibly be correct. Chomsky argues that the only way that these structures could develop is if there is an innate basis for them in the human mind.

(2) Conscious Awareness

We are not aware of most of the knowledge that we possess. For example, most of the principles of language are beyond our conscious awareness. In broad terms, the modern innatist position is very much like that of the rationalist philosophers (Descartes, Leibniz). Probably the biggest single difference (besides the extensive detailed technical developments in the modern period) is that the philosophers generally seem to have believed that the principles of mind were available to conscious introspection. It also does not seem unreasonable to claim that even behaviourists would only invoke principles of explanation of which they were consciously aware, although they did not explicitly state this. According to the modern view, although principles of knowledge are not necessarily available to consciousness, they are still in the mind, and thus a matter of individual psychology. Giving up the assumption of the necessity of conscious awareness of principles of mind is a liberating force in learning theory, for it makes possible the development of theoretical constructs which traditionally would have been immediately ruled out on the basis of introspection.

(3) Domain-Specific and Species-Specific Principles

The modern view violates the cardinal principle of the traditional view, that all knowledge except for some simple principles of association is learned. But it also violates the two subsidiary principles, that learning principles do not depend on the species or on the domain of knowledge. Principles of learning differ from species to species. Animals do not learn language, because the principles of language only occur in humans. Some scholars are quite willing to accept the innate character of principles of learning, but believe that these principles operate in all domains of knowledge. That is, the principles are some kind of complicated hypothesis-formation ability. But the modern view holds that there are different principles in different domains of knowledge. Thus those which underlie our ability to recognize objects are different from those which enable us to use language. This latter view has come to be called the *modular* view of cognition. In the entire history of learning theory, there are really only two general kinds of ideas about learning: the formation of associations, and some kind of hypothesis-formation. With the development of the modern view of domain-specific principles, it is possible to have a much more delineated learning theory with particular principles for particular domains of knowledge. Of course it is an open and empirical question whether more general principles of cognition and learning underlie the specific principles which have been discovered. On the evidence to date, it appears unlikely that the domains will be completely unified. For example, visual perception and language just *look* different.

(4) Reinforcement

In many traditional views of learning, an organism could only learn if properly reinforced. For example, a child was supposed to learn a response better if given a piece of candy when he made the correct response. The modern view, based on considerable evidence, is that reinforcement appears much less necessary for learning, although it may still be an effective motivator. Skinner (1957) argued that children learned to speak grammatically by being positively reinforced for correct sentences and negatively reinforced for incorrect sentences. But Brown and Hanlon (1970) and other investigators have shown that parents do not differentially reinforce grammatical and non-grammatical utterances of young children in the language learning period. Thus reinforcement does not appear to play a significant role in language learning, from the standpoint of giving information to the child. Its role as a motivator is more difficult to assess precisely.

(5) Instruction

One of the surprising discoveries of the modern period is the degree to which children spontaneously develop cognitive abilities, with no special arrangements of the environment. The field of language acquisition, and cognitive development more generally, is replete with examples. It is clear that the rules of language, for example, are not taught to children. People in general do not know the rules, although they use them implicitly, so how could they teach them? Some scholars believe that although parents do not teach the rules of language, they nevertheless provide special instruction by presenting children with a particular simplified language that is 'fine-tuned' to their levels of ability (Snow and Ferguson, 1977). But the best evidence (Newport, Gleitman and Gleitman, 1977) seems to show that there is no such fine-tuning.

Certain abilities unfold naturally, with no special instruction. Language appears to be one of these. Principles of visual perception also follow this outline. The same may be true for certain basic principles of counting, although not for the learning of the names of numbers (Gelman and Gallistel, 1978). Other abilities seem to stretch the ordinary limits of the human mind, and seem to demand instruction in the usual case. The learning of advanced mathematics, or many other subjects, seems to follow this pattern.

(6) Learnability and Feasibility

It has proved possible to define mathematically the question of the possibility of learning. Gold (1967) provided one of the first useful formalizations. Wexler and Culicover (1980) investigated the question of learnabililty for systems of natural language and showed that linguistic systems could be learned if language-specific constraints were invoked. They further investigated the problem of feasibility, that is, learnability under realistic conditions. Specific constraints can be invoked which allow for feasible learning systems, specifically, very complex systems which can nevertheless be learned from simple input. This would seem to mirror the situation for a child, who learns an essentially infinite system (say language) from exposure to only a fairly small part of the system.

(7) Animal Research

We have concentrated on learning in humans, especially the learning of language, the ability most centrally related to the human species. However, extensive modern research on animal learning also questions the traditional assumptions. It appears that traditional learning theory is not an adequate theory for animals.

(8) Social Implications

The assumption of innate principles of human cognition does *not* imply that there are innate differences between individuals or races. The central idea of the modern view is that the innate principles are part of the shared human endowment, just as the innate existence of a heart is. In fact, the existence of the innate principles of mind may be thought of as helping to define human nature, an old concept generally out of favour in the social sciences. Contemporary social scientists in general founded their theories of society and politics on a psychology closely associated with traditional learning theory. Thus, children are 'socialized' into the values of their society. But it is conceivable that there are principles of mind (of human nature) which relate to the structure of society (or to interpersonal relations, or ethics). If so, the modern view of learning might one day be expanded to include these principles, and there may conceivably be a social science founded on the modern view of learning.

Kenneth Wexler
University of California, Irvine

References
Brown, R. and Hanlon, C. (1970), 'Derivational complexity and the order of acquisition of child speech', in J. R. Hayes (ed.), *Cognition and the Development of Language*, New York.
Chomsky, N. (1965), *Aspects of the Theory of Syntax*, Cambridge, Mass.
Chomsky, N. (1975), *Reflections on Language*, New York.
Gelman, R. and Gallistel, C. R. (1978), *The Child's Understanding of Number*, Cambridge, Mass.
Gold, E. M. (1967), 'Language identification in the limit', *Information and Control*, 10.
Newport, E., Gleitman, H. and Gleitman, L. R. (1977), 'Mother I'd rather do it myself: some effects and non-

effects of maternal speech style', in C. E. Snow and C. A. Ferguson (eds), *Talking to Children*, Cambridge.

Skinner, B. F. (1957), *The Behavior of Organisms*, New York.

Snow, C. E. and Ferguson, C. A. (eds) (1977), *Talking to Children: Language Input and Acquisition*, Cambridge.

Wexler, K. and Culicover, P. W. (1980), *Formal Principles of Language Acquisition*, Cambridge, Mass.

Further Reading

Piatelli-Palmarini, M. (ed.) (1980), *Language and Learning*, Cambridge, Mass.

See also: *associationism; behaviourism; conditioning; Hull; language development.*

Life-Span Development

Life-span development is the study of individual change (ontogeny) throughout the course of life, in an effort to obtain knowledge about both general principles and individual variation. Although life-span considerations have enjoyed a long history, it is only during the last two decades that researchers have begun to take this approach seriously, following the lead of twentieth-century psychologists such as Bühler, Erikson, Hall and Jung (Baltes, Reese and Lipsitt, 1980; Featherman, 1983).

Life-span development is less a theory than an orientation, containing several unique propositions about development. These are: (1) There is considerable inter-individual variation in development. Whereas child developmentalists have sought unidirectional, universally applicable laws, adult developmentalists have noted greater diversity and plasticity (adaptability) of developmental patterns. (2) Historical changes affect the path development takes. The role of historical change has been studied, for example, with the use of age/cohort sequential methodology, where individuals from two or more cohorts (generations) are followed over a long period of time (Schaie, 1979). (3) Interdisciplinary collaboration is necessary in order to describe fully individual development within a changing world. Featherman (1983) illustrates the usefulness of such an interdisciplinary approach in the fields of psychology, sociology and economics. Jointly considered, these three propositions advanced in life-span research have necessitated an emphasis on the interactive relationships between individual development and historical change, resulting in a dialectical (Riegel, 1976) and contextualist (Lerner *et al.*, 1983) conception of human development.

Life-span researchers propose several frameworks for conceptualizing the direction and patterning of development. One framework emphasizes generalized (normative) patterns of development, as illustrated in Havighurst's work on developmental tasks and Erikson's on life-long sequences of personality themes and goals. Another framework considers variability and plasticity in human development (for example, Brim and Kagan, 1980; Schaie, 1979). To account for such variability, Baltes and his colleagues have described three interacting systems of influences on development: age-graded, history-graded, and non-normative (Baltes *et al.*, 1980). All these systems take into account both biological and environmental factors.

Age-correlated factors have been the major focus of mainstream developmental psychology, particularly child-developmental. History-graded influences refer to biocultural changes in the conditions (for example, health status, resources, tasks, roles, expectations) that may influence the development of particular subgroups, as evidenced, for example, in generation or cohort membership; these have been a hallmark of sociological work on the life course (Elder, 1975; Riley, 1984). Finally, non-normative influences refer to unique biological and environmental events that are not representative of the experiences of the majority of individuals of a given cohort or time period (for example, winning a lottery, contracting a serious illness at an early age, immigrating to a new culture). Explication of the combined operation of age-graded, history-graded, and non-normative life events permits the specification of both commonalities (for example, age-graded) and differences (such as history-graded, non-normative) in life-span development.

Let us consider the development of intelligence across the life span as a substantive example (Labouvie-Vief, 1984; Schaie, 1979). Research has pointed to inter-individual differences in the patterns of growth, maintenance and/or decline of intellectual skills. On the one hand, such variability is the result of differences in life history such as those associated with educational and occupational status. More highly educated individuals, for example, maintain their intellectual skills into old age better than less educated individuals. On the other hand, such variability also involves differences between abilities. For example, measures of fluid intelligence (an index of basic information processing and reasoning presumably independent of specific learning) are more susceptible to deterioration with age, while those of crystallized intelligence (an index of acquired knowledge) may even improve into old age. Furthermore, there is much plasticity in life-long development since, depending on which cognitive processes are exercised or not, the level and rate of intellectual development can vary widely. Even in old age, intellectual capacity remains plastic to some extent.

Life-span developmental research forces us to consider the plurality of factors involved in development. It has provided us with a more dynamic view of human development, and has re-evaluated the more traditional ideas of development across the course of the life which largely depicted behaviour as deterministic and unchanging. The emphasis on flexibility inherent in this view is another important perspective (Featherman, 1983). Such flexibility has implications for child development as well, where the traditional view of childhood as the major determining force in later behaviour has been challenged (Brim and Kagan, 1980). We now know that childhood does not necessarily set the stage for irreversible behaviour patterns in adulthood. A key task of future work on life-span development is to sort out conditions for both universal and particular laws and phenomena of development.

Deirdre A. Kramer
Paul B. Baltes
Max Planck Institute for Human Development and Education,
Berlin

References

Baltes, P. B., Reese, H. W. and Lipsitt, L. P. (1980), 'Life-span developmental psychology', *Annual Review of Psychology*, 31.

Brim, O. G., Jr and Kagan, J. (1980), *Constancy and Change in Human Development*, Cambridge, Mass.

Elder, G. H., Jr (1975), 'Age-differentiation in life course perspective', *Annual Review of Sociology*, 1.

Featherman, D. L. (1983), 'The life-span perspective in social science research', in P. B. Baltes and O. G. Brim, Jr (eds), *Life-Span Development and Behavior*, vol. 5, New York.

Labouvie-Vief, G. (1984), 'Intelligence and cognition', in J. E. Birren and K. W. Schaie (eds), *Handbook of the Psychology of Aging*, 2nd edn, New York.

Lerner, R. M., Hultsch, D. F. and Dixon, R. A. (1983), 'Contextualism and the characteristic of developmental psychology in the 1970's', *Annals of the New York Academy of Sciences*.

Riegel, K. F. (1976), 'The dialectics of human development', *American Psychologist*, 31.

Riley, M. W. (1984), 'Age strata in social systems', in R. H. Binstock and E. Shanas (eds), *Handbook of Aging and the Social Sciences* (revised edn), New York.

Schaie, K. W. (1979), 'The primary mental abilities in adulthood: an exploration in the development of psychometric intelligence', in P. B. Baltes and O. G. Brim, Jr (eds), *Life-span Development and Behavior*, vol. 2, New York.

See also: *ageing; developmental psychology*.

Luria, Alexander Romanovich (1902–1977)

Alexander Romanovich Luria, the Russian pioneer of neuro-psychology, was born in Kazan in Soviet Central Asia, and died in Moscow. After graduating in social sciences from the University of Kazan in 1921, he entered the Kazan medical school. However, he had already become interested in psychology, and in 1923 he took up a position at the Institute of Psychology at Moscow State University. His earliest work used measures of word association and motor reaction to study the effects of stress and anxiety upon the expression of affective states. His account of this research sought to integrate an objective, behaviouristic approach with psychoanalytic notions about personality dynamics (Luria, 1932; 1979).

In 1924 Luria was joined by Lev Vygotsky, who was formulating his ideas on the role of language and other culturally transmitted devices in the mediation of higher mental functions. From then until Vygotsky's death in 1934 they carried out research together with Alexei Leontiev on the nature of conscious mental processes, on the social aspects of intellectual development and on the effects of brain damage upon cognitive function. Following the Marxist-Leninist thesis that consciousness is the product of sociohistorical processes, they stressed that human cognition evolved at both the individual and the societal level within a historical context. Moreover, this development should be reflected in the cerebral organization of cognition function and in the patterns of dysfunction associated with neurological damage (Luria, 1979).

In 1931 and 1932 Luria led two expeditions to Uzbekistan and Kirghizia to examine the intellectual abilities of peasant communities under the impact of collectivization. Their findings were generally consistent with Levy-Bruhl's notion that sociocultural differences in cognitive behaviour reflected different stages of intellectual development. Brief reports of these expeditions appeared in Western journals. However, in the USSR it was felt undesirable that such research should be published when the central government was trying to get these communities to participate in the national economy, and fuller accounts did not appear until the 1970s (Luria, 1976b; 1979).

The same ideological perspective led to an interest in the relative importance of biological and environmental determinants of behaviour. Luria and others at the Medico-Genetic Institute in Moscow investigated this in many studies comparing twins who received different methods of instruction. But these studies, too, were felt to be politically controversial, and Luria's own findings once again remained largely unpublished.

Vygotsky, Luria, and many of their colleagues were also attacked during the early 1930s because of their association with the mental testing movement and their promotion of Western psychological traditions in contrast to the work of Pavlov and the 'reflexologists'. Although they set up an alternative centre for teaching and research in Kharkhov, in 1936 Luria decided to return full time to his medical training, which he had been doing on a part-time basis since the late 1920s. He graduated from the First Moscow Medical School in 1937, and then specialized in neurology. Following on his earlier work with Vygotsky, he focused on studying psychological consequences of neurological damage and disease, the discipline now known as clinical neuropsychology, and especially upon the typology of acquired speech disorders.

After the outbreak of the Second World War, in 1941 Luria became head of a rehabilitation hospital in the southern Urals for patients with brain injuries. His extensive experience before and during the War resulted in two major books on traumatic aphasia (Luria, 1970) and on recovery from neurological damage (Luria, 1963a). In these books, and in all his subsequent work, he emphasized the detailed symptomatology of individual patients. In 1945 he was appointed professor of psychology at Moscow State University, and continued his work at the Bourdenko Institute of Neurosurgery on the impairment of higher mental functions following local brain lesions. He explored the nature of both normal and abnormal cognitive function and the representation of such function in the human brain (Luria, 1966b).

Soviet academic life experienced a considerable upheaval in the late 1940s and early 1950s. Although Luria had followed Pavlov and Bekhterev in emphasizing neural plasticity and the possibility of functional reorganization within the damaged brain, his own work once again came under criticism for paying insufficient regard to Pavlovian principles, and in 1950 he was dismissed from his post at the Institute of Neurosurgery. But since he had been elected to the Russian Academy of Pedagogical Sciences in 1947, he was able to take up a position at the Academy's Institute of Defectology. During the 1950s he studied mentally handicapped children. He hypothesized that they were retarded because in their case speech had failed to assume its normal regulative functions (Luria, 1963b; 1979). He was also able to publish a study done in the 1930s of a pair of identical twins with retarded speech and behaviour (Luria & Yudovich, 1959); this has since become very influential among teachers and educationalists in Western Europe.

In the late 1950s Luria was allowed to return to the Institute of Neurosurgery to continue his work in clinical neuropsychology. During the last twenty years of his life, in a series of books, Luria developed a comprehensive theory on the systematic organization of higher cognitive functions (Luria, 1966a, 1966b, 1973, 1976c, 1981). This built upon Vygotsky's ideas concerning the role of language in the development of cerebral control over behaviour (reflected in his interest in the neurophysiology of the frontal lobes), and upon Pavlov's notion of cerebral reflexes as the basic elements of behaviour. The theory also had close affinities to the information-processing accounts of human cognition prevalent in the West during the same period. His basic assertion was that the brain should be regarded as 'a *complex functional system*, embracing different levels and different components each making its own contribution to the final structure of mental activity' (Luria, 1973). While there were undoubted differences in functional organization among different parts of the brain, there was nevertheless considerable 'equipotentiality' within relatively large anatomical regions. In his work, he emphasized careful qualitative description rather than detailed quantitative assessment. This was very much in the tradition of classical neurological examination.

Two studies published in the 1960s based on case material extending back more than 25 years attempt to revive the traditions of 'romantic science' in opposition to the reductionism of 'classical' science. *The Mind of a Mnemonist* (Luria, 1968) described an individual with a remarkable ability to remember specific experiences and episodes, but who nevertheless was not able to abstract meaning from those experiences; and *The Man with a Shattered World* (Luria, 1972) described the rehabilitation of a case of severe brain damage from the Second World War by means of extracts from the patient's own diary.

Towards the end of his life, Luria returned to the analysis of the particular disorders of language function resulting from local brain damage. Influenced directly by Roman Jakobson's ideas on the structure of language, he attempted to provide a comprehensive neuropsychological analysis of the comprehension and production of both spoken and written language and a rigorous classification of aphasic disorders (Luria, 1976a). While taking note of recent developments in semiotics, linguistics, and psycholinguistics, he considered that he was taking 'the first steps towards a general scheme of a new branch of science – that of neurolinguistics, using observations on disturbances of language and speech in patients with local brain lesions as a method for a better understanding of some components of language itself'.

John T. E. Richardson
Brunel University, Uxbridge

References

Luria, A. R., (1932 [1930]), *The Nature of Human Conflicts; or Emotion, Conflict, and Will: An Objective Study of Disorganization and Control of Human Behavior* (ed. and trans., W. H. Gantt), New York.

Luria, A. R. (1936), 'The development of mental functions in twins', *Character and Personality*, 5.

Luria, A. R. (1963a [1948]), *Restoration of Function after Brain Injury* (B. Haigh, trans.; O. L. Zangwill, Ed.), Oxford.

Luria, A. R. (ed.) (1963b), *The Mentally Retarded Child: Essays Based on a Study of the Peculiarities of the Higher Nervous Functioning of Child-Oligophrenics* (W. P. Robinson, trans.; B. Kirman, ed.), Oxford.

Luria, A. R. (1966a [1962]), *Higher Cortical Functions in Man* (B. Haigh, trans.), New York.

Luria, A. R. (1966b [1963]), *Human Brain and Psychological Processes* (B. Haigh, trans.), New York.

Luria, A. R. (1968 [1965]), *The Mind of a Mnemonist: A Little Book About a Vast Memory* (L. Solotaroff, trans.), New York.

Luria, A. R. (1969), 'The neuropsychological study of brain lesions and restoration of damaged brain function', in M.

Cole & I. Maltzman (eds.) *A Handbook of Contemporary Soviet Psychology* (pp. 277–301), New York.

Luria, A. R. (1970 [1947]), *Traumatic Aphasia* (D. Bowden, trans.), The Hague.

Luria, A. R. (1972 [1971]), *The Man with a Shattered World: The History of a Brain Wound* (L. Solotaroff, trans.), New York.

Luria, A. R. (1973), *The Working Brain* (B. Haigh, trans.), Harmondsworth.

Luria, A. R. (1976a [1975]), *Basic Problems of Neurolinguistics* (B. Haigh, trans.), The Hague.

Luria, A. R. (1976b [1974]), *Cognitive Development: Its Cultural and Social Foundations* (M. Lopez-Morillas & L. Solotaroff, trans.; M. Cole, ed.), Cambridge, Mass.

Luria, A. R. (1976c [1974; 1976]), *The Neuropsychology of Memory*, New York.

Luria, A. R. (1979), *The Making of Mind: A Personal Account of Soviet Psychology* (M. Cole & S. Cole, eds.), Cambridge, Mass.

Luria, A. R. (1981 [1978]), *Language and Cognition* (J. V. Wertsch, ed.), New York.

Luria, A. R. and Yudovich, F. I. (1959 [1956]), *Speech and the Development of Mental Processes in the Child* (O. Kovasc and J. Simon, trans. J. Simon, ed.), London.

Memory

Memory involves the storage of information and its subsequent retrieval. Despite being referred to by a single term, memory comprises a collection of subsystems rather than a single faculty. It can be divided into three components: sensory memory, short-term or working memory, and long-term memory, each of which can be further subdivided.

(1) *Sensory memory.* Part of the process of perception involves the brief storage of sensory information. In the case of vision the term 'iconic memory' is used to refer to this temporary store. The cinema is dependent on such a system. Without it we would see a film as a series of briefly presented still pictures rather than as a continuous image. Similarly, a brief auditory memory, sometimes termed 'echoic memory' is involved in perceiving speech.

(2) *Short-term or working memory.* If one is required to multiply 27 by 5 in one's head, one needs to make use of a good deal of temporary storage, not only of the sum itself but of the intervening steps such as carrying. Such temporary storage is also involved in reasoning, in learning and comprehending, where one may, for example, need to retain a relatively precise record of the beginning of a sentence in order to interpret the end. The term 'working memory' is used for this system which in turn comprises a number of subcomponents. For instance, if asked to remember a postal code long enough to copy it on an envelope, one is likely to use some form of verbal coding, probably repeating it under one's breath. In contrast, if A asks B to remember how many windows there are in B's present house, B will probably create in his 'mind's eye' a temporary image of his house, and perhaps imagine himself wandering around and counting the windows. This type of imagery appears to involve a rather separate component of working memory. These and other components are integrated by an attentional system that selects and manipulates information from the subsystems.

(3) *Long-term memory.* In contrast to the two previous systems, long-term memory is concerned with the relatively permanent storage of information. It can be regarded as analogous to a library, in which information is entered, stored and subsequently retrieved. Like a good library, organization is essential, and organization on the basis of the meaning of the material to be remembered is particularly important. Forgetting occurs over time, although whether this is due to memory traces being destroyed, or simply becoming mislaid, is a matter of some controversy.

It is certainly the case that some forgetting is due to difficulties in locating a memory trace rather than its destruction. Most people have the experience of knowing a name which is on 'the tip of their tongue' but cannot be recalled. Typically such a name would be recognized immediately from a list of plausible alternatives, indicating that the information had been mislaid rather than destroyed.

In general, reinstating the conditions operating during learning is likely to enhance retrieval (the *encoding specificity principle*). For example, material that is learnt in one physical environment or mood is best recalled in that same environment, hence deep-sea divers who learnt something underwater were best able to recall it underwater, while in another experiment, subjects who were presented with a list of words when sad recalled more of them on a subsequent occasion when sadness was induced than when they were happy, and vice versa.

A further distinction within long-term memory is between semantic and episodic memory. The term semantic memory refers to knowledge of the world. It comprises the sort of memory that is needed to answer questions such as 'What is the capital of France?', 'What is the chemical formula for salt?' and 'How many legs does a crocodile have?'. Episodic memory is the ability to remember specific personally experienced events such as what one had for breakfast or whom one met on holiday last year.

There is general agreement that the distinction between semantic and episodic memory is useful theoretically, but there is disagreement on whether the two rely on separate parts of the brain. The distinction between working memory and long-term memory, on the other hand, does appear to reflect different areas of the brain. Studies of brain-damaged patients indicate that a deficit of long-term memory can occur in a patient with normal working memory, and vice versa.

Alan Baddeley
MRC, Applied Psychology Unit, Cambridge

Further Reading
Baddeley, A. D. (1983), *Your Memory: A User's Guide*,
  Harmondsworth.
See also: *sensation and perception; thinking; time.*

Mental Disorders

Descriptions of psychological behaviour and intellectual disturbances have existed in the literature of Western civilizations since ancient times. Disturbances associated with the ageing process were among the first to be recorded. There are also descriptions of alcoholic deterioration, as well as phenomena which today would be called delirium, affective disorder, or psychoses. Depending upon the *Zeitgeist*, however, the phenomena were interpreted in many ways. Galen's Doctrine of the Four Humours was invoked as an explanation of psychological and behavioural disturbances well into the seventeeth century, while theories of the occult strongly influenced views of mental disturbances throughout the eighteenth century and into the early nineteenth century.

The origin of modern scientific psychiatry can be traced to the Enlightenment. During this era, the notion of mental disturbances as illnesses began to take hold with some intellectual force. By creating a climate which encouraged people to look upon the mental illnesses as natural phenomena, the rationalism of the age made the phenomena more accessible to systematic inquiry through observation, experimentation, and classification. As with any scientific endeavours to study the human condition, efforts to delineate the mental disorders were influenced by: (1) the dominant intellectual assumptions and attitudes which determine what data will receive attention and how the data will be ordered; (2) the technologies and methodologies available for gathering the data; and (3) the setting or social context delimiting the universe of phenomena accessible to study.

(1) Organic Versus Functional Mental Disorders
In the early nineteenth century, the care of the mentally disturbed gradually became the responsibility of the medical rather than the law enforcement or religious arms of society. Asylums and mental hospitals of the day became the primary sites for the conduct of scientific inquiry. As a result, the phenomena under study represented the most severe examples of behavioural or psychological disturbances. A materialistic philosophical orientation dominated medical thinking. Research in the fields of physiology, bacteriology and pathology were quite productive in delineating the pathophysiology and aetiology of physical illnesses. The philosophical perspective and technological advances tended to promote a view of mental

disorder as the expression of physical disease or biological disease processes.

The notion of biological causality was, and remains, a major orienting principle in efforts to understand the nature of mental illness. Then, as today, the existing technology was not adequate to the task of defining an invariable relationship between the behavioural and psychological phenomena under study and either anatomical lesions or pathophysiological processes. A useful convention was adopted, however, by segregating the organic from the functional mental disorders. This dichotomy is based upon an aetiological distinction – the presence or absence of a biological abnormality or dysfunction that fully accounts for the condition.

(2) Psychotic Versus Non-Psychotic Functional Disorders

Since an aetiological distinction based on biological causality could not be used as the basis for differentiating the functional mental disorders, a phenomenological approach was used. Essentially qualitative, the approach involved the careful observation of a clinical picture on a case-by-case basis. From the observations, relatively unique configurations of symptoms and symptom clusters were identified that suggested natural groupings of phenomena. In this manner, conditions where the dominant feature was a profound disturbance of mood were segregated from those where the dominant feature was a disturbance in the process and content of thought. This distinction between disorders of mood and disorders of thought received further corroboration when longitudinal data indicated that the course of the disorders also differed. Disorders of mood were more likely to remit, while those of thought were associated with progressive deterioration. For many years, these characteristics formed the primary basis for a distinction between what we today call the schizophrenic and the manic depressive disorders.

Regardless of the characteristics differentiating the disorders of thought and mood, individuals with both disorders shared three characteristics: (a) behaviour that grossly violated social norms; (b) the incorrect valuation of the accuracy of thoughts or perceptions; and (c) the marked tendency to draw false inferences about external reality even in the face of incontrovertible evidence to the contrary. These latter two features constitute what is referred to as impaired reality testing. This impaired reality testing, together with bizarre, disorganized behaviour well beyond the pale of social acceptability became the cardinal features for designating functional disorders as psychotic rather than non-psychotic. The utility of this dichotomy as the basis for classification is currently a major source of debate within psychiatry; nevertheless, it still remains a useful convention for differentiating the most severe mental disorders – the schizophrenic disorders, the major affective disorders, and the paranoid disorders – from the other non-organic psychological and behavioural phenomena that constitute the functional mental disorders.

(3) Neurotic Personality and Stress-Related Disorders

The further elaboration of conditions constituting the functional mental disorders was stimulated by two occurrences of particular importance in the field of psychiatry: the shift of the centre of academic inquiry from the asylum to the university psychiatric clinic, and the emergence of psychoanalysis. The former made an increasingly broad range of phenomena acceptable and accessible to study; the latter brought a conceptual framework and methodology for studying the psychogenic origins of disordered behaviour. In addition, the growing interaction among the clinical, behavioural, social and biological sciences that began at the end of the nineteenth century and has carried through to the present, generated a number of useful paradigms. While facilitating an examination of the psychological and social origins of the mental disorders, these paradigms contributed to the demarcation of three major clusters of non-psychotic functional mental disorders: the neurotic, the personality, and the stress-related disorders.

(a) The neurotic disorders

Just as the invention of the microscope expanded the scope of biology, so the techniques of medical hypnosis and free association opened new avenues for exploring mental functioning and rendered the unconscious accessible to scientific inquiry. An important corollary of these methodological advances was the identification of psychological process. This process is characterized by the existence of conflict within an individual, perceived as a potential threat or danger, which calls into play response patterns called defence mechanisms. These three events occur outside of the individual's conscious awareness. When the events lead to the formation of symptoms or symptom complexes that are distressing, recognized as unacceptable, and experienced as unhealthy or foreign, the outcome is a neurotic disorder.

Not everyone accepts the scientific validity of evidence derived through applying the psychoanalytic method. They question the aetiologic paradigm described above and have offered other models, frequently based on learning theory, to explain the neuroses. Even so, few dispute the importance of psychological mechanisms in the genesis of these disorders. Further, evidence from the clinical and epidemiologic literature indicates that the neurotic disorders can be found in very different cultures, findings which support the view of the phenomena as a discrete class of mental disorders.

The neurotic disorders are identified primarily in terms of their mode of symptomatic or behavioural expression (for example, anxiety disorder, hypochondriasis, dissociative state). While some of the behaviours at times appear bizarre, as in the case of the obsessive, compulsive or phobic disorders, they do not grossly violate social norms. This circumstance, together with the absence of impaired reality testing, provides a basis for distinguishing the neurotic from the psychotic functional mental disorders.

(b) The personality disorders

Originally, personality disorders were identified on the basis of overt behaviour that was associated with, or could lead to, frank violations of the formal rules and conventions established within a society to maintain social order. Criminal, sexually perverse and addictive behaviours fell most easily under this rubric, particularly in those instances where the individual manifesting the behaviours was not psychotic or neurotic, and did not suffer significant subjective distress.

The delineation of personality disorders solely on the basis of rule-breaking behaviour seemed well off the mark as more came to be understood about the social, cultural and psychological processes shaping personality development. Personality came to be viewed as a product of social interaction and individual experiences in a cultural environment. This notion led to a definition of personality as deeply ingrained patterns of behaviour that determine how individuals relate to, perceive, and think about themselves and the environment. Personality disorder, on the other hand, was defined as the existence of persistent, inflexible and maladaptive patterns of behaviour that consistently and predictably were (i) in violation of the rights of others; (ii) denigrating to oneself or others; (iii) destructive to interpersonal and social relationships or vocational performance; or (iv) undermining of the ability to meet day-to-day obligations or achieve life goals. Although conditions characterized primarily by socially deviant behaviour (such as the perversions or anti-social personality disorder) are still considered personality disorders, so too are conditions where interpersonal relationships are significantly compromised (such as the schizoid or explosive personality disorders), or where personality absorption is the dominant feature (such as the aesthenic or inadequate personality disorders).

(c) The stress-related disorders

The interest in the relationship between stress and mental illness, an outgrowth of the experience of military psychiatry in World War I, has been sustained throughout the twentieth century. In the social sciences, research has focused on natural disasters; in the epidemiologic and clinical sciences, on life events and mental disorder; in the behavioural sciences, the emphasis is on coping and adaptation, and in the biological sciences, on homeostasis. A firmer understanding has developed about psychological vulnerability occurring during transitional states as well as normal developmental phases. In turn, the general systems theory has facilitated an examination of psychological factors as stressors that generate pathophysiological responses.

A related group of clinical phenomena was identified, not on the basis of their symptomatic manifestations (which are legion in their variations) but on the basis of the precipitants. These stress-related disorders include: (i) acute catastrophic stress reactions with clear environmental precipitants, such as war or natural disaster; (ii) post-traumatic stress disorders characterized by a re-experiencing of the trauma, reduced involvement with the external world, and a variety of autonomic, dysphoric or cognitive symptoms; (iii) the adjustment disorders precipitated by an array of life events, family factors, developmental crises and the like, which act as psychosocial stressors; (iv) psychophysiological malfunctions of psychogenic origin which occur in the absence of tissue damage or a demonstrable disease process (for example, hyperventilation, neurocirculatory aesthenia or dysmenorrhoea); and (v) psychic factors associated with physical disease – a category which conveys the notion that psychologically meaningful environmental stimuli can initiate or exacerbate certain physical disorders such as asthma, rheumatoid arthritis or ulcerative colitis.

Conclusion

By any criteria, the past century and a half has witnessed enormous strides in the delineation of the mental disorders. With the exception of the organic mental disorders, however, a knowledge of aetiology remains quite primitive. Behavioural, social and neuroscientists are searching for aetiologic factors. To the extent that the demonstration of aetiology allows us to make sharper distinctions among the mental disorders than does a strictly descriptive approach, these efforts, if successful, would undoubtedly lead to further modification of our definitions of the mental disorders.

Gary L. Tischler
Yale University

Further Reading

Alexander, E. S. and Selasnick, S. T. (1966), *The History of Psychiatry*, New York.

American Psychiatric Association (1980), *DSM-III: Diagnostic and Statistical Manual of Mental Disorders*, 3rd edn, Washington D.C.

Brenner, C. (1973), *An Elementary Textbook of Psychoanalysis*, New York.

Gunderson, E. K. E. and Rahe, R. H. (1974), *Life Stress and Illness*, Springfield, Ill.

Kraepelin, E. (1909), *Psychiatrie*, 8th edn, Leipzig.

Levy, R. (1982), *The New Language of Psychiatry*, Boston.

Nichols, A. M. (1978), *The Harvard Guide to Modern Psychiatry*, Cambridge, Mass.

Paykel, E. S. (1982), *Handbook of Affective Disorders*, New York.

Wang, J., Cooper, J. and Sartorius, N. (1974), *The Measurement and Classification of Psychiatric Symptoms*, Cambridge, Mass.

Woodruff, R. A., Goodwin, D. W. and Guze, S. B. (1974), *Psychiatric Diagnosis*, New York.

See also: *character disorders; DSM III; mental health; neurosis.*

Mental Health

The categories of mental health and mental illness have to be understood against the backdrop of the social institutions and practices which gave rise to them; and to do this, we need to set the whole in historical context.

Mental illness replaced earlier nineteenth-century concepts of 'madness' or 'insanity'. This was not primarily because of changing beliefs about the cause of mental disturbances, but because the medical profession had gained control of their management. Psychiatry arose hand in hand with the asylum system, but at the outset the latter was conceived as a social remedy for a social problem: if anything, doctors captured this territory *despite* their association with physical theories and treatments, not because of it. Thus, the concepts of mental health and illness were not closely tied to a physical approach to mental disorders. In the nineteenth century, indeed, the most significant feature of mental illness was not its cause but its treatment – incarceration in an asylum. Mental patients, at this time, were defined as a group primarily by the danger they were seen to pose to themselves or others, a danger which could not be contained in any other way.

The asylum became in practice a last resort when no hope remained for the patient, but in this century the fight against mental illness was taken outside its walls and into the home, work-place and school, where interventions could be made before problems had become intractable. The invention of psychological theories and treatments, in which Freud played a key role, greatly facilitated this spread. Treatment moved from the asylum to the consulting-room, and the meanings of mental illness and mental health shifted accordingly. A new range of illnesses (most importantly, the neuroses) was reco- gnized, and a new range of professions – social work, psycho- therapy and the various branches of psychology – arose along- side psychiatry.

Rather than being seen as dangerous, the mental patient was now primarily someone who could not cope with his allotted tasks in life: mental illness was seen as partial and reversible (Armstrong, 1980). Mental health, in the rhetoric of the influ- ential 'mental hygiene movement' founded in America in 1909, became equated with productiveness, social adjustment, and contentment – 'the good life' itself.

The promise of this approach as a panacea for all human ills, coupled with the enormous potential market it opened up to professionals, led to a huge increase in mental health services by the middle of this century. A key factor in the creation of this 'therapeutic state' was the adoption by the mental health professions of a 'scientific' image: in this way, their interventions came to be seen as applications of a value-free, ideologically neutral technology, after the fashion of Comte's 'positivism'.

Social scientists have approached mental health in two main ways. The first is to explore the connection between mental illnesses and aspects of the social environment. Classic studies in this mould are those of Hollingshead and Redlich (1958), who found an increased incidence of mental illness in lower social classes; Brenner (1973), who associated mental illness

and economic cycles; and Brown and Harris (1978), who identified predisposing and precipitating factors in women's
depression. Though this approach can be seen as merely an
extension of the psychiatric enterprise, it nevertheless suggests
that to treat environmentally-related conditions as cases of individual malfunctioning may be a form of 'blaming the victim'
(Ryan, 1972). In this light, the role of psychiatrists emerges
as a fundamentally conservative one: to alleviate the stresses
inherent in the social order, while removing any threat to that
order itself. It is implicit in the psychiatric concept of
'maladjustment' that it is the individual who has to adapt to
society, and not the other way round.

Nevertheless, in the heyday of psychiatric expansionism in
the US (the 1950s and early 1960s), some psychiatrists argued
that the reform of adverse social conditions was a valid part of
psychiatry's mandate after all. Yet financial cutbacks,
professional inhibitions, and a political shift to the right soon
nipped this 'preventive' psychiatry in the bud.

The second approach adopted by social scientists challenges
the very notion of mental illness, and questions the motives
that lie behind professional interventions. (Such questioning
is invited by the seemingly arbitrary variations in psychiatric
nosology, diagnosis and treatment between different times,
places and practitioners.) One line of argument focuses on the
way in which the field has been shaped by professional self-
interest and financial or political factors (for example, profite-
ering by the drug companies): this critique runs parallel to that
made by Illich (1977) and Freidson (1970) of physical medicine.
Such an approach has been adopted by historians who have
set out to correct the 'triumphalist' picture which professions
tend to present of their own history – a picture in which the
cumulative victories of reason and humanity culminate inevitably in the achievements of the present.

Other commentators, however, take the argument a step
further: they treat mental health as an ideological concept,
concealing highly problematic notions about how people should
live, and regard the professions that deal with it as agencies of
social control. This critique came to the fore in the 1960s, via

the work of Foucault (1961), Szasz (1961), Goffman (1961), Scheff (1966) and 'anti-psychiatrists' such as Laing (1960). These writers were not simply claiming that the labelling of certain conditions as 'pathological' was value-laden and culture-bound, for, as Sedgwick (1982) pointed out, the same is true of physical conditions. The critique of psychiatry went further, in claiming that the so-called 'symptoms' were in fact meaningful and freely-chosen acts.

This criticism seems warranted when psychiatry stops people from doing what they want, by means of physical or chemical intervention – for example, political dissidents in the Soviet Union, homosexuals in the West, or (according to Shrag and Divoky, 1975) the million or so American schoolchildren kept under permanent sedation to prevent 'hyperactivity'. Such an analysis seems inapplicable, however, when treatment is actively sought by people anxious to get rid of their 'symptoms'. Moreover, some treatments (especially psychotherapy) claim to increase autonomy, not to diminish it. To treat mental illness as deviance pure and simple is to ignore essential distinctions between 'mad' and 'bad' behaviour – chiefly, the fact that the former is regarded as not making sense, and not under the control of the individual. A straightforward social control model of the mental health professions is therefore limited in its applications.

This is not to say, however, that the remaining instances lack any political significance and are purely therapeutic in character. Behind the concept of mental health lie numerous presuppositions about norms of work, education and family life; and the mental health professions are probably instrumental in maintaining these norms, by influencing not just problem cases but our way of making sense of the world. (Feminists, for example, have argued that psychiatry powerfully reinforces women's traditional role in society (Chessler, 1972).) But if this is a social control mechanism, it is one which has been largely internalized by the population itself. Foucault (1980) goes further, arguing that the power of this mechanism is not 'repressive' but 'productive', since it actually *creates* forms of subjectivity and social life.

Plenty of instances still remain of repression in the name of mental health – as the activities of civil rights organizations and patients' groups testify – and the most convincing analysis is perhaps that of Castel *et al.* (1982), who see the 'hard' and 'soft' methods of treatment as an ensemble, each depending on the other to be fully effective. Although this idea has obvious validity, it is doubtful whether an adequate understanding of the place of mental health in modern society will ever be achieved by trying to impose the same model on such diverse phenomena as lobotomy, forcible incarceration, marital counselling, psychoanalysis and encounter groups.

David Ingleby
University of Utrecht

References

Armstrong, D. (1980), 'Madness and coping', *Sociology of Health and Illness*, 2.

Brenner, H. (1973), *Mental Illness and the Economy*, Cambridge, Mass.

Brown, G. and Harris, T. (1978), *Social Origins of Depression*, London.

Castel, F., Castel, R. and Lovell, A. (1982), *The Psychiatric Society*, New York.

Chessler, P. (1972), *Women and Madness*, New York.

Foucault, M. (1971), *Madness and Civilization*, New York. (Original French, *Histoire de la folie*, Paris, 1961.)

Foucault, M. (1980), 'Truth and power', in *Power/Knowledge: Selected Interviews and Other Writings 1972–1977*, Hassocks.

Freidson, E. (1970), *Professional Dominance*, New York.

Goffman, E. (1961), *Asylums: Essays on the Social Situation of Mental Patients and Other Inmates*, New York.

Hollingshead, A. B. and Redlich, F. C. (1958), *Social Class and Mental Illness*, New York.

Illich, I. (1977), *Disabling Professions*, London.

Laing, R. D. (1960), *The Divided Self*, London.

Ryan, W. (1972), *Blaming the Victim*, New York.

Scheff, T. (1966), *Being Mentally Ill: A Sociological Theory*, London.

Sedgwick, P. (1982), *Psycho Politics*, London.

Shrag, P. and Divoky, D. (1975), *The Myth of the Hyperactive Child and Other Means of Child Control*, New York.

Szasz, T. (1961), *The Myth of Mental Illness*, New York.

Further Reading
Ingleby, D. (ed.) (1980), *Critical Psychiatry: The Politics of Mental Health*, New York.
See also: *mental disorders; psychiatry; stigma.*

Mental Retardation

Mental retardation is identified by intellectual subnormality, which is associated with deficits in adaptive behaviour originating during the developmental period. It is a joint product of the individual's biological make-up and successive encounters with his physical and social-psychological environments.

Intelligent behaviour depends both on an intact and developed central nervous system and on facilitating and supportive environmental interactions. There is a continuum of disability in intelligent behaviour, ranging from those who manifest neurological impairments and other components of organic disease, including severe forms of intellectual impairment, to persons with no recognizable underlying organic disease but who nevertheless manifest some intellectual impairment and find it difficult to master academic activities in school situations. The phenotypic trait of intelligence is due in part to many genes, each of which adds a little to the development of the trait of intelligence (Haywood and Wachs, 1981; Scarr-Salapatek, 1975).

Lewis (1933), Penrose (1963) and Zigler and Balla (1981) categorize two subpopulations with reduced intelligence: (1) The 'pathological' or organically-retarded who show demonstrable disease and pathology. These represent the organically-diseased variants of the general population. (2) The 'subcultural' or psychosocially retarded with no demonstrable diseases.

These represent the lower end of the nonpathological variation in intelligence found in the general population.

Many categories of severe retardation involve biological syndromes that disfigure the whole body. Gargoylism, anencephaly, meningomyelocele and hydrocephaly are examples, as are many types of brain damage resulting from such adverse prenatal influences as undernutrition, rubella, cytomegalic inclusion disease, radiation and lead poisoning. Organically-retarded persons usually have IQ scores under 50 (American Association on Mental Deficiency, 1977). These cases occur almost equally in all social classes and constitute nearly 25 per cent of the mentally-retarded population (Clarke and Clarke, 1977). The psychosocially retarded are primarily from the lower social classes and usually have IQs of between 50 and 70. They constitute about 75 per cent of the mentally-retarded population (Clarke and Clarke, 1977; Zigler, 1967).

Evidence has been accumulating (Weisz and Zigler, 1969) that the mentally retarded go through the same stages of cognitive development as the nonretarded. However, the mentally retarded develop at a much slower rate, and ultimately reach a lower level of cognitive development. The more severe the mental retardation, the slower the rate and ultimate level of cognitive development. Within a Piagetian model of cognitive development, the mildly retarded might attain the concrete operation stage, the moderately retarded the preoperation stage, the severely retarded the fringes of the preoperation stage, while the profoundly retarded might approach the limits of the sensorimotor stage.

Mentally-retarded persons perform more poorly on a wide variety of tasks than would be predicted from their general level of cognitive ability, as defined by their mental ages. One might expect that retarded and younger nonretarded persons matched on mental age should perform at about the same level and use similar cognitive processes on a wide variety of tasks that require intelligent behaviour. However, the retarded members of such matches do less well than do their nonretarded, but younger, peers. They manifest a mental-age deficit. This mental-age deficit in performance between retarded and nonre-

tarded groups has been interpreted as partly the result of differences in motivation between the two groups.

Haywood and his students (Haywood *et al.*, 1982) have identified a broad trait variable, task-intrinsic motivational orientation, that is associated with individual differences in the
efficiency of learning and performance. They define 'intrinsi-
cally-motivated' persons as those who characteristically seek
their principal satisfactions through task achievement, learning,
responsibility, creativity, and aesthetic aspects of tasks. Extrinsically-motivated persons, rather than seek satisfactions,
concentrate on avoiding dissatisfactions through nontask
aspects of the environment such as ease, comfort, safety,
security, practicality, material gain, and avoidance of effort.
Mildly and moderately-retarded children who are relatively
intrinsically motivated, have significantly higher school achievement scores than extrinsically-motivated children of the same
age, sex and IQ. They can learn a visual-size discrimination
problem in fewer trials and more efficiently; they persist longer
and work more vigorously at a simple motor task for a 'task-
intrinsic' incentive – merely the opportunity to do more work;
they can work harder under self-monitored than under exter-
nally-imposed reinforcement, and they set 'leaner' reinforcement schedules for themselves than under the self-monitored
condition. The mental-age deficit often observed in mentally-
retarded groups may be due in part to decreased task-intrinsic
motivation.

Zigler and his students (Zigler and Balla, 1981) have conceptualized the motivational problems of retarded persons as being
due partly to deficient effectance motivation, and a lack of
concern for the intrinsic motivation that is inherent in being
correct, regardless of whether or not an external agent dispenses
the reinforcer. Ziglar believes that the socially-depriving life
histories of psychosocially-retarded children, their cognitive
deficiencies, and their related failure experience all lead to an
attenuation of effectance motivation with a concomitant
increase in extrinsically-motivated behaviour.

Harter and Zigler (1974) constructed measures of several
aspects of effectance motivation including variation seeking,

curiosity, mastery for the sake of competence, and preference for challenging as compared to nonchallenging tasks. Intellectually average, noninstitutionalized retarded, and institutionalized retarded children of comparable mental age were tested. On all components of effectance motivation measured, the intellectually-average children showed more effectance motivation than did the retarded children. Institutionalized retarded children also displayed less curiosity than did noninstitutionalized retarded children.

However, it has been demonstrated that the motivational systems of retarded persons can be improved and their performances facilitated by various early educational intervention programmes such as Project Head Start (Gray *et al.*, 1981; Seitz *et al.*, 1981), the Milwaukee Project (Garber and Heber, 1977) and the Abecedarian Project (Ramey and Hawkins, 1981). Suggestions for changing 'task-extrinsic' motivational orientations into 'task-intrinsic' ones are to be found in Harter (1981).

Harvey N. Switzky
Northern Illinois University, DeKalb, Illinois

References

American Association on Mental Deficiency (1977), *Manual on Terminology and Classification in Mental Retardation*, Washington.

Clarke, A. B. D. and Clarke, A. M. (1977), 'Prospects for prevention and amelioration of mental retardation: a guest editorial', *American Journal of Mental Deficiency*, 81.

Garber, H. and Heber, R. (1977), 'The Milwaukee Project', in P. Mittler (ed.), *Research to Practice in Mental Retardation*, Baltimore.

Gray, S. W., Ramsey, B. K. and Klaus, R. A. (1981), *From 3 to 20: The Early Training Project*, Baltimore.

Harter, S. (1981), 'A model of intrinsic mastery motivation in children: individual differences and development change', in W. A. Collins (ed.), *Minnesota Symposium on Child Psychology*, 14, Hillsdale, N.J.

Harter, S. and Zigler, E. (1974), 'The assessment of effectance motivation in normal and retarded children', *Developmental Psychology*, 10.

Haywood, H. C. (1968), 'Motivational orientation of overachieving and underachieving elementary school children', *American Journal of Mental Deficiency*, 72.

Haywood, H. C. and Wachs, T. (1981), 'Intelligence, cognition, and individual differences', in M. J. Begab *et al.* (eds), *Issues and Theories in Development*, Baltimore.

Haywood, H. C., Meyers, C. E. and Switzky, H. N. (1982), 'Mental retardation', *Annual Review of Psychology*, Palo Alto.

Lewis, E. O. (1933), 'Types of mental deficiency and their social significance', *Journal of Mental Science*, 79.

Penrose, L. S. (1963), *The Biology of Mental Deficiency*, London.

Ramey, C . T. and Hawkins, R. (1981), 'The causes and treatment of school failure; insights from the Carolina Abecedarian Project', in M. J. Begab *et al.* (eds), *Prevention of Retarded Development in Psychosocially Disadvantaged*, Baltimore.

Scarr-Salapatek, S. (1975), 'Genetics and the development of intelligence', in F. P. Horowitz, *Review of Child Development Research*, 4.

Seitz, V., Aptel, N. H. and Rosenbaum, L. (1981), 'Projects Headstart and Follow Through: a longitudinal evaluation of adolescents', in M. J. Begab *et al.* (eds), Baltimore.

Weisz, J. R. and Zigler, E. (1969), 'Developmental versus difference theories of mental retardation', *American Journal of Mental Deficiency*, 73.

Zigler, E. (1967), 'Familial mental retardation: a continuing dilemma', *Science*, 155.

Zigler, E. and Balla, D. (1981), 'Issues in personality and motivation in mentally retarded persons', in M. J. Begab *et al.* (eds), Baltimore.

Further Reading

Ellis, N. R. (ed.) (1979), *Handbook of Mental Deficiency*, 2nd edn, Hillsdale, N.J.

Haywood, H. C., Meyers, C. E. and Switzky, H. N. (1982),

'Mental retardation', *Annual Review of Psychology*, Palo Alto, CA.

Inhelder, B. (1968), *The Diagnosis of Reasoning in the Mentally Retarded*, New York.

Kavoly, P. and Kanfer, F. H. (1982), *Self-Management and Behavior Change*, New York.

Sternberg, R. J. (ed.) (1982), *Handbook of Human Intelligence*, New York.

Switzky, H. N. and Haywood, H. C. (1984), 'A biosocial ecological perspective on mental retardation', in N. Endle and J. M. V. Hunt (eds), *Personality and Behaviour Disorders*, 2nd edn, New York.

See also: *developmental psychology; intelligence; learning; nervous system.*

Mind

'Mind' is derived from old Teutonic *gamundi* meaning to think, remember, intend. These various senses are apparent in current phrases such as: to bear in mind, remind, give one's mind to, make up or change one's mind. Most verbal forms are now obsolete or dialectal but remain in such phrases as 'never mind' or 'mind how you go' in the sense of attend. Traditionally 'mind' has been used to refer collectively to mental abilities such as perceiving, imagining, remembering, thinking, believing, feeling, desiring, deciding, intending. Sometimes an agent is implied: 'Mind is the mysterious something which feels and thinks' (Mill, 1843); sometimes not: 'What we call mind is nothing but a heap or collection of different perceptions, united together by certain relations' (Hume, 1740).

In classical Greece, questions about the mind were inter-woven with those about the soul or spirit, as was the case in medieval Europe, where theological concerns predominated. Plato's tripartite division of the mind into cognitive, conative and affective functions lasted at least until the nineteenth century. Numerous classifications of mental faculties were offered in the eighteenth and nineteenth centuries. Although these were generally speculative, artificial and non-explanatory, they laid the ground for later work in psychometrics and cortical localization of function (McFie, 1972).

Diverse criteria have been offered for distinguishing the mental from the physical (Feigl, 1958). According to the first, mental phenomena are private whereas physical phenomena are public. However, public evidence is in fact intersubjective. Descartes (1641) claimed that body occupied space and was subject to deterministic laws, whereas mind was nonspatial and free. Neither of these criteria are without problems. Quantum mechanics and relativity cast doubt on space as a simple concept in physics. Mental phenomena such as images have spatial properties, and if mind-brain identity theory is accepted, the denial of spatial properties to mental phenomena may become an outmoded convention. Indeterminism has been found to apply to physical phenomena at the subatomic level and it is assumed by psychologists that mental phenomena are determined. Criteria in terms of mnemic properties (Russell, 1921) or purposiveness (McDougall, 1912) are probably too weak. Fairly simple machines are capable of memory and goal direction. Whether purpose implies conscious agency is more difficult to decide. Brentano (1874) suggested intensionality as characteristic of the mental: perceiving, thinking and desiring imply objects which may have no objective existence. This feature of symbolic representation is central to artificial intelligence. Contrasts betwen qualitative and quantitative, holistic and atomistic, or emergent and compositional are inadequate. They represent alternative descriptions rather than distinctions of substance. Attempts have been made to distinguish mental and physical in terms of different logics, for example, intensional and extensional (Chisholm, 1967), or linguistic conventions (Ryle, 1949). The current view is that mental descriptions are compatible with, but logically irreducible to, physical descriptions (Boden, 1972).

Traditionally the mind has been identified with conscious experience: 'Consciousness . . . is the condition or accompaniment of every mental operation' (Fleming, 1858); 'No proposition can be said to be in the Mind which it was never yet conscious of' (Locke, 1690). However, this proposition seems to be patently false. Neurophysiologists and clinicians in the nineteenth century recognized different levels of functioning in the nervous system and acknowledged unconscious mental activity, although the idea has a much more venerable history dating back at least to classical Greek times. William James (1890) pointed out that it is only the perchings and not the flights of thought that are available to consciousness. The majority of mental processes take place outside awareness, for instance, large parts of perception, retrieval, skills and creative thinking. This fact is made even more obvious by consideration of such phenomena as hypnosis, subliminal perception, learning without awareness, split personality and blindsight (a clinical condition in which patients with damage to the occipital lobes may report no experience of seeing and yet be able to make correct discriminations in a forced choice situation).

In Western philosophy a distinction has generally been drawn between mind and body, largely as a result of the influence of Descartes. If such a distinction is made (dualism) the problem of their relation arises, to which various solutions have been offered. Psychophysical parallelism asserts that mental and physical events are correlated but causally independent. This is somewhat unparsimonious and leaves the correlation unexplained. Interaction postulates two-way causal dependence. This accords with common sense, but the problem is how there could be causal relations between two systems so distinctively different; for example, how could bodily causes produce mental effects if the latter are defined as nondetermined? The principles of conservation of energy and matter are contravened: if physical causes are sufficient, mental causes can hardly be necessary. Epiphenomenalism posits causal dependence of mental on physical events but not vice versa. This is an extrapolation, possibly unwarranted, from cases where conscious processes are inefficacious. It is difficult, if not impossible, to test because conscious processes are always accompanied by physical ones. Monist solutions attempt to reduce one set of events to the other or assert that both are aspects of some fundamental neutral stuff (double aspect theory). This last is superficially attractive but vague, and leaves the fundamental stuff unknowable. Idealism claims that all physical events can be reduced to mental: matter is the 'permanent possibililty of sensation' (Mill, 1843). Prima facie this is compelling but encounters difficulties when trying to account for the consistency of experience. Materialism attempts to reduce mental events to physical and has been held in many different forms. Logical behaviourism claims that mental descriptions can be analysed in terms of physical ones such as dispositions to behave. It is false because mental descriptions are not identical in meaning to physical descriptions. Experiences cannot be identified with the behavioural and physiological evidence for them. Thus, supporters of the mind-brain identity theory claim that the identity which holds between conscious experiences and brain states is contingent rather than conceptual: it is a matter for empirical discovery. This is a parsimonious theory which has the advantage that mental states can be assigned a genuinely causal role. However, there are difficulties in specifying the level at which the identity holds. Functionalism is based on the recognition that mental processes are independent of a particular physical realization: what characterizes the mental is its functional organization rather than its material constitution. According to the computer analogy, mind is the program of software, and brain is the hardware. Mental states are defined in terms of the operations of a Turing machine. Functionalism cannot provide a satisfactory analysis of qualitative differences in experience, for example, where experiences of red and green are interchanged (the 'inverted spectrum') but behaviour remains the same.

Nevertheless the computer analogy has been extremely fruitful in cognitive science. The underlying assumption is that theories of the mind can be expressed in computational terms. Complex operations can be broken down into simple ones, such as composition, primitive recursion and minimization (Johnson-Laird, 1983). The contribution of artificial intelligence is to enable the specification of possible mechanisms at an appropriate level of abstraction and to examine their feasibility.

The mind can be modelled by a hierarchy of multiple parallel processors, enabling speed and flexibility, with interactions and dependencies within and between levels. At the lowest level they govern sensory and motor interactions with the external world. At the highest level overall goals are monitored. Some modules may be fairly general in function; the majority are probably relatively specialized. The evidence suggests a broad division of labour between those specialized for verbal processing and those specialized for spatial processing. A small subset of results, but not the inner workings, are available to consciousness in a limited capacity serial processor which interrelates products of parallel processors. The system can construct models of the external world (including one of itself), which influence its input and output. The contents of the mind appear to be images, propositions, models and procedures for carrying out actions. It is clear that 'mind' is a term which is too vague to be useful. The tools are now becoming available for the detailed specification of its functions, which will require the combined efforts of work in artificial intelligence, empirical psychology and neurophysiology.

E. R. Valentine
Royal Holloway and Bedford New College
University of London

References

Boden, M. (1972), *Purposive Explanation in Psychology*, Cambridge, Mass.

Brentano, F. (1874), *Psychologie vom empirischen Standpunkt*, Leipzig.

Chisholm, R. M. (1967), 'Intentionality', in P. Edwards (ed.), *The Encyclopaedia of Philosophy IV*, New York.

Descartes, R. (1953 [1641]), *Discourse on Method*, trans., London.

Feigl, H. (1958), 'The "mental" and the "physical" ', in H. Feigl *et al.* (eds), *Concepts, Theories and the Mind-Body Problem*, Minneapolis.

Fleming, W. (1858), *The Vocabulary of Philosophy*, London.

Hume, D. (1740), *Treatise of Human Nature*, London.

James, W. (1890), *Principles of Psychology*, New York.

Johnson-Laird, P. N. (1983), *Mental Models*, Cambridge.

Locke, J. (1690), *Essay Concerning Human Understanding*, London.

McDougall, W. (1912), *Psychology: The Study of Behaviour*, London.

McFie, J. (1972), 'Factors in the brain', *Bulletin of the British Psychological Society*, 25.

Mill J. S. (1843), *A System of Logic*, London.

Russell, B. (1921), *The Analysis of Mind*, London.

Ryle, G. (1949), *The Concept of Mind*, London.

Further Reading
Valentine, E. R. (1982), *Conceptual Issues in Psychology*, London.
See also: *artificial intelligence; nervous system; sensation and perception; thinking.*

Motivation

Motivation, as the word implies, is what *moves* people. If most of psychology deals with 'How' questions, like 'How do people perceive?' or 'How do people learn habits?' the field of motivation is concerned with more fundamental 'Why?' questions. The most basic of these include: 'Why does the organism behave at all?'; 'Why does this behaviour lead in one direction rather than another at a particular time?'; and 'Why does the intensity or persistence of the behaviour vary at different times?'

The main types of answers which have been given to these sorts of questions in the last hundred years or so can be listed roughly chronologically in terms of when they were first proposed. Although each approach was developed to some extent in reaction to what went before, and was seen by its adherents as superior in some respect to its predecessors, proponents of all these approaches will be found in one form or another in present-day psychology.

(1) The earliest approach was that of *hedonism*, which said simply that people behave in such a way as to maximize pleasure and minimize pain. From this perspective man was seen as being an essentially rational being, making sensible

decisions about what courses of action to take in the light of their likely consequences in relation to pleasure or pain.

(2) The development of *psychoanalysis* from the turn of the century onwards marked a break with this 'commonsense' view. Freud argued that man is irrational and that his behaviour is largely determined by the outcome of the continual struggle between the powerful unconscious urges of the id (especially the sexual drive, or eros) and the individual's conscience, or super-ego, representing the dictates of society (see especially, Freud, 1933). Every subsequent form of depth psychology has had at least this in common with Freud's original version: that man is seen as being to some extent at the mercy of psychological forces which are outside his conscious control, and that he is usually unaware of the real reasons for his actions.

(3) *Instinct* theorists, like William McDougall (1908), also emphasized the nonrational side of human nature, bringing out the continuity between animal and human motivation, and answering the 'Why' questions in the context of Darwinian biology. This general approach has been adopted again more recently by ethologists like Tinbergen (1951), although the research techniques and interests of ethologists are remote from those of McDougall.

(4) As laboratory experimental work with animals came to dominate psychology, so another motivational concept began to hold sway: that of *drive*. This concept was introduced by Woodworth (1918) to describe the strength of internal forces which impel the organism into action. The main advantage of this concept was that drive could be defined operationally, for example by the number of hours of food deprivation; in this way motivation could be quantified and made more amenable to rigorous scientific investigation. There was broad agreement that such biological drives existed as a hunger drive, a thirst drive and a sexual drive, and later some theorists added various social drives and even such drives an an exploratory drive. The use of the concept probably reached its high point in the elaborate learning theory of Clark Hull (1943), one of the basic ideas of which was that the aim of all behaviour is 'drive-reduction', this being 'reinforcing' to the organism.

(5) A major problem with the notion of drive-reduction was that the organism, especially the human organism, often seems to be engaged in attempts to increase its stimulation and to present itself with challenges, rather than always to maintain drive at as low a level as possible. This problem was overcome with *optimal arousal theory*, originally proposed by Hebb (1955), which suggested that the organism is seeking to attain, and maintain, some level of arousal which is intermediate on the arousal dimension. Thus, the organism is provoked into action not just when arousal is too high but also when it is too low (the latter being experienced, for example, by feelings of boredom). A further advantage of this theory was that the arousal concept provided a way of linking psychological and physiological research.

(6) A completely different approach to motivation was taken by Maslow (1954), with his notion of *self-actualization*, a concept which has subsequently become one of the mainstays of humanistic psychology. The general idea is that people have a fundamental need to grow psychologically in such a way that they become fully individual and fulfil their own potentials. According to Maslow there is a need hierarchy which ascends from physiological and safety needs, up through the need to belong and love and the need for self-esteem, to the highest level which is that of self-actualization itself. Living involves a kind of snakes-and-ladders course up and down this hierarchy, but the aim is always to reach the top, success in which is marked by so-called 'peak experiences'.

(7) A recent theory, known as *'reversal theory'* (Apter, 1982), makes a radical challenge to the basic assumption on which all the other theories of motivation are based: namely, that of homeostasis (in its broadest systems-theory sense). This implies that there is some single preferred state which the organism attempts at all times to achieve, and to maintain once achieved. This may be, for example, low drive, intermediate arousal or the top of a need hierarchy. However it is defined, it remains a relatively unchanging end-point for the organism to strive towards. Reversal theory argues that this is an absurd oversimplification and that, at least in the human case, people want

quite contrary things at different times and are in this respect inherently inconsistent. To give just one example, sometimes people want extremely low arousal (for example, when very tired), and at other times they want extremely high arousal (such as during sexual intercourse, or while watching sport). The end-point, therefore, is dynamic rather than static, and the overall situation is better characterized as one of multistability than homeostasis.

Michael J. Apter
University College Cardiff

References
Apter, M. J. (1982), *The Experience of Motivation: The Theory of Psychological Reversals*, London.
Freud, S. (1933), *New Introductory Lectures on Psychoanalysis*, New York.
Hebb, D. O. (1955), 'Drives and the C.N.S. (Conceptual Nervous System)', *Psychological Review*, 62.
Hull, C. L. (1943), *Principles of Behavior*, New York.
Maslow, A. H. (1954), *Motivation and Personality*, New York.
McDougall, W. (1908), *An Introduction to Social Psychology*, London.
Tinbergen, N. (1951), *The Study of Instinct*, London.
Woodworth, R. S. (1918), *Dynamic Psychology*, New York.

Further Reading
Franken, R. E. (1982), *Human Motivation*, Monterey, Calif.
Jung, J. (1978), *Understanding Human Motivation: A Cognitive Approach*, New York.
See also: *learning; psychoanalysis*.

Nervous System

The nervous system has long been recognized as the locus of the control of human action, but the nature of its contribution and the mechanisms by which this is achieved are still a matter of active debate. The main thrust of investigation has been empirical, and has been initiated from two fields within psychology – physiological psychology and human neuropsychology.

(1) *Physiological Psychology* has investigated the influence of general physiological systems upon the fundamental aspects of behaviour, and has concentrated on affective and conative mechanisms rather than cognitive processes. Because the site of these mechanisms is in the central subcortical parts of the head, and in lower brain systems, they have generally been studied in animal preparations, for the survival of human cases with damage to these areas is relatively poor. Research has identified three major functional systems: (i) The limbic system, which includes the cingulate gyrus, the septal region, the fornix, the hippocampus and the amygdala, is involved in the evaluation of experience as punishing or rewarding. It also maintains a memory of these evaluations, so that behaviour can be adaptive and appropriate to its context. Rage and fear, taming, flight and attack are all associated with this region, as is the regulation of psychological mood. (ii) The medial forebrain bundle, grouped around the hypothalamus, is involved in the basic motivational systems for hunger, thirst and sexual behaviour. It can be convenient to think of subsystems within the hypothalamus which turn such drives 'on' or 'off', although the system is in reality more complex. Related structures subserve the effects of reward and punishment, and also exert control on the endocrine system of hormones, and on the autonomic nervous system involved in emotion and anxiety. If pleasure is generated anywhere within the brain, it is here. (iii) The system in the brainstem governs the operation of reflex responses and maintains the general level of alertness and attention within the rest of the nervous system.

(2) The other, and more recently prominent, field is that of *Human Neuropsychology*. This has mainly investigated cognitive functions, and in the cerebral cortex of human subjects. Its origins are in clinical neuropsychology, the study of patients with damage to the central nervous system. From the latter half of the nineteenth century, investigators recognized that fairly discrete behavioural defects could be associated with relatively localized injuries to the surface of the brain. This study of focal

brain lesions, promoted by the observation of those injured in both World Wars, laid the basis of modern neuropsychology as both a research area and an applied clinical discipline. The most widely adopted functional model derived from this work is that of regional equipotentiality within an interactionist theory. Interactionist theory, originating with Hughlings Jackson and more recently developed by Luria and Geschwind, proposes that higher abilities are built up from a number of more basic component skills which are themselves relatively localized. Regional equipotentiality argues for localization only within certain rather loosely defined regions. That higher functions appear incompletely localized in the brain may be due to the flexibility of cognitive systems in employing basic components in complex performance.

Three main approaches are adopted in modern clinical neuropsychology: (i) Behavioural neurology, derived from the work of Luria and most widely practised in the Soviet Union, is individual-centred and aims at a qualitative analysis and description of the patient's problems rather than a quantitative assessment. The focus of interest is not only the level of performance, but also the way in which a given task is performed. (ii) An approach, popular in the United States, concentrates on the use of test batteries. The two currently most important are the Halstead-Reitan and the Luria-Nebraska Neuropsychological Batteries. Such batteries, composed of a large number of standard tests, seek to give a complete description of the patient's level of performance across the whole spectrum of abilities, and use statistical methods. Diagnostic indicators are also usually a feature of the results. (iii) The individual-centred, normative approach is most commonly practised in Britain. It relies to some extent upon formal psychometric assessment, but emphasizes the need to tailor the assessment to the nature of a particular patient's difficulties. The aim is an accurate description of the dysfunction being investigated, going beyond a simple diagnostic classification to an understanding in cognitive psychological terms. This approach is more efficient in terms of time and resources, but makes greater demands upon professional skill and clinical insight. The approaches are, of course, rather less distinct in clinical practice.

The clinical tradition in neuropsychology has developed in the past two decades through important contributions from cognitive experimental psychology. The stimulus for this development was undoubtedly the study of the commissurotomy or 'split-brain' patients by Sperry and Gazzaniga in the early 1960s. These patients, in whom the two lateral hemispheres of the cortex had been surgically separated for the treatment of epilepsy, provided a unique opportunity to study the functions of each hemisphere operating alone. It was demonstrated that each was capable of perceiving, learning and remembering, and that there were in addition relative specializations characteristic of each hemisphere: the left subserved speech and verbal, symbolic, logical and serial operations, while the right undertook spatial-perceptual, holistic and parallel processes. The split-brain patients also provided a milieu for the empirical investigation of the seat of consciousness, although the conclusions to be drawn are still very much a matter of debate. However, apart from the research findings directly derived from the split-brain patients which are sometimes difficult to interpret, this work demonstrated that methods already employed in a different context in experimental psychology could be used to investigate brain organization in normal intact human adults. These methods all rely upon presenting information to the nervous system so that by virtue of the arrangement of sensory pathways it is projected initially to only one hemisphere. This may be in vision (divided visual field presentation), in hearing (dichotic listening), or in touch (haptic presentation). Subsequent human performance, in terms of speed or accuracy of response, can then be analysed as a function of which hemisphere received the information. An enormous literature has now built up around these techniques, and the results, although far from unanimous, broadly support the conclusion derived from the split-brain patients. This is that the hemispheres possess relative specializations for cognitive function. While it was at one time thought that this might relate to the type of material processed, or the response mechanisms employed, it is now thought that the nature of the processing determines the relative proficiency of each hemisphere. No one specification of the relevant processing characteristics has yet been widely accepted.

Alongside these developments in experimental neuro-psychology has been a renewed interest in electrophysiological processes. The new technology of averaged evoked response recording, and new ways of looking at the ongoing electrical activity of the brain (EEG), have both produced significant advances in directly linking cognitive events in the psycho-logical domain to observable concurrent events in the physio-logical domain. While this research is difficult in technological and methodological terms, it holds the promise of being able to identify accurately, with good temporal resolution, the concomitants of cognitive processes within the physiological activity of the brain. Despite inventive research, this promise is some way from being fulfilled. At the same time, psychophysiological studies, which have a longer history, have continued into the psychological correlates of autonomic nervous system functions. Much has been learned of the periph-eral changes in heart rate, electrodermal response, respiration, blood pressure and vascular changes which accompany changes in emotion and mood, but the problems of individual and situ-ational variability, and the poor temporal association between mental and physiological states because of the slow response of the autonomic processes, have led to a decline in interest in recent years.

A number of fundamental problems face the apparently successful study of brain-behaviour relationships: (1) The philo-sophical issue of the mind-body problem. Most neuroscientists adopt a position of psychoneural monism, assuming that some identity can be established between mental and physiological events. This, of course, may be a conceptual error. It is possible that developments in electrophysiology may provide a means for the empirical investigation of this issue, till now primarily the domain of philosophers. (2) Much of experimental neuro-psychology proceeds by inference to, rather than direct obser-vation of, physiological processes, so placing great importance upon methodological rigour. (3) It has to be admitted that we still have no real idea of how the brain operates to produce high-level cognition. A rather vague cybernetic-electronic model is often assumed, but there is no real certainty that this in any way reflects the actual principles of operation within the brain. (4) The nervous system is a very complex set of highly integrated subsystems. It is unlikely that significant progress will be made in our understanding of it until more adequate models can be developed, both of the physiological performance of large neural systems and of the psychological structure of cognitive abilities.

J. Graham Beaumont
University of Leicester

Further Reading
Beaumont, J. G. (1983), *Introduction to Neuropsychology*, Oxford.
Bradshaw, J. L. and Nettleton, N. C. (1983), *Human Cerebral Asymmetry*, Englewood Cliffs, N.J.
Carlson, N. R. (1981), *Physiology of Behavior*, 2nd edn, Boston, Mass.
Dimond, S. J. (1980), *Neuropsychology*, London.
Heilman, K. M. and Valenstein, E. (eds) (1979), *Clinical Neuropsychology*, New York.
See also: *biological psychiatry; mind; physiological psychology; vision.*

Neuroses

Historically, the neuroses or psychoneuroses have constituted a major category of mental disorders in psychiatry and psychoanalysis. The term neuroses evolved from the belief that the symptoms of these disorders originate in neural disturbances. Later the term psychoneuroses came into being to reflect the understanding that most neurotic symptoms have psychic or emotional origins. The two terms are nowadays used interchangeably. In fact, the *Diagnostic and Statistical Manual of Mental Disorders* (DSM–III) of the American Psychiatric Association – the organization's official manual for nomenclature published in 1980 – omits the classification of 'neuroses'; instead, the neuroses are included under the affective, anxiety, somatoform, dissociative, and psychosexual disorders.

Traditionally, the neuroses have been categorized according to the symptoms or manifestations of anxiety, which is considered their common source. In these illnesses, the predominant disturbance is a symptom or a group of symptoms which cause distress to the individual and are recognized as unacceptable and alien. However, reality testing remains grossly intact and there is no demonstrable organic aetiology. Thus, a neurotic individual's behaviour remains largely normal. Without treatment, these conditions are relatively enduring or recurrent.

Because the definition of normality or health is difficult, one can assume that everyone is a potential neurotic. A person may be considered neurotic when his ego defences are quantitively excessive and disruptive to usual patterns of adaptive functioning. The neurotic process hinders one's freedom to change, limits the capacity to sustain effort, and reduces flexibility in the areas of thinking, behaviour and emotions. Neuroses can be circumscribed, affecting only one of these areas, or they may be more widespread, touching on several areas in the individual's life.

Psychoanalysts and dynamically-oriented psychiatrists believe that the neuroses are caused by conflicts between the sexual and aggressive id drives and ego forces that are attempting to control and modify the drives. Neuroses may also arise from conflicts between the super-ego, or conscience, and the ego. Object relations theorists contend that neurotic conflicts may arise from incongruous self-representations within the ego and super-ego and their internal interactions, as well as from their interactions with the external environment.

According to the classic dynamic formulation, symptom formation is a consequence of the emergence into consciousness of the instinctual derivatives and memory traces producing anxiety. A danger is created, calling forth repression and other defensive mechanisms to ward off the anxiety. If these mechanisms are unsuccessful in containing anxiety, symptoms emerge which represent substitute expressions of the instinctual drives.

The symptoms can be understood as compromise formations or attempts of the ego to integrate ego drives, super-ego, and reality.

The appearance of a neurosis in a person usually indicates a fixation or regression to an earlier phase of infantile development. These illnesses may be precipitated by realistic situations that correspond to earlier traumatic life experiences. Unconscious fantasies and feelings are stirred up, activating the original conflict. While there is no definite evidence of biogenetic factors in the production of neurotic disorders, constitutional differences may be contributory.

Originally, Freud classified hysteria, phobias, and the obsessive-compulsive neuroses under the heading 'transference neuroses', because patients with these conditions repeat childhood neurotic patterns within the transference during treatment. Since patients with melancholia and schizophrenia did not exhibit the same tendency in treatment, these entities were termed *narcissistic neuroses*. The term *symptom neuroses* corresponds to the present-day neurotic disorder, while *character neuroses* is roughly equivalent to the concept of personality disorder.

Freud's classification of neuroses was based both on his psychoanalytic understanding of the condition and his experience of those patients' responses to the treatment situation. The psychiatric establishment, unwilling to accept Freud's approach, found a compromise and classified the neuroses as different patterns for dealing with anxiety. Thus, hysterical neurosis, conversion type, implied that anxiety had been converted into a physical symptom, for example, a paralysis. Phobia assumed that anxiety was compartmentalized, and so on.

The more recent psychiatric classification, DSM III has moved still further away from any theory of the underlying dynamics. Instead, the focus is descriptive and behavioural. The current diagnosis of what were once designated neuroses are: panic disorder, generalized anxiety disorder, conversion disorder, psychogenic pain disorder, psychogenic amnesia, psychogenic fugue, multiple personality, sleepwalking disorder (in childhood), simple phobia, social phobia, agoraphobia with panic attacks, agoraphobia without panic attacks, separation anxiety disorder (in childhood), obsessive compulsive disorder, depersonalization disorder, and hypochondriasis. As this list demonstrates, the emphasis is not on the theory of aetiology; rather, classification depends on careful description of the symptoms of the disorder. In addition, two new classifications have been introduced: somatization disorder, and acute and chronic post-traumatic stress disorders.

Nevertheless, it is still true that in these conditions the individual experiences anxiety, directly or indirectly, in addition to one or several recognizable defence mechanisms that serve to identify the disorder. An example would be an obsessive-compulsive disorder in which the person is troubled by involuntary recurrent, persistent ideas, thoughts, images, or impulses that are ego-dystonic (obsessions) and engages in repetitive and seemingly purposeful behaviours performed according to certain rules, or in a stereotyped fashion (compulsions). The individual recognizes that these obsessions and compulsions are senseless or unreasonable, but mounting tension ensues when he attempts to resist the compulsion or to ignore the obsession. Common obsessions include thoughts of violence, contamination, and doubt, while common compulsions are handwashing, checking, counting, and touching.

The neuroses have responded well to psychoanalysis and other forms of dynamic psychotherapy such as individual reconstructive psychotherapy, supportive therapy, and psychoanalytic group psychotherapy. Other modalities used in treatment of neuroses include behaviour modification, hypnosis, psychotropic medications, and various nondynamic approaches.

Normund Wong
Menninger Foundation
University of Kansas

References
Freud, S. (1959 [1926]), *Inhibitions, Symptoms and Anxiety* (Standard edition of *Complete Psychological Works of Sigmund*

Freud, Vol. xx), London. (Original German, *Hemmung, Symptom und Angst*.)

Shapiro, D. (1965), *Neurotic Styles*, New York.

See also: *anxiety; hysteria; obsessive-compulsive disorder; phobia*.

Obsessive-Compulsive Disorder

It is common human experience to have an idea or an image come to mind seemingly of its own accord. When this happens repeatedly and the ideas and images are disturbing, they are called obsessions. Paradoxically, ordinary language describes as obsessed a person who voluntarily fixes on some single idea or goal. Thus, the concept of obsession expresses a dialectical opposition of voluntary and involuntary preoccupation. Adding to the semantic confusion is the practice of using the phrase compulsive (that is involuntary) thoughts interchangeably with obsessions.

The simple technical rule is to limit obsessions to mental events, and compulsions to behaviour. Symptomatic compulsive behaviours are repetitive and stereotyped irrational attempts to produce or prevent some imagined result. The diagnostic term obsessive-compulsive disorder captures a typical pattern. Some obsessive thought comes to mind which is magically prevented by some compulsive ritual. The essence of the obsessive-compulsive disorder is captured in the children's rhyme, 'step on a crack, break your mother's back'. The child then may have a momentary compulsion to avoid stepping on cracks.

Psychoanalysts interpret obsessive phenomena as unconscious ideas coming into consciousness. Typical obsessional ideas have to do with violence, as in the children's rhyme. Another common theme is contamination, leading to hand-washing compulsion. Freud emphasized the similarities between obsessive-compulsive phenomena, superstition, and religious ritual.

Severe obsessive-compulsive disorders can be quite disabling. They are often associated with obvious depression or are thought to mask an underlying depression. French psychiatrists have described a related condition, '*Folie du doute*', the madness of doubting. This condition suggests yet another sense of obsession. The person endlessly ruminates about the remote consequences of any action and becomes immobilized by indecision and uncertainty. Although obsessive-compulsive disorder is not ordinarily associated with actual violence, in rare cases the person acts out the violence or other impulse. Compulsive ritual activity in very young children is often an indication of extreme psychopathology.

Alan A. Stone
Harvard University

See also: *depressive disorders; neuroses; phobia.*

Occupational Psychology

Occupational psychology is a somewhat catch-all title for an area which has variously been called industrial psychology, organizational psychology, vocational psychology and personnel psychology. Industrial psychology perhaps carries a hint of psychology in the interests of management; organizational psychology limits the field to a particular context; vocational psychology tends to deal with individual careers outside the organizational context in which they are usually conducted, while personnel psychology possibly ignores the non-organizational context. Thus occupational psychology is a useful label, since it incorporates all of these emphases.

Historically, we can view the development of occupational psychology as a product of the social, economic, and cultural changes in Western industrial society. Sometimes, these effects were mediated through parallel developments in mainstream psychology. A few examples may make these relationships clearer.

The biological determinism of the nineteenth century, exemplified in Galton's researches into the supposed hereditary basis of outstanding intellectual ability, coincided with the growth of 'scientific management'. As expounded by F. W. Taylor, this approach assumed that work could be broken down into tasks for which specific abilities were required. The First World War led to the development of psychometric tests to select for military functions, so the ideological justification and the practical tools were available for the growth of the psychometric testing movement for purposes of occupational selection. That this tradition lives on is evident from the following quotation from the doyen of American applied psychologists, Marvin Dunnette (1976): 'Human attributes do indeed exist to a sufficiently consistent degree across situations so that the prediction of human work performance can realistically be undertaken on the basis of tested aptitudes and skills apart from situational modifiers.' This statement clearly implies the assumptions that individuals possess lasting characteristics; that these character-istics hold true across situations; that they are related to particular aspects of jobs, and that jobs are definable in terms of the tasks they involve.

A second influence upon occupational psychology has been the emphasis during the first half of the twentieth century on the importance of the small group. Again, the evidence of the Second World War indicated the value of group cohesiveness in achieving certain sorts of objectives. The military idea of leadership and the post-war emphasis upon skills of man–management led to increased study of work groups. The concept of the working group as dependent for its success upon easy interpersonal relationships gained credence, and managers were seen as oriented towards the maintenance of these relationships as well as towards the achievement of organizational goals. Hence the leadership theories of Fred Fiedler, and the theory x and theory y typology of management propounded by David McGregor fitted in well with the current *zeitgeist*.

The third wave of development in occupational psychology related to the strong cultural influence of humanism in the 1960s, exemplified in the popular text *The Greening of America* (1970) by Theodore Reich. Self-actualization, the reaching of one's full potential, and other slogans gained support of such mainstream psychologists as Carl Rogers and Abraham Maslow. Their influence spilled over into occupational psychology in the form of various types of group training in management development programmes. The objective of many of these programmes was to help individuals to get in touch with their 'real selves' and as a consequence realize more of their true potential as individuals.

The history of occupational psychology can cynically be seen as a response to the opportunity to make the most out of each current ephemeral cultural fad. An alternative point of view might suggest that psychologists have been used for practical purposes when it was thought by the authorities that they could be of use.

Social psychology has much to say about the relationship between organizations and individuals in the theory of roles; about the meaning of work in the phenomenological approaches to cognition; about life careers in the life-span theories of human development; and about the relationships between organizations and between nation states in the theories of conflict and negotiation. The focus today is less upon individuals in isolation from their context, and also less upon the primary working group. The organizational context of work, together with the values and image it implies, are much more to the fore. So too is the environment of organizations, to which they must continuously adapt if they are to survive. In particular, labour relations and economic and technological change are being brought into psychological focus. Cross-cultural studies are beginning to demonstrate how ethnocentric our theories have hitherto been, and how irrelevant they are to the needs of developing nations. Only if a broad perspective proves stronger than a parochial professionalism will occupational psychology come into its own.

Peter Herriot
Birkbeck College, University of London

Reference
Dunnette, M. (ed.) (1976), *Handbook of Industrial and Organizational Psychology*, Chicago.

Further Reading
Bass, B. M. and Barrett, G. V. (1981), *People, Work and Organizations*, 3rd edn, Boston.

Katz, D. and Kahn, R. L. (1978), *The Social Psychology of Organizations*, 2nd edn, New York.
See also: *aptitude tests; industrial and organizational psychology; vocational career and development*.

Pain

Pain research and therapy have long been dominated by specificity theory, which proposes that pain is a specific sensation subserved by a straight-through transmission system from skin to brain, and that intensity of pain is proportional to the extent of tissue damage. Recent evidence, however, shows that pain is not simply a function of the amount of bodily damage alone, but is influenced by attention, anxiety, suggestion, prior conditioning, and other psychological variables (Melzack and Wall, 1982). Moreover, the results of neurosurgical operations which cut the so-called pain pathway – a natural outcome of specificity theory – have been disappointing, particularly for chronic pain syndromes. Not only does the pain tend to return in a substantial proportion of patients, but new pains may appear. The psychological and neurological data, then, refute the concept of a simple, straight-through pain transmission system.

In recent years the evidence on pain has moved in the direction of recognizing the plasticity and modifiability of events in the central nervous system. Pain is a complex perceptual and affective experience determined by the unique past history of the individual, by the meaning of the stimulus to him, by his 'state of mind' at the moment, as well as by the sensory nerve patterns evoked by physical injury or pathology.

In the light of this understanding of pain processes, Melzack and Wall (1965) proposed the gate-control theory of pain. Basically, the theory states that neural mechanisms in the dorsal horn of the spinal cord act like a gate which can increase or decrease the flow of nerve impulses from peripheral fibres to the spinal cord cells that project to the brain. Somatic input is therefore subjected to the modulating influence of the gate *before* it evokes pain perception and response. The theory suggests that large-fibre inputs tend to close the gate while small-fibre inputs generally open it, and that the gate is also profoundly influenced by descending influences from the brain. It further proposes that the sensory input is modulated at successive synapses throughout its projection from the spinal cord to the brain areas responsible for pain experience and response. Pain occurs when the number of nerve impulses that arrives at these areas exceeds a critical level.

Melzack and Wall (1982) have recently assessed the present-day status of the gate-control theory in the light of new physiological research. The theory is clearly alive and well despite considerable controversy and conflicting evidence. Although some of the physiological details may need revision, the concept of gating (or input modulation) is stronger than ever.

The subjective experience of pain has well-known sensory qualities, such as burning, shooting and sharp. In addition, it has a distinctly unpleasant, affective quality. It becomes overwhelming, demands immediate attention, and disrupts ongoing behaviour and thought. It motivates or drives the organism into activity aimed at stopping the pain as quickly as possible. On the basis of these considerations, Melzack and Casey (1968) proposed that there are three major psychological dimensions of pain: sensory-discriminative, motivational-affective, and cognitive-evaluative. Recent physiological evidence suggests that each is subserved by a physiologically specialized system in the brain. Recognition of the multidimensional nature of pain experience has led to the development of a paper-and-pencil questionnaire (the McGill Pain Question-naire) to obtain numerical measures of the intensity and qualities of pain (Melzack, 1975).

Many new methods to control pain have been developed in recent years (Melzack and Wall, 1982). Sensory modulation techniques such as transcutaneous electrical nerve stimulation and ice massage are widely used in the attempt to activate inhibitory neural mechanisms to suppress pain. Psychological techniques have also been developed which allow patients to achieve some degree of control over their pain. These techniques include biofeedback, hypnosis, distraction, behaviour modification, and the use of imagery and other cognitive activities to modulate the transmission of the nerve-impulse patterns that subserve pain. A large body of research demonstrates that several of these techniques employed at the same time – 'multiple convergent therapy' – are often highly effective for the control of chronic pain states, particularly those such as low back pain which have prominent elements of tension, depression and anxiety.

Ronald Melzack
McGill University

References

Melzack, R. (1975), 'The McGill Pain Questionnaire: major properties and scoring methods', *Pain*, 1.

Melzack, R. and Casey, K. L. (1968), 'Sensory, motivational and central control determinants of pain: a new conceptual model', in D. Kenshalo (ed.), *The Skin Senses*, Springfield, Ill.

Melzack, R. and Wall, P. D. (1965), 'Pain mechanisms: a new theory', *Science*, 150.

Melzack, R. and Wall, P. D. (1982), *The Challenge of Pain*, Harmondsworth.

See also: *nervous system.*

Paranoid Reactions

Paranoid reactions are a group of pathological responses to emotional stress. They may stand alone, be mixed with other psychopathological states, and even be found in everyday life.

The core of the paranoid reaction is the psychological defence of projection. The essence of this defence is the attribution to the external world of those wishes, impulses, feelings and thoughts that are unacceptable to the individual, though emerging from within him. For example, a person experiencing unacceptable hostility towards other people may project (attribute outward) this feeling and believe himself to be the *object* of hostility or persecution from without.

These reactions, like many mental symptoms, have a restitutive function; that is, they serve a reparative purpose in the mental economy of the individual. An example might be a person suffering from intolerable depression through loneliness, who may project his wish for company in a disguised way by viewing himself as the object of a great deal of attention (though not necessarily benign attention) from others, thus: 'The FBI is following me everywhere, tapping my phone, reading my mail and sending signals through the TV.' As this last example shows, paranoid reactions may become extreme and elaborate, encompassing hallucinations and delusions, which may occasionally be grandiose.

The example also hints at a very common form of paranoid reaction, the false belief that one is the subject of an interaction that has no actual relation at all to oneself; formally, this delusion that a neutral event refers to oneself is termed an 'idea of reference'. Other hallmarks of paranoid reactions are suspicion, mistrust, and guardedness of manner, understandable as reflections of a person's mistrust of his *own* feelings, projected onto others.

Thomas G. Gutheil
Harvard University
Program in Psychiatry and Law, Boston

Further Reading

Freud, S. (1911), 'Psychoanalytic notes upon an autobiographical account of a case of paranoia', *Collected Papers, Volume III*, ed. J. Strachey, London.

Knight, R. (1940), 'The relationship of latent homosexuality to the mechanism of paranoid delusions', *Bulletin of the Menninger Clinic*, 4.

Waelder, R. (1951), 'The structure of paranoid ideas', *International Journal of Psychoanalysis*, 32.

Parapsychology

Parapsychology in general is concerned with paranormal events – events which cannot be explained according to the usual laws of science. Such events range widely, from the Lochness monster to UFOs (unidentified flying objects), astrological predictions and ghosts. However, the term parapsychology is usually employed in a rather more limited sense, to refer to four major phenomena. These are: (1) *telepathy*: the acquisition of information about another person, at a distant place, by means not involving the known senses or logical inference; (2) *clairvoyance*: similar to telepathy, clairvoyance involves the acquisition of information about an object or event, rather than a person; (3) *precognition*: this refers to a similar kind of information acquisition, but of information which will only exist in the future, such as knowledge about a person's death two weeks ahead, or an accident to take place in the future; (4) *psychokinesis*: the influence of the human mind, by direct action of will, on another person, or event, not mediated by any physical force yet known.

Spontaneous parapsychological phenomena have been reported over centuries, but in the nature of things are hard to submit to scientific scrutiny. This is due to the impossibility of treating the data statistically. A person may dream that a particular horse would win the Derby, or a particular team the cup final; if the horse, or the team, actually succeeds, this might be interpreted as indicating precognition. However, it is not known how many people may have dreamed about the wrong horse, or team, coming out in front, nor do we know much about the actual probability of the given horse, or team, winning. Such stories are intuitively convincing to some people, but have no scientific value. Another difficulty is that such stories are usually only publicized after the event; there is no guarantee that the dream predicting the event actually happened. It would require written notification before the event in order to take the dream seriously as evidence of precognition.

Such reports do exist. Consider the Aberfan disaster in 1966, when 128 children and adults died in a cataclysm, a coal tip sliding down the mountain side and engulfing a South Wales mining town. A number of people reported precognitively, and in the presence of witnesses, having had dreams or other premonitions accurately describing the disaster. Many other authenticated cases have been described in the literature, making spontaneous parapsychological events acceptable to scientific study.

Much more convincing scientifically would of course be experimental evidence collected in the laboratory. The first to do this on any large scale was an American biologist, Joseph Banks Rhine, who started the first parapsychological laboratory at Duke University. Most of his work was done using packs of twenty-five cards, each bearing one of five different symbols (circle, star, wavy line, plus sign and square). Subjects were asked to guess the symbol on each card, under many different kinds of conditions. The probability of guessing correctly is of course one in five, and it is possible statistically to evaluate the chances of guessing at a higher rate than that. Conditions of testing might be with the experimenter looking at a given card, and the subject guessing (telepathy); or the stack of cards lying in front of the subject, but with no one looking at the faces of the cards, and the subject calling out the sequence (clairvoyance). In precognition trials the subject might have to call out the sequence of the twenty-five cards, as this would be after shuffling; having recorded the subject's calls, the experimenter would then shuffle the cards, and compare the resulting sequence with the calls made by the subject before the shuffle. There are many combinations and subtle changes in these procedures, but on the whole there is much evidence that extra-chance results can be obtained, particularly by a small number of specially gifted subjects.

Psychokinesis was tested by Rhine and his associates by means of a dice, either thrown by the experimenter or in an automatically revolving box. Subjects would try to influence the dice to come at either with a high or a low (6 or 1) number, and again the data published in the literature suggest that extra-chance results have been obtained in many cases. These data might be called the *direct* evidence in favour of parapsychological events, also sometimes called ESP (extrasensory perception), or PSI.

There are indirect types of evidence showing phenomena predictable from well-known psychological laws. Thus it has been found that a general tendency exists for scoring rates in all these types of test to decline over time; in other words, a kind of fatigue effect. Motivational factors have been shown to be important, as has personality and attitude. Extroverts tend to do better than introverts, and people who believe in the existence of PSI tend to do better than people who disbelieve it.

A tremendous amount of research has been done since the days of Rhine's early pioneering work, and much of this has been concerned with devising automating procedures and making them foolproof. Thus, to take one example, Helmut Schmidt generated random targets, registered subject's guesses and recorded all relevant data in a computerized manner. The radioactive decay of the isotope strontium-90 was used to generate random targets for use in PSI-testing, and with the help of his machine Schmidt showed that many people were able to guess when such emissions would or would not take place. The completely automatic nature of the data-gathering and analysing precluded any accidental or wilful errors which might have caused departures from chance.

Critics of parapsychological beliefs have pointed out the ever-present possibility of fraud, the lack of foolproof laboratory procedure that always generates positive data; the possibilities of errors in transcription and analysing; the difficulties inherent in statistical analysis of such data; and the apparent waxing and waning of the parapsychological abilities of even the best subjects. Recent advances have overcome many of these criticisms, and there is now no doubt about the statistics used by parapsychologists, the experimental controls exerted, or the abolition of errors through automation. Fraud is an ever-present danger in all scientific experiments, and there certainly have been cases where fraud has been proved to have occurred in parapsychological experiments. However, it seems unlikely that hundreds of well-known scientists, with a reputation to consider, would risk their good standing in order to fabricate meaningless data, or intentionally defraud the public. On this point, of course, every student of the subject must decide for himself.

H. J. Eysenck
Institute of Psychiatry
University of London

Further Reading
Eysenck, H. J. and Sargent, C. (1982), *Explaining the Unexplained*, London.

Pavlov, Ivan Petrovich (1849–1936)

The great Russian physiologist and founder of the study of conditioned reflexes, I. P. Pavlov, was the great-grandson of a freed serf and son and grandson of village priests. His sixty-two years of continuous and active research on what he came to call 'Higher Nervous Activity' profoundly and immutably altered the course of scientific study and conceptualization of the behaviour of living organisms, and for the first time established appropriate contact between philosophical empiricism and associationism and laboratory science. The young Pavlov won a gold medal for his second experiment ('The nerve supply of the pancreas'), one of eleven publications before his graduation in 1879 from the Imperial Medico-Surgical Academy in St Petersburg. After completing his doctoral dissertation ('Efferent nerves of the heart') in 1883, he was appointed lecturer in physiology, spent two years in postdoctoral research with Ludwig in Leipzig and Haidenhain in Breslau, became professor of pharmacology in the Academy and director of the Physiological Laboratory of the new St Petersburg Institute of Experimental Medicine in 1890, and, in 1895, professor of physiology in the Academy. In 1924 he was appointed director of a new Institute of Physiology, created by the Soviet Academy of Sciences especially for his burgeoning research enterprise. He remained in this post until his death, in Leningrad, in 1936.

Pavlov was fifty-five when in 1904 he won the Nobel Prize for his work on neural regulation of digestive secretion – the first given to a Russian and to a physiologist. A special surgical technique he developed during this period, the Pavlov Pouch, is still used. This technique exemplifies a cardinal principle in his work – he disdained the artificiality of 'acute' preparations used by his contemporaries in their stimulation and extirpation research, preferring to study an intact and physiologically 'normal' animal whose life need not be 'sacrificed' after the experiment. Not long after receiving the Nobel award, Pavlov abruptly shifted to the topic for which we remember him: conditioning. Here, too, he emphasized the chronic preparation, studying some dogs for many years, yet always maintaining sound physiological standards (Rule 1. Control of all stimulation, experimental as well as surrounding; Rule 2. Reliable quantitative measures).

Then, already over seventy and famous, he again shifted his emphasis, this time to the study of psychopathology, beginning with laboratory-produced experimental neurosis but also including work with actual patients in mental hospitals and psychiatric clinics.

The basic terminology and research strategies employed today in research on animal conditioning and human behaviour modification originated mainly in Pavlov's laboratory. Modern psychiatry and clinical psychology depend substantially upon ideas and methods, not to mention the myriad of facts, growing out of his work. From behaviour therapy to biofeedback, from the study of how worms and fish learn to the theory and treatment of neurotic anxiety, Pavlov's stubbornly objective and pervasively materialistic application of the scientific method in the study of the nervous system's control of all of the functions of life, including its most adaptive feature – its plasticity – have continued to prove fruitful if not essential.

H. D. Kimmel
University of South Florida

Further Reading
Babkin, B. P. (1949), *Pavlov: A Biography*, Chicago.

Gray, J. A. (1979), *Pavlov*, London.

Pavlov, I. P. (1960 [1927]), *Conditioned Reflexes: An Investigation of the Physiological Activity of the Cerebral Cortex*, New York.

Pavlov, I. P. (1940–9), *Polnoe Sobranie Trudov [Complete Works]*, Moscow.

See also: *behaviourism; conditioning.*

Personal Construct Theory

Personal construct theory appeared on the psychological scene unheralded but complete in Kelly (1955). What distinguished it from traditional psychological theories was its central model of *person-as-scientist*. Historically, psychology has mimicked the natural sciences in distinguishing between the purposeful and understanding scientist and the scientist's ignorant and mechanical subject matter. Kelly insisted that all people are scientists/psychologists in that they theorize about their own nature and the nature of the world: their behaviour is a continuous experiment based on expectations they derive from their theories, and they modify their theories in the light of the relationship between their expectations and unfolding events.

People's theories take the form of personal construct systems. 'Personal' indicates that since we cannot directly apprehend reality, we must interpret it, and no two persons have identical ways of interpreting their world. Though we may communicate our experience and society provides a common interpretative base, we still live in unique personal worlds. 'Construct' refers to the *bipolar discrimination* we use to make sense of the world (nice-nasty, east-west, plus-minus, expensive-cheap, coloured-plain and myriads more). Our constructs are neither all conscious nor verbally labelled but they are part of a 'system'. They are organized hierarchically and, since they are linked, every act of construing is an act of prediction (if, for you, the construct female-male is positively linked to the construct gentle-harsh then you will anticipate gentle behaviour from females).

Kelly's fundamental postulate argued that 'a person's processes are psychologically channelized by the ways in which he or she anticipates events'. Since to construe is to anticipate, then unfolding events may prove you to be right or wrong or perhaps irrelevant. It is in terms of such varying validational fortunes that a person's construct system will change, both in its organizational structure and in its content.

Kelly made a further radical break with traditional psychology in refusing to distinguish between 'thought' and 'emotion'. The affect-cognition distinction is ancient in human culture and has dominated modern psychology to the extent of producing not one psychology but *psychologies of thought* and *psychologies of feeling*. Kelly integrated the two by arguing that 'feeling' is our awareness that our construct system is in transition; it is elaborating or breaking down or threatened by movement. Thus we may be resisting movement and showing hostility which is defined as 'an attempt to extort validational evidence from a kind of social prediction which is already proving a failure'; we may be anxious, that is 'aware of being confronted by elements which lie mostly outside the range of convenience of our construct system'; we may feel guilty, 'aware of imminent dislodgement from core role construing' (our construing of self) and so forth. In spite of Kelly's clarity on this issue his theory is often wrongly categorized as a *cognitive* theory of personality and criticized as 'mentalistic'.

Kelly demonstrated the practical value of his theory in the field of psychotherapy and, up to his death in 1967, clinical psychology remained its primary field of application. Since then the theory has been vigorously taken up in broad professional fields such as educational and industrial psychology and applied to areas as diverse as architecture, child development, politics, cross-cultural differences, personal relationships, religion, language and so forth. Much research has made use of instruments developed by Kelly directly from construct theory, such as self-characterization, fixed-role therapy and repertory grid technique (Kelly, 1979). A repertory grid is a series of judgements made by a person, using his constructs, on some aspect of the world. The pattern of judgements is statistically analysed so as to show how the person's constructs are defined, related and changing.

D. Bannister
Medical Research Council
External Scientific Staff

References
Kelly, G. A. (1955), *The Psychology of Personal Constructs*, vols I & II, New York.

Kelly, G. A. (1979), *Clinical Psychology and Personality: the Selected Essays of George Kelly*, ed. B. A. Maher, New York.

Further Reading
Bannister, D. and Fransella, F. (1985), *Inquiring Man*, Beckenham.

Personality

Personality (from the Latin *persona*, an actor's mask) is an ill-defined concept embracing the entire constellation of psychological characteristics that differentiate people from one another. There is no consensus on its precise definition: in 1937 Gordon W. Allport quoted more than fifty distinct definitions, and the list has grown considerably since then. The underlying assumptions common to all definitions are that people have more or less stable patterns of behaviour across certain situations, and that these behaviour patterns differ from one person to the next. Whereas most areas of psychological research are concerned with universal aspects of behaviour and mental experience, the study of personality focuses specifically on individual differences.

The earliest personality theory of note, uncertainly attributed to Hippocrates (*c*. 400 BC) and Galen (AD *c*. 170) and widely accepted throughout the Middle Ages, is the doctrine of the four temperaments. According to this theory, people can be classified into four personality types according to the balance of humours or fluids in their bodies. Optimistic people are governed by blood (*sanguis*), depressive people by black bile (*melas chole*), short-tempered people by yellow bile (*chole*), and apathetic people by phlegm (*phlegma*). The physiological basis of this theory collapsed during the Renaissance with advances in biological knowledge, but the underlying typology survived in some modern personality theories.

The first systematic investigation of individual differences using modern empirical methods was Francis Galton's study of intelligence in England in 1884. A more reliable method of measuring intelligence, developed by the French psychologists Alfred Binet and Theodore Simon in 1905, stimulated research into other kinds of individual differences. Work on intelligence continued to flourish independently and is still (illogically) excluded from most academic discussions of personality.

The simplest personality theories focus on single traits or characteristics. Among the most extensively researched of the single-trait theories are those concerned with authoritarianism, field dependence, and locus of control.

Field dependence is a personality trait, first identified by Witkin in 1949, associated with the way in which people perceive themselves in relation to the environment. A field dependent person is strongly influenced by the environment and tends to assimilate information non-selectively; a field independent person, in contrast, is more reliant on internally generated cues and more discriminating in the use of external information. The trait was originally investigated with the rod and frame test, in which the subject, seated in a darkened room, tries to adjust a luminous rod to the vertical position within a tilted rectangular frame. Field dependent people are unduly influenced by the tilted frame, whereas field independent people are more able to discount the frame and concentrate on internal gravitational cues in judging the vertical. Researchers later developed more convenient measures of field dependence, notably the paper-and-pencil embedded figures test, which involves the identification of simple geometric figures embedded in larger, more complex diagrams. Scores on these tests are predictive of behaviour across a wide range of situations. Witkin and Goodenough (1977) concluded from the voluminous published research that field independent people are especially adept at certain forms of logical thinking, tend to gravitate towards occupations such as engineering, architecture, science teaching, and experimental psychology, and are often regarded by others as ambitious, inconsiderate, and opportunistic. Field dependent people, on the other hand, excel at interpersonal relations and are generally considered to be popular, friendly, warm, and sensitive; they are most usefully employed in such occupations as social work, elementary school teaching, and clinical psychology. Field dependence generally declines with age, and women are more field dependent, on average, than men.

Locus of control is a personality trait first described by Phares in 1957, and incorporated by Rotter into his social learning theory in 1966. It indicates the degree to which people consider their lives to be under their own personal control. It is measured on a continuum from *internal* to *external* by means of questionnaires constructed by Rotter and others. People whose locus of control is internal tend to believe that they are largely responsible for their own destinies, whereas those whose locus is external tend to attribute their successes and failures to the influence of other people and uncontrollable chance events. According to Rotter and his followers, a person's locus of control affects the way that person will perceive most situations and influences behaviour in predictable ways. Research has consistently shown that people whose locus of control is internal, as compared to those whose locus is external, are more likely to adopt health-promoting activities such as weight-watching, giving up smoking, visiting dentists regularly, and taking exercise; they are relatively resistant to social influence and persuasion, and are generally better adjusted and less anxious than those whose locus of control is external. Mental disorders such as schizophrenia and depression are generally associated with external locus of control.

More ambitious multi-trait theories of personality are intended to account for human personality as a whole rather than just one aspect of it. Their aim is to identify the constellation of fundamental traits that constitute the structure of personality, and to explain differences between people according to their location on these dimensions. Allport and Odbert (1936) found 4,500 words denoting personality traits in a standard English dictionary. The first task of any multi-trait theory is to identify the most important of these, taking into account the considerable overlap between them. A statistical technique designed for this purpose, called factor analysis, reduces the measured correlations between a large number of traits to a relatively small number of dimensions or factors. These primary factors, which will generally be found to correlate with one another, can then be reduced to a still smaller number of higher-order factors. This is analogous to reducing the multitude of distinguishable shades of colour to the three dimensions of hue, saturation, and brightness, which suffice to explain all the differences. The most influential multi-trait theories are those of Raymond B. Cattell, who has concentrated mainly on primary factors, and Hans J. Eysenck, who prefers higher-order factors.

Cattell's theory (Cattell and Kline, 1977), which he outlined in the 1940s and elaborated over the succeeding decades, is based on 171 traits that are intended to encompass the entire sphere of personality. They represent the list of dictionary traits after the elimination of synonyms and the addition of a handful of technical terms. Factor analytic studies of ratings and questionnaires reduced the list to sixteen primary factors or source traits, measured by a standardized paper-and-pencil test called the Sixteen Personality Factor (16PF) questionnaire. They include easily recognizable characteristics such as intelligence, excitability, submissiveness/dominance, and forthrightness/shrewdness, together with several others for which Cattell invented neologisms, such as sizia, threcta, and zeppia.

An important aspect of personality in Cattell's theory, in addition to the temperament and ability factors that determine *how* people behave, is the analysis of motivational factors determining *why* they behave as they do. According to the theory, the ultimate sources of motivation, called ergs, are biologically based and culturally universal factors such as food-seeking, mating, gregariousness, and acquisitiveness. The means by which they are satisfied are called sentiments; these are culturally variable and include such activities as sport, religion, and work. Five ergs and five sentiments are measured by the Motivational Analysis Test (MAT). Factor analysis has revealed three basic dimensions of motivation, corresponding roughly to Freud's id, ego, and superego. If a person is motivated to read a particular book, for example, this may be because of impulsive desire (id interest), rational choice (ego interest), or a sense of obligation (superego interest).

Eysenck's theory (Eysenck, 1967), which he has developed steadily since the 1940s, is simpler than Cattell's, partly because it is based on higher-order factors. The three major factors or dimensions of personality in this theory are extraversion (E), neuroticism (N), and psychoticism (P). They are measured by standardized scales such as the Eysenck Personality Questionnaire (EPQ). Traits associated with the extraversion factor are sociability, friendliness, enjoyment of excitement, talkativeness, impulsiveness, cheerfulness, activity, and spontaneity. Traits associated with neuroticism include worrying, moodiness, tenseness, nervousness, and anxiety. Psychoticism involves feelings of persecution, irrational thinking, a liking for very strong physical sensations, inhumane cruelty, and lack of empathy.

According to Eysenck's theory, the location of a person on these three independent factors explains a great deal about that person's everyday behaviour. The theory also accounts for psychological disorders. Low E, high N, and low P, for example, is suggestive of obsessional neurosis; high E, high N, and low P points to hysteria; low E, low N, and high P is characteristic of schizophrenia; and so on. Most people, of course, fall somewhere between the extremes on all three scales. Eysenck believes that the three factors are biologically based and largely hereditary, and he has devoted a great deal of attention to their possible locations in the brain and central nervous system.

One of Eysenck's most controversial applications of his theory is to the explanation of crime and antisocial behaviour (Eysenck, 1977). He has argued that extreme extraversion, associated with a low level of arousal in the reticular formation of the brain stem, results in weak susceptibility to conditioning, which in turn leads to inadequate socialization and conscience development. Added to this, low arousal produces sensation-seeking behaviour. For both reasons, Eysenck believes, a great deal of criminal and antisocial behaviour is explicable in terms of the biologically based and largely hereditary extraversion factor in his personality theory.

The most important controversy in the field of personality, initiated by Mischel in 1968, centres on the issue of consistency. Mischel summarized an impressive array of evidence that seemed to cast doubt on one of the underlying assumptions of all personality theories – that people display more or less stable patterns of behaviour across situations. He drew particular attention to the low correlations between personality test scores and behaviour, and concluded that behaviour can be more reliably predicted from past behaviour than from personality test scores. This suggestion implies that behaviour is merely predictive of itself, and that theories of personality are futile, at least for predicting behaviour. Mischel recommended that personality research should be abandoned in favour of the investigation of situational factors that influence behaviour.

The situationist (or contextualist) critique of personality generated a considerable amount of debate and research, much of it appearing to refute Mischel's arguments and evidence. The debate is unresolved, but the views of most authorities since the mid-1970s have tended towards interactionism. According to this view, human behaviour is dependent partly on internal personality factors, partly on external situational factors, and partly on interactions (in the statistical sense) between personality and situational factors.

Andrew M. Colman
University of Leicester

References

Allport, G. W. (1937), *Personality: A Psychological Interpretation*, New York.

Cattell, R. B. and Kline, P. (1977), *The Scientific Analysis of Personality and Motivation*, London.

Eysenck, H. J. (1967), *The Biological Basis of Personality*, Springfield, IL.

Eysenck, H. J. (1977), *Crime and Personality*, London.

Mischel, W. (1968), *Personality and Assessment*, New York.

Phares, E. J. (1957), 'Expectancy changes in skill and chance situations', *Journal of Abnormal and Social Psychology*, 54.

Rotter, J. B. (1966), 'Generalized expectancies for internal versus external control of reinforcement', *Psychological Monographs*, 80, Whole No. 609.

Witkin, H. A. and Goodenough, D. R. (1977), 'Field dependence and interpersonal behavior', *Psychological Bulletin*, 84.

Further Reading

Hall, C. S. and Lindzey, G. (1978), *Theories of Personality*, 3rd edn, New York.

Hampson, S. (1982), *The Construction of Personality: An Introduction*, London.

See also: *authoritarianism and the authoritarian personality; culture and personality; Eysenck; personality assessment.*

Personality Assessment

There is little agreement among psychologists concerning the meaning of personality. However, one definition which under-pins this article is that personality is the sum of an individual's attributes. The task of personality assessment is, therefore, to measure these attributes.

There are two basic approaches to the measurement of personality – the nomothetic and the idiographic. The former is concerned with the measurement of traits that are to be found in more or less degree among all individuals; the latter seeks to measure that which is specific to the individual concerned. Cutting across the nomethetic and idiographic distinction are the different methods of personality measurement. There are three basic methods which we shall discuss separately below, together with some more general procedures which are, some-times unwisely, used in personality assessment. The three types of personality test are (1) the inventory or questionnaire; (2) the projective technique, and (3) the objective test. Good measurement demands of tests high reliability (the capability of giving the same scores to individuals on repeated testing, and also internal consistency) and high validity (that is, the test clearly measures what it claims to measure). In addition to these methods, it is possible to use interviews, rating-scales, semantic differentials and repertory grids, although these are not common in personality assessment.

(1) *Personality inventories* consist of items, phrases or sentences about behaviour, to which subjects have to respond Yes/No, True/False, Like/Dislike, for example. The items are selected by two methods. In the first, criterion keying, items are selected if they can discriminate one group from another, for instance,

schizophrenics from normals. A well-known test thus constructed is the MMPI, the Minnesota Multiphasic Personality Inventory. The second method uses factor analysis to select the items. Factor analysis is a statistical technique which can evaluate dimensions underlying correlations (in this case between test items). Thus a factor analytic test, *ipso facto*, measures a dimension. The best-known examples of these are Cattell's 16PF test, Eysenck's EPQ and the Personality Inventories constructed by Guilford. Personality inventories are reliable and reasonably valid, and have been found useful in industrial and educational psychology for guidance and selection. From these nomothetic tests two variables stand clear: extraversion and anxiety.

(2) *Projective tests* generally consist of ambiguous stimuli to which subjects have to respond more or less freely. There is much argument over their reliability and validity. Essentially idiographic techniques, the Rorschach test, consisting of series of inkblots, is perhaps the most famous example.

(3) *Objective tests* are a recent development in personality assessment stemming mainly from Cattell. They are defined as tests which can be objectively scored and whose purpose cannot be guessed, thus making them highly useful in selection. However, as yet there is little evidence concerning the validity of these nomothetic measures and thus they are definitely at the experimental stage only. Typical tests are: the fidgetometer, a chair which measures movement, for example, during an interview, the slow line drawing test, handwriting pressure test and a balloon blowing measure.

Finally, rating scales and interviews and other methods as mentioned above are usually shown to be lacking in both reliability and validity. Personality tests are much to be preferred, allowing quantification for applied and research purposes.

Paul Kline
University of Exeter

Further Reading
Cattell, R. B. and Kline, P. (1977), *The Scientific Analysis of Personality and Motivation*, London.
Kline, P. (1979), *Psychometrics and Psychology*, London.
Vernon, P. E. (1964), *Personality Assessment*, London.
See also: *personality; projective methods*.

Phobia

A phobia is a pathological fear of a situation, object or living thing; the fear is understood to be out of proportion, or inappropriate, to the fear-inspiring properties inherent in the external focus. Phobias tend to promote avoidance of the object of the fear.

Phobias may range from mild and non-impairing (for example, a person with a flying phobia may continue to travel by air, although feeling anxious), to totally immobilizing (for example, someone with a very common fear, agoraphobia – fear of going outdoors alone – may be totally house-bound). Phobias may exist within, or in conjunction with, other psychopathological states.

At present, three major explanatory theories and three major treatment approaches pertain to phobias: (1) Dynamic psychiatrists view phobias as symbolic expressions of feared unconscious neurotic material (internal) which is magically warded off by avoidance of the phobia's (external) target. For example, a person disturbed by sexual impulses and resultant guilt may develop a germ phobia and take elaborate sanitary measures to avoid (ward off) 'contamination' (here to be understood symbolically as representing sexual guilt). This phobia, by the way, may be distinguished from a close psychological cousin, a cleanliness compulsion, by noting that the phobia is usually aimed at self-protection; the compulsion is aimed at protection of others from infection. Stekel, one of the earliest psychoanalysts, expressed this as, 'The phobic is self-ill, the compulsive is object-ill.' Clinicians of this school treat phobias with dynamic psychotherapy.

(2) Behaviourists see phobic avoidance as a learned response that may develop in reaction to extremely subtle cues, and they

treat it with a variety of behavioural techniques, including desensitization.

(3) Recently, a pharmacotherapy of phobias has emerged, featuring use of so-called 'minor tranquillizers', anti-depressants, and drugs that block the beta-adrenergic nervous system. Based on the effectiveness of anti-depressant treatments, biologically-oriented psychiatrists now understand certain phobias as symptoms of an underlying depression.

Thomas G. Gutheil
Harvard University
Program in Psychiatry and Law, Boston

Further Reading

Birk, L. (1978), 'Behavior therapy and behavioral psychotherapy', in A. M. Nicholi (ed.), *Harvard Guide to Modern Psychiatry*, Cambridge, Mass.

Marks, I. N. (1978), *Living with Fear*, New York.

Nemiah, J. C. (1978), 'Psychoneurotic disorders', in A. M. Nicholi (ed.), *Harvard Guide to Modern Psychiatry*, Cambridge, Mass.

Sheehan, D. V. (1979), 'The efficient treatment of phobic disorders', in T. C. Manschreck (ed.), *Psychiatric Medicine Update, Massachusetts General Hospital Review for Physicians*, New York.

See also: *obsessive-compulsive disorders.*

Physiological Psychology

Before 1879, when Wundt founded his psychological laboratory in Germany and initiated the contemporary era of scientific psychology as a distinct academic discipline, psychological issues had been investigated within the framework of physiology by pioneering sensory physiologists such as Helmholtz. Even Wundt – and many of his European and American followers – primarily regarded themselves as physiological psychologists, in that they were concerned with elucidating how the human brain and mind are related. Modern physiological psychology, however, relies heavily on the application of physiological measures and manipulations of animals (and particularly animal models of human psychology). For this reason, Thompson (1967) traces the subject's origins as a distinct psychological subdiscipline to Shepherd Franz's 1902 publication on the effects of frontal lobe lesions on simple animal learning tasks, devised by Thorndike at the turn of the century.

Then, as now, the subject was construed as the study of how the brain and endocrine system control those behaviours associated with perception, emotion, motivation, attention, thinking, language, learning and memory. For many years, because of the influence of Watsonian behaviourism, it suffered from a general unwillingness to postulate psychological processes mediating observable behaviour. This neglect, which arose from a justified mistrust of introspection as the royal road to the mind, has been criticized by Hebb (1980), who argued that mental operations are essentially unconscious and can only be inferred from patterns of behavioural and related brain activity. As such inferences are hard to make, there exists an opposing tendency among physiological psychologists, in which, instead of making no theoretical postulates, they explain brain–mind relationships in terms of overly general intuitive psychological concepts, like attention. Success in the enterprise therefore requires both an adequate technology for influencing and measuring brain processes, and also methods for measuring and interpreting behaviour. Exciting developments in techniques for exploring brain processes over the past thirty years have not yet been matched by improvements in analysing behavioural processes, although these may come as artificial intelligence research has increasing impact.

The central issues of physiological psychology concern the extent to which the control of psychological functions is localized in the brain, how these functions are mediated, and how this control emerges in phylogeny and ontogeny. The first two of these issues have been polemical since the late eighteenth century with the emergence of phrenology, over a century before Franz began his research. The phrenologists believed that the control of complex psychological functions, such as philoprogenitiveness, was highly localized in the brain and that their degree of development was indicated by bumps on the overlying skull. Some nineteenth-century researchers, like Flourens (who lesioned pigeon brains to see what functions were lost), adopted a holistic position and argued that functional control was distributed, not localized. Others, such as the neurologists Broca and Wernicke, who found that specific left cortical lesions causes selective verbal impairments, argued that complex functions are indeed controlled by small brain regions. The controversy continued into this century when Karl Lashley formulated an influential holistic viewpoint, based on studies of the effects of lesions on learning in the rat, defined by his principles of mass action (efficiency of a given function depends on the amount of available brain tissue) and equipotentiability (widely distributed brain regions have equivalent function).

The longevity of the holistic v. localized dispute depended partly on an inadequate analysis of the nature of complex psychological functions, such as memory, and partly on the crudeness of physiological techniques before World War II. As Luria (1973) indicated, psychological goals, like remembering, may be achieved through a variety of routes, each using somewhat different subprocesses. Blocking a preferred route by a specific brain lesion may cause a less preferred one to be adopted and different (spared) subprocesses used. How the brain controls these subprocesses is the key issue. Componential analysis of complex behaviours into their functional atoms is based on criteria lacking universal agreement. This uncertainty permits the existence of a range of views about the reasons why partial recovery may occur after brain damage. Some propose that there is always functional loss so that 'recovered' behaviours are performed differently, whereas others argue that functions genuinely recover and are mediated by surviving brain tissue (Stein, Finger and Hart, 1983). The uncertainty also explains the inchoate state of understanding of three other major issues: (1) It relates to why early brain lesions sometimes have different effects than adult lesions. For example, does the fact that early left hemisphere lesions disturb verbal behaviour much less than adult lesions mean that certain processes have not yet been irreversibly assigned to that hemisphere, or that in early life verbal behaviour is achieved differently? (2) It relates to the issue of how different is the organization of people's brains. For example, Ojemann (1983) has reported that the ability to name things is disturbed by electrically stimulating different cortical regions in distinct individuals. Are their subprocesses differently located, or do they name in different ways? (3) The same question arises with the last issue, cross-species comparisons. Do species with radically differing brains, who can perform similar complex tasks, do so by using distinct systems of subprocesses?

The use of improved physiological techniques have, however, made clear that functions are more localized than Lashley believed. The brain is now seen as an enormous interlinked set of modules, each acting as a special-purpose computer. Roughly, the neocortex comprises a functional mosaic of modules, which process distinct aspects of sensory information in series and in parallel so that meaning can be extracted and spatial representations constructed by cross-modal integration. This information is stored mainly in the neocortex when further subcortical systems are activated. Further neocortical and subcortical modules programme appropriate behaviour, based on such sensory analysis and a determination (made largely subcortically) of the motivational significance of the information.

Detailed parts of this framework have sprung from the application of physiological techniques. These techniques are now sophisticated. Animal lesions can be precisely placed and identified, and accidental human lesions can now be better located in life using computed axial tomography, cerebral blood flow measurement and positron-emission computed tomography. The last technique, in particular, makes it possible to measure a lesion-induced disturbance of apparently healthy tissue. This bears on a major problem with lesion studies: a function may be lost either because it was controlled by destroyed tissue or because the destruction makes healthy tissue act abnormally. The difficulty can only be resolved by the supplementary use of other techniques like electrical or chemical stimulation of tissue, or recording electrophysiological, metabolic or biochemical activity of neurons whilst an animal (or human) subject is performing a selected task. If the use of these techniques yields consistent and convergent implications, an interpretation can be made of the function of a given brain region. Confidence in such interpretations can be further increased by improved knowledge of the brain's microanatomy and connections. Modern techniques have led to a massive surge in this knowledge, giving rise to the hope that by the turn of the century it will be possible to make detailed computer simulations of how activity in well-described brain regions mediates complex psychological abilities, such as the visual perception of objects.

Andrew Mayes
University of Manchester

References

Hebb, D. O. (1980), *Essay on Mind*, Hillsdale, N.J.

Luria, A. R. (1973), *The Working Brain*, Harmondsworth.

Ojemann, G. A. (1983), 'Brain organization for language from the perspective of electrical stimulation mapping', *The Behavioral and Brain Sciences*, 6.

Stein, D. G., Finger, S. and Hart, T. (1983), 'Brain damage and recovery: problems and perspectives', *Behavioral and Neural Biology*, 37.

Thompson, R. (1967), *Foundations of Physiological Psychology*, London.

Further Reading

Carlson, N. R. (1981), *Physiology of Behavior*, 2nd edn, Boston.

Carlson, N. R. (1979), *The Brain: A Scientific American Book*, Oxford.

Kolb, B. and Whishaw, I. Q. (1980), *Fundamentals of Human Neuropsychology*, San Francisco.

Oatley, K. (1978), *Perceptions and Representations*, London.

See also: *biological psychiatry; nervous system*.

Piaget, Jean (1896–1980)

Jean Piaget, the Swiss psychologist, biologist and philosopher, was professor of experimental psychology at the University of Geneva (1940–1971) and of developmental psychology at the Sorbonne in Paris (1952–1963). As a psychologist, Piaget was influenced by Freud, Janet, J. M. Baldwin and Claparède. Piaget's theories and experiments, which he published in innumerable books and articles, place him among the foremost psychologists of the century.

Piaget's lifelong quest was for the origins of knowledge. Trained as a biologist, and initially influenced by Bergson's evolutionary philosophy, he sought to explain the conditions of knowledge by studying its genesis. Evolutionary theory, the developmental psychology of children's intelligence and the history of science were to provide the scientific underpinnings of this epistemological project.

In his early work (1923–36), Piaget tried to gain insight into children's logic by studying their verbally expressed thought. Using a free method of interrogation, the 'clinical method', Piaget investigated children's reasoning about everyday phenomena, causality and moral problems. A leading idea expressed in Piaget's early books is that of egocentrism in early childhood and its gradual replacement by socialized, and therefore logical, thinking. Young children's egocentrism is revealed in their incapacity to differentiate between their own point of view and that of another. Neither experience nor the influence of adults are sufficient grounds for the attainment of logical thinking. Instead, Piaget explained the abandonment of egocentricism by the child's desire and need to communicate with children of the same age.

In the late 1920s and early 1930s Piaget made extensive observations of his own children as babies and elaborated his theory of sensorimotor intelligence in infancy. Contrary to contemporary conceptions, he considered babies as actively and spontaneously oriented towards their environment. As they 'assimilate' things to their action patterns, they at the same time have to 'accommodate' these patterns to the exigencies of the external world. In this process of interaction with the environment the child's innate reflexes and patterns of behaviour are altered, differentiated and mutually co-ordinated. The organization of action patterns gives rise to a 'logic of actions'. In his account of the development of the object concept, Piaget states that initially children do not appear to recognize a world existing independently of their actions upon it. A baby playing with a toy does not search for it when it is covered; according to Piaget, it ceases to exist for the baby. The concept of an independently existing world is gradually constructed during infancy and is attained only at about 18 months when the child becomes capable of representing things mentally.

The existence of a logic in action, demonstrated in the baby studies, made Piaget revise his earlier theories of the origins of logical thinking in early and middle childhood. Logical operations are prepared in sensorimotor intelligence and the former are the result of internalization of the latter. The attainment of logical thinking, therefore, is not the result of verbal interactions with other children, but of the child's reconstruction of the action logic on a new, mental plane. Piaget now viewed cognitive development as resulting in stages, characterized by a dynamic equilibrium between the child's cognitive structures and the environment. Development is the result of a process of equilibration, in which equilibria of a progressively more stable kind are sought and attained. Piaget distinguished three stages: the sensorimotor stage (0–about 18 months), the stage of concrete operations (about 7–11 years) and the stage of formal operations (from about 11 years). In each of these three stages children's thinking is characterized by its own kind of logic: an action logic in the sensorimotor stage, a logic applied to concrete situations in the concrete operational stage, and a logic applied to statements of a symbolic or verbal kind in the formal operational stage.

In the period between the sensorimotor and the concrete operational stage (which Piaget called the preoperational period) the child's thinking lacks the possibility to carry out operations, that is, reversible mental actions. Piaget and his collaborators demonstrated in many simple yet elegant experiments the transition from preoperational to concrete thinking about concepts such as number, velocity, space, and physical causality. In these experiments they no longer restricted themselves to verbal interaction, but introduced materials which the child could manipulate. In the famous conservation task, the child must judge whether the amount of fluid poured into a glass of different proportions changes or does not change. Preoperational children are characteristically misled by the perceptual appearance of the situation. Only concrete operational children can reverse the transfer in thought and give the correct answer.

From 1950 onward Piaget wrote his great epistemological studies, in which he rejected empiricism and rationalism. Consequently he opposed behaviourism, maturational theories of development and nativist ideas in Gestalt psychology. The newborn child is neither a *tabula rasa*, ready to receive the impression of the environment, nor endowed with a priori knowledge about the world. Piaget showed himself a pupil of Kant by assuming that our knowledge of the world is mediated by cognitive structures. But, unlike Kant, he did not consider these as fundamental ideas given at birth: he showed them to be the products of a lengthy process of construction in the interaction of subject and environment. He therefore coined his epistemology a *genetic* epistemology.

The aim of genetic epistemology is to reconstruct the development of knowledge from its most elementary biological forms up to its highest achievements, scientific thinking included. Psychology has a place in this project, in so far as it studies the development of biological structures in the human baby into sensorimotor and operational intelligence. But the enterprise is essentially a biological one, as the development of intelligence is conceived of as an extension of biological adaptation. Intelligence is the specific product in humans of the same biological principles applying to all living nature: adaptation resulting in structural reorganizations and in equilibria of increasing stability.

Piaget saw psychology as a necessary but limited part of his epistemology, and he always regretted the exclusive interest for the psychological component of his work. In the International

Centre for Genetic Epistemology, which he founded at the
University of Geneva in 1955 and to which he attracted specialists in all fields of study, he stimulated the interdisciplinary
study of epistemology. But the acclaim for his epistemological
ideas was never more than a shadow of the universal enthusiasm
for the *psychologist* Piaget.

Piaget's influence on developmental psychology can hardly
be overestimated. His ideas were seen as a help in supplanting
behaviouristic and psychoanalytic theories in psychology. He
set the margins for discussions in cognitive developmental
psychology from the 1960s up to the present time. But his ideas
and methods have always been the object of sharp criticism.
Many developmental psychologists think that Piaget under-
rated the cognitive capacities of young children, and he is repro-
ached for neglecting in his later studies the social context of
development in favour of an isolated epistemic subject. Therefore, many now go beyond the mature Piaget and find inspiration in his early works.

Ed Elbers
University of Leiden

Further Reading

(A) Works by Piaget
Piaget, J. (1923), *Le Langage et la pensée chez l'enfant*, Neuchâtel.
   (*The Language and Thought of the Child*, London, 1926.)
Piaget, J. (1932), *Le Jugement moral chez l'enfant*, Paris. (*The
   Moral Judgment of the Child*, London, 1932.)
Piaget, J. (1936), *La Naissance de l'intelligence chez l'enfant*,
   Neuchâtel. (*The Origin of Intelligence in the Child*, London,
   1952.)
Piaget, J. and Inhelder, B. (1948), *La Représentation de l'espace
   chez l'enfant*, Paris. (*The Child's Conception of Space*, London,
   1956.)
Piaget, J. (1950), *Introduction à l'épistémologie génétique*, Vols 1–3,
   Paris.
Piaget, J. and Inhelder, B, (1959), *La Génèse des structures logiques*

élémentaires, Neuchâtel. (*The Early Growth of Logic in the Child*, London, 1964.)

Piaget, J. and Inhelder, B. (1966), *La Psychologie de l'enfant*, Paris. (*The Psychology of the Child*, London, 1969.)

Piaget, J. (1967), *Biologie et connaissance*, Paris. (*Biology and Knowledge*, London, 1971.)

Piaget, J. (1974), *La Prise de conscience*, Paris. (*The Grasp of Consciousness*, London, 1976.)

Piaget, J. (1975), *L'Equilibration des structures cognitives*, Paris. (*The Development of Thought: Equilibration of Cognitive Structures*, Oxford, 1977.)

(B) General

Boden, M. (1979), *Piaget*, London.

Flavell, J. H. (1963), *The Developmental Psychology of Jean Piaget*, Princeton.

Gruber, H. E. and Vonèche, J. J. (eds) (1977), *The Essential Piaget: An Interpretive Reference and Guide*, London.

Rotman, B. (1977), *Jean Piaget: Psychologist of the Real*, Hassocks.

See also: *developmental psychology*.

Play

Easily recognized in children or young domestic animals, play has been impossible to define clearly. It is most frequent in immature creatures and consists of motor patterns belonging to feeding, agonistic, sexual, fleeing or comfort behaviours, but without leading to their usual biological ends. Sequences in play may be highly unlikely, such as fleeing, reclining, and fleeing following one another.

Solitary, parallel, and social play can be distinguished. In parallel play an animal or child observes, copies or is influenced by another playing individual without direct interaction, which is characteristic of social play. Object play can be solitary or social.

Some definitions of play are descriptive: 'Play behavior consists of elements drawn from other types of behavior and rearranged in new patterns of timing and sequence' (Marler and Hamilton, 1966). Others infer processes of behaviour development: 'In mammals, play is comprised largely of rehearsals performed in a nonfunctional context of the serious activities of searching, fighting, courtship, hunting, and copulation' (Wilson, 1971). Assumed proximate causation may be part of a definition: '[Play is] any action which is performed as an outlet for surplus energy which is not required by the animal for its immediate vital activities . . .' (Bolwig, 1963). Similarly, play has been seen as 'behavioural fat' engineered into the behaviour repertoire of a growing animal. It can be dropped without harm to other activities in times of energetic stress (Muller-Schwarze, 1978).

Many short- and long-term *functions* of play have been postulated. These range from general exercise of the cardiovascular and neuromuscular-skeletal systems to learning of specific, especially social, skills such as effective communication or handling of agonistic interactions. Motor development in preambulatory infants has been accelerated by rotational vestibular stimulation as would occur in vigorous play (Clark *et al.*, 1977).

The *evolution* of play clearly parellels that of brain size and function. Primates play more and in more diverse ways than other mammals, and those in turn more than birds. Among birds, play is most prevalent in the larger-brained corvids, whose behaviour is more generalized. Antecedents of play may be found in lower vertebrates but defy recognition and definition.

Sex differences in play have been clearly demonstrated (reviewed by Fagen, 1981). Fagen proposes the study of play in the context of life-history strategies, a confluence of evolutionary and development considerations. Its importance can be measured by the price an animal pays in terms of time, energy and risk to be able to play at certain ages. This price can be viewed as investment in delayed benefits – ultimately improved inclusive fitness.

The occurrence and quality of play can be evaluated in terms of mental and physical health. Social play has been used for rehabilitation of socially isolated rhesus monkeys (Cummins and Suomi, 1976). Hospitalized children benefit from object play, supervised by a play specialist (Jolly, 1968).

Dietland Muller-Schwarze
State University of New York, Syracuse

References
Bolwig, N. (1963), 'Bringing up a young monkey (*Erythrocebus patas*)', *Behaviour*, 21.
Clark, D. L., Kreutzberg, J. R. and Chee, F. K. W. (1977), 'Vestibular stimulation influence on motor development in infants', *Science*, 196.
Cummins, M. S. and Suomi, S. J. (1976), 'Longterm effects of social rehabilitation in rhesus monkeys', *Primates*, 17.
Fagen, R. (1981), *Animal Play Behavior*, New York.
Jolly, H. (1968), 'Play and the sick child: a comparative study of its role in a teaching hospital in London and one in Ghana', *Lancet*, 2.
Marler, P. and Hamilton, W. J. III (1966), *Mechanisms of Animal Behavior*, New York.
Muller-Schwarze, D. (ed.) (1978), *Evolution of Play Behavior*, Stroudsburg, Pennsylvania.
Wilson, E. O. (1971), *The Insect Societies*, Cambridge, Mass.

Prejudice

The word prejudice means pre-judgement, implying that a prejudiced person is someone who has made up his mind about a certain topic before assessing the relevant information. This sense of pre-judgement has formed an important part of the social psychological concept of prejudice. In addition, three other features are associated with prejudiced beliefs: (1) Prejudice typically refers to beliefs about social groups; it can refer also to judgements about individuals, where an individual is evaluated on the basis of being a member of a particular social group. (2) The belief or judgement is essentially an unfavourable one. Whereas it is logically possible to be prejudiced *in favour* of a group, prejudice usually denotes a negative or hostile attitude *against* a group: racist, anti-semitic and sexist attitudes would all be considered prime examples of prejudice. (3) A prejudiced belief is assumed to be erroneous or liable to lead the believer into error. A prejudice is not based on a realistic assessment of a social group, nor is contact with the group likely to overturn the prejudices. Thus Allport, in his classic discussion of prejudice, wrote 'pre-judgements become prejudices only if they are not reversible when exposed to new knowledge' (1958).

Part of the prejudiced person's error derives from a tendency to think about social groups in terms of stereotypes. In one of the first social psychological investigations of stereotypes, Katz and Braly (1935) found amongst American college students a widespread tendency to ascribe clichéd descriptions to different social groups: thus the stereotype of Blacks included the traits of being 'superstitious' and 'lazy', that of Jews as 'mercenary' and 'grasping', that of Turks as 'cruel' and 'treacherous', and so on. By thinking in such stereotypes, the prejudiced person not only has an unfavourable concept of the groups as a whole but he also exaggerates the percentage of individuals who might happen to possess the stereotyped trait; in the case of extreme prejudice, he will believe that *all* Jews or *all* Blacks possess the unfavourable traits in question.

Early research into prejudice assumed a direct relation between holding prejudiced beliefs and behaving in a discriminatory way to members of the relevant outgroup. For example, the Bogardus Distance Scale asked respondents whether they would entertain having close relations (such as marriage) or less close relations (such as working in the same place) with particular outgroups. It was assumed that the respondent's replies would predict actual behaviour towards members of outgroups. However, research into attitude theory in general has revealed that the views expressed in attitude questionnaires do not necessarily reflect behaviour.

In consequence, it is now recognized that the relations between prejudice and discrimination are more complex than was formerly thought.

Among the many theories used to explain the psychological roots of prejudice, it is possible to distinguish between motivational and learning theories. Motivational theories have sought to relate prejudiced attitudes to personality defects or to unfulfilled yearnings within the individual. These are often called 'scapegoat' theories in that they assume that the victims of prejudice are being irrationally blamed for ills that reside within the prejudiced person. One such scapegoat theory is the frustration–aggression theory (originally proposed by Dollard *et al.* (1939) and reformulated by Berkowitz (1962)). It asserts that prejudice arises when an individual has been angered by some frustration and is unable, for some reason or other, to direct this anger back on to the source of the frustration. Instead, the anger is displaced onto an innocent target. This theory has been employed, for instance, to explain why minority groups may become targets of increased prejudice in times of economic deprivation. Another motivational theory is that of Adorno *et al.* (1950) which seeks to account for prejudice in terms of the repressed hostility of authoritarian-type personalities: such people, it is argued, direct their hostilities on to weak outgroups because of their own personal inadequacies.

Motivational theories as general theories of prejudice are limited. For example, they fail to explain why particular targets are chosen for prejudice and not others; they also tend to understate the extent to which prejudiced beliefs might be the product of learning. Pettigrew's comparison of the different levels of prejudice in South Africa and the United States showed that personality factors were less important than the existence of cultural traditions (Pettigrew, 1958). In the case of White South Africans these traditions had resulted in prejudiced beliefs, which were so widely accepted that they had become normative and, by contrast, tolerance was regarded as socially deviant. Thus, within such a prejudiced society, children are likely to be socialized through learning into acquiring prejudiced beliefs; the displacement of underlying motivations need not feature in the process.

Much of the recent research in social psychology has concentrated upon the cognitive aspects of prejudice and investigates prejudice in terms of the ways people generally perceive and make sense of the world. This research suggests that a large degree of prejudiced thinking is not the result of 'abnormal' psychological processes. Jerome Bruner (1958) and Henri Tajfel (1981) have indicated that people are not passive recipients of information; rather, they try to make sense of incoming stimuli. Thus 'normal' perception involves a certain amount of error and simplification as information is categorized and assessed according to pre-judgements, which in turn determine what is perceived or experienced. Stereotyped thinking represents an extreme case of such processes, with the stereotype influencing what aspects of the social world are selected for attention and how these aspects are interpreted. For example, a person who views a particular group as lazy will often unconsciously seek confirmation of his stereotype and ignore contradictory evidence. In addition, ambiguous evidence will be interpreted in support of the idea that the group is lazy, and the result will be a perception of that group with a systematic distortion which appears to confirm the stereotype. If the stereotype is widely held within a society, then not only will it pass as common sense, and social pressures will promote the stereotype, but cognitive processes may prevent believers from becoming aware of their own biases.

Michael Billig
Loughborough University

References

Adorno, T. W., Frenkel-Brunswik, E., Levinson, D. J. and Sanford, R. N. (1950), *The Authoritarian Personality*, New York.

Allport, G. W. (1958), *The Nature of Prejudice*, Garden City, N.Y.

Berkowitz, L. (1962), *Aggression: A Social Psychological Analysis*, New York.

Bruner, J. S. (1958), 'Social psychology and perception', in E. E. Maccoby, T. W. Newcomb and E. L. Hartley (eds), *Readings in Social Psychology*, London.

Dollard, J. L., Doob, W., Miller, N. E., Mowrer, O. H. and Sears, R. R. (1939), *Frustration and Aggression*, New Haven.

Katz, D. and Braly, K. W. (1935), 'Racial prejudice and racial stereotypes', *Journal of Abnormal and Social Psychology*, 30.

Pettigrew, T. F. (1958), 'Personality and sociocultural factors in intergroup attitudes: a cross national comparison', *Journal of Conflict Resolution*, 2.

Tajfel, H. (1981), *Human Groups and Social Categories*, Cambridge,

Further Reading

Hamilton, D. L. (1979), 'A cognitive-attributional analysis of stereotyping', in L. Berkowitz (ed.), *Advances in Experimental Social Psychology*.

See also: *attitudes; authoritarian personality; stereotypes.*

Problem Solving

Problem solving is a major function of thought and has long been researched in cognitive psychology. Since the information-processing approach to cognitive psychology became theoretically dominant in the early 1960s, thinking has generally been regarded as a serial symbol manipulation process that makes use of a very limited working memory, supported by an extensive long-term memory. This approach has been fruitful and, by emphasizing both analysis and organization, largely avoids the dangers of elementarism and vagueness which had beset the earlier behaviourist and Gestalt approaches. Much of the recent research on problem solving has focused on 'move' and reasoning tasks which I discuss in this article.

Move Problems

In this class of well-defined tasks, objects or quantities have to be manipulated (in reality or symbolically) in order to change some given starting configuration into a goal configuration. Normally, the available moves or actions are specified for the would-be solver at the start. Move problems may or may not involve an adversary. Non adversary move problems, especially small-scale, artificial puzzles, have been extensively investigated. The importance of prior experience with the problem area has clearly emerged in the study of adversary move problems. De Groot (1965) found that both amateur and grand master level chess players searched mentally to similar extents when asked to choose the best next move in a given board position; but, the grand masters always came up with a better move. A series of studies involving memory for realistic and randomly arranged chess boards showed that grand masters have developed a very extensive network of familiar patterns in terms of which they can efficiently encode new positions (De Groot, 1965; Chase and Simon, 1973). Similar results regarding expertise have also been found in the games of GO (Eisenstadt and Kareev, 1977) and Bridge (Charness, 1979).

Reasoning Problems

Deductive and inductive reasoning problems have recently been the focus of considerable attention. In the deductive area, the syllogism has been a favourite experimental task. The somewhat venerable 'atmosphere' hypothesis, according to which the presence of particulars or negatives in the premises colours the conclusions reached (Woodworth and Sells, 1935), still seems to be *descriptively* useful in summarizing error patterns (Begg and Denny, 1969), although the explanation for these patterns is still controversial, for the following reasons:

(1) The arguments of Henle (1962) for human rationality, which stressed the discrepancies between experimenters' and subjects' interpretations of syllogistic tasks, have been very influential. (2) Phenomena that are not accounted for by the atmosphere hypothesis have been uncovered, for example, Johnson-Laird's (1975) finding that the order of the premises affects the nature of the conclusion drawn. Johnson-Laird and Steedman (1978) were able to account for this 'figural bias' effect and for other fine grain results with a computer simulation that embodied a very promising 'analogical' model of reasoning.

Inductive reasoning has been intensively studied, especially in the contexts of concept learning and Wason's 4-card task. In the case of concept learning, Bruner, Goodnow and Austin (1956) noticed a reluctance among their subjects to attempt falsification of current hypotheses, and this apparent 'set' for verification was the starting point for a long series of studies by Wason and others using the 4-card task. In this task, subjects have to say which cards need to be turned over to test a conditional rule relating the showing and the not-showing faces of the cards. For example, the rule might be 'if there is an "A" on one side there is a "4" on the other side'. Given cards showing A, B, 4 and 7, which need be turned over? (Answer, A and 7). Most subjects do not choose the potentially falsifying '7' card. Johnson-Laird and Wason (1970) interpreted this result as showing 'verification bias'. A number of subsequent studies found improved performance if the materials were thematic rather than abstract (Wason and Shapiro, 1971; but see Manktelow and Evans, 1979, for a cautionary note). Facilitation was also found if the rules were of dubious truth-value (Pollard and Evans, 1981) or if certain ambiguities in the standard task were clarified (Smalley, 1974). While many have interpreted the above pattern of results in a manner akin to Henle's analysis of interpretation factors in syllogistic reasoning, Evans (1980) proposed that most responses to the standard form of the task are due to an unconscious, nonrational, 'matching bias'. Supporting evidence comes from the high success rates found with negative 'if-then' rules, coupled with zero transfer to positive rules.

Concluding Comments

Overall, the results of recent research on problem solving are consistent with the standard information-processing assumptions of serial processing, limited working memory and vast long-term memory. Perhaps not surprisingly, data from studies of daydreaming and creative thinking suggest, however, that more complex models will be required to explain thought in general (Gilhooly, 1982) than seem required for the special case of 'problem solving'.

K. J. Gilhooly
University of Aberdeen

References

Begg, I. and Denny, J. P. (1969), 'Empirical reconciliation of atmosphere and conversion interpretations of syllogistic reasoning errors', *Journal of Experimental Psychology*, 81.

Bruner, J. S., Goodnow, J. J. and Austin, G. A. (1956), *A Study of Thinking*, New York.

Charness, N. (1979), 'Components of skill in bridge', *Canadian Journal of Psychology*, 33.

Chase, W. G. and Simon, H. A. (1973), 'Perception in chess', *Cognitive Psychology*, 4.

De Groot, A. D. (1965), *Thought and Choice in Chess*, The Hague.

Eisenstadt, M. and Kareev, Y. (1977), 'Perception in game playing', in P. N. Johnson-Laird and P. C. Wason (eds), *Thinking*, Cambridge.

Evans, J. St B. T. (1980), 'Current issues in the psychology of reasoning', *British Journal of Psychology*, 71.

Gilhooly, K. J. (1982), *Thinking: Directed, Undirected and Creative*, London.

Henle, M. (1962), 'On the relation between logic and thinking', *Psychology Review*, 69.

Johnson-Laird, P. N. (1975), 'Models of deduction', in R. C. Falmagne (ed.), *Reasoning: Representation and Process*, Hillsdale, N.J.

Johnson-Laird, P. N. and Steedman, M. (1978), 'The psychology of syllogisms', *Cognitive Psychology*, 10.

Johnson-Laird, P. N. and Wason, P. C. (1970), 'A theoretical analysis of insight into a reasoning task', *Cognitive Psychology*, 1.

Manktelow, K. I. and Evans, J. St B. T. (1979), 'Facilitation of reasoning by realism: effect or non-effect?', *British Journal of Psychology*, 70.

Pollard, P. and Evans, J. St B. T. (1981), 'The effects of prior beliefs in reasoning: an associational interpretation', *British Journal of Psychology*, 72.

Smalley, N. S. (1974), 'Evaluating a rule against possible instances', *British Journal of Psychology*, 65.

Wason, P. C. and Shapiro, D. (1971), 'Natural and contrived

experience in a reasoning problem', *Quarterly Journal of Experimental Psychology*, 23.

Woodworth, R. S. and Sells, S. B. (1935), 'An atmosphere effect in formal syllogistic reasoning', *Journal of Experimental Psychology*, 18.

Further Reading

Mayer, R. E. (1983), *Thinking, Problem Solving, Cognition*, San Francisco.

See also: *thinking*.

Projective Methods

Projective methods encompass a wide range of approaches to the assessment of individuals and share the following characteristics: (1) stimulus ambiguity-projective techniques consist of materials that can be interpreted, structured, or responded to in a great many different plausible ways; (2) lack of any one correct or true answer – projective stimuli are not designed to represent or resemble any one specific object of experience; and (3) open-ended, complex, and individualized responses – the subject does not usually provide a simple yes-no or true-false answer, but is given the opportunity to organize or structure his response in a personal or individualized way. Projective methods represent an indirect approach to the assessment of a person. Personality characteristics are revealed while the person is ostensibly doing something else, such as telling a story about a picture, or drawing a person. Proponents of projective techniques claim that the person's subjective experience is revealed through these responses; in this manner, the mainsprings of his social behaviour are expressed.

The term projective methods was coined by Lawrence K. Frank, more than thirty years after projective techniques were introduced. Upon surveying the growing number of these techniques and trying to establish what they had in common, Frank concluded that projective methods provide 'a field with relatively little structure and cultural patterning, so that the personality can project upon that plastic field his way of seeing life, his meanings, significances, patterns, and especially his feelings'

(Frank, 1939). This is accomplished by means of projection, that is, attributing one's own traits and characteristics to external stimuli. Frank also spelled out several implications of this position: (1) Projection takes place with a minimum of awareness or conscious control. The person transcends the limits of his self-knowledge and reveals more than he is capable of communicating directly. (2) The ambiguous stimuli of projective techniques serve mainly as stepping stones for self-expression. Their specific characteristics are relatively unimportant. (3) The responses to projective techniques are little influenced by the social situation in which they are presented or by the person's current psychological state; they are based on his enduring personality characteristics.

This conceptualization of projective methods is compatible with psychodynamic theories of personality, such as those of Freud and Jung, which emphasize the importance of unconscious impulses and motives. Responses to projective methods lend themselves easily to interpretation in terms of unconscious drives, intrapsychic conflicts, defences against them, and symbolic representation of these forces.

More recent theoretical formulations have attempted to look at projective techniques from other points of view. Bruner (1948) forged links between responses to projective stimuli and the principles of the 'hypothesis theory' of perception. In Bruner's view, responses to ambiguous stimuli reflect hypotheses, based on past experience and present expectations. Fulkerson's (1965) point of departure was decision making under conditions of uncertainty. Uncertainty in responding to projective methods is of two kinds: stimulus ambiguity, amply emphasized by Frank and other traditional theorists, and situational ambiguity, somewhat glossed over in these formulations. Fulkerson stressed the conscious choices open to the person: to emit or to withhold a response and how to present or communicate it to the examiner, all on the basis of the person's subjective understanding of the context and purpose of projective examination. Epstein integrated responses to projective stimuli with conflict theory. The situation with which the person is confronted in responding to projective materials arouses a conflict of expression versus inhibition of various drive states. This conflict can result in verbal expression of the impulse in question, its suppression, or various compromise reactions, for example, expressing the drive symbolically, partially, or indirectly.

Since 1900, a multitude of projective techniques have been developed. Of these, four varieties have become prominent: inkblot tests, which require the person to impose meaning upon, and to interpret, inkblots or portions thereof; story-telling tests in which the person is asked to provide an imaginative, dramatic account of a picture; graphic techniques, in which the task is to produce a drawing, of a person, or a house, for example, with a minimum of further specifications; and completion techniques, exemplified by sentence completion in which the person is asked to complete a sentence stem, for example, 'Last summer . . .', 'Whenever I get angry . . .'. Projective techniques have preponderantly relied upon the visual modality for the presentation or production of stimuli. Auditory techniques consisting of vague sounds difficult to recognize or structure have been repeatedly proposed, but have not gained wide acceptance. The same is true of several projective techniques that require tactile exploration of stimuli.

Inkblots were introduced by Hermann Rorschach of Switzerland who developed a test consisting of 10 cards. Rorschach devised a multidimensional scoring system based on content (for example, animal, human, plant, object) as well as determinants (for example, form, movement, colour, shading) and location (for example, whole, large, small, or tiny detail). In the ensuing decades, this test was widely used in clinical and research settings; a reasearch literature came into being numbering by now several thousand studies. Not unexpectedly, the results of this work were divergent and complex; some of it supported. and some of it refuted, Rorschach's and other proponents' claims. In 1961, Wayne Holtzman at the University of Texas succeeded in developing a modern and statistically streamlined inkblot test. Consisting of two forms of 45 inkblots each, it allows only one response per card, makes possible determination of test-retest reliability, and exhibits improved objectivity in scoring. Remarkably, it has supplemented, especially as a research tool, but has not replaced, the Rorschach which its proponents continue to prefer because of its allegedly superior clinical sensitivity and ease of administration.

The most prominent exemplar of the story-telling format is the Thematic Apperception Test introduced in 1935 by Henry A. Murray at Harvard University. Twenty cards are administered to the person who is asked not only to describe what he sees, but to extend the story beyond the present into both past and future and to relate the actions, thoughts and feelings of the people depicted. The resulting imaginative production, in Murray's words, reflects person's 'regnant preoccupations', his characteristic motives, feelings and fantasies. The voluminous literature about the T.A.T. has demonstrated, but not really explained adequately, how its content relates to overt, observable behaviour.

Graphic approaches are best illustrated by the Draw-a-person and House-Tree-Person techniques. Their rationale rests on the assumption that the person's own characteristics are reflected, or projected, in response to the minimally brief instructions, such as, 'Draw a person, any kind of a person.'

In the completion techniques, more structure is provided and the person's contribution is concentrated upon a 'gap-filling' activity, as in completing an incomplete sentence or story. Despite its manifest transparency and the ease with which it can be faked, sentence completion, in light of accumulated research, has proved valuable as an auxiliary avenue for assessing personality.

After over eight decades of use, projective techniques remain controversial. In general, they stand in a nonrandom, but highly imperfect, relationship to their nontest referents. They work better in identifying broad and general tendencies of behaviour than in predicting specific acts. Their continued use and study, despite some loss of popularity in the 1970s, is linked to views which emphasize the importance of a person's subjective experience not only as a determinant of his behaviour, but also as a worthy subject of knowledge in its own right.

Juris G. Draguns
Pennsylvania State University

References

Bruner, J. S. (1948), 'Perceptual theory and the Rorschach test', *Journal of Personality*, 17.

Epstein, S. (1966), 'Some theoretical considerations on the nature of ambiguity and the use of stimulus dimensions in projective techniques', *Journal of Consulting Psychology*, 30.

Frank, L. K. (1939), 'Projective methods for the study of personality', *Journal of Psychology*, 8.

Fulkerson, S. C. (1965). 'Some implications of the new cognitive theory for projective tests', *Journal of Consulting Psychology*, 29.

Further Reading

Rabin, A. J. (ed.) (1981), *Assessment with Projective Techniques: A Concise Introduction*, New York.

Semeonoff, B. (1976), *Projective Techniques*, London.

Psychiatry

Psychiatry is a speciality of medicine concerned with the diagnosis, treatment and study of mental diseases or disorders. Its practitioners are psychiatrists (in the United States, physicians who complete four years of approved training following their graduation from medical school). A number of professionals from other disciplines treat patients with psychiatric disorders. The most important of these are clinical psychologists, psychiatric social workers and psychiatric nurses. They commonly refer to those who seek help as 'clients' rather than 'patients'. These professionals may work in various collaborative relationships with psychiatrists or as independent practitioners. They employ the same verbal therapies as psychiatrists. Psychiatry differs from these specialities in being a medical discipline whose practitioners are physicians. As such, psychiatrists are specifically trained to (1) make precise syndromal or aetiological diagnoses, whenever possible, and distinguish one syndrome from another; (2) diagnose (or know when to refer to other physicians) those organic conditions which mimic psychiatric disorders. such as brain tumour, cancer of the pancreas, and hyperthyroidism (these conditions can present as anxiety or depressive disorders); (3) treat particular psychiatric disorders with psychotropic medications or other somatic treatments; (4) manage untoward psychological reactions to medical illness; and (5) integrate the biological with the psychological and social dimensions of mental disorders. In addition, the psychiatrist's training in medicine may encourage a research career in the biology of mental disorders. American psychiatrists as a whole have a high level of expertise in psychological treatments, particularly the psychodynamic approach. This is due to the impact of psychoanalytic theory on academic psychiatry especially since 1945, when many distinguished psychoanalysts assumed the chairs of academic departments.

Psychiatry relates closely to other medical specialities such as internal medicine, family medicine, neurology and pediatrics as well as to many scientific disciplines that contribute to the understanding of mental disorders. These include psychology, epidemiology, anthropology, sociology, genetics, and biochemistry.

The Range of Psychiatric Disorders
Although abnormal states of thinking, feeling, and behaving may be studied and treated in isolation, more often they are understood as part of specific syndromes, disorders, or diseases. In the US the most widely accepted classification of psychiatric disorders is presented in the American Psychiatric Association's third edition of the Diagnostic and Statistical Manual of Mental Disorders (DSM-III). Although developed by psychiatrists in the United States, this classification is widely used by psychiatrists in other countries, and by other mental health professionals. The classification attempts to provide a comprehensive description of the manifestations of mental disorders while remaining atheoretical with regard to aetiology. A related

classification of mental disorders with broad international acceptance is the ninth edition of the International Classification of Disease (ICD-9).

The following are the major categories of psychiatric disorders according to DSM-III:
- Disorders Usually First Evident in Infancy, Childhood, or Adolescence
- Organic Mental Disorders
- Substance Abuse Disorders
- Schizophrenic Disorders
- Paranoid Disorders
- Psychotic Disorders Not Elsewhere Classified
- Affective Disorders
- Anxiety Disorders
- Somatoform Disorders
- Dissociative Disorders
- Psychosexual Disorders
- Factitious Disorders
- Disorders of Impulse Control Not Elsewhere Classified
- Adjustment Disorders
- Psychological Factors Affecting Physical Condition
- Personality Disorders

The manual describes subcategories of the above major categories together with specific defining criteria for each disorder. There is a high degree of reliability for most of the disorders; that is, two observers of the same patient are likely to agree on the diagnosis. There is considerable variability in the established validity of these diagnostic categories.

Family and couple therapists criticize DSM-III on the grounds that they regard the couple or the family, not the patient, as the pathologic unit. Behaviour therapists criticize DSM-III on grounds that it is the thought, feeling, or behaviour, not the syndrome or disease, that is the pathologic unit. Psychodynamic clinicians are apt to view psychopathology as part of a continuum based on the concept of 'developmental lines', rather than as discrete disease entities. In addition, they believe that each patient can be described only by a unique and complex formulation. Diagnostic categories are regarded therefore as both conceptually incorrect as well as oversimplifications of human problems. Despite these criticisms, there is a growing consensus amongst US psychiatrists that DSM-III will prevail and continue to grow in importance through future editions.

There are two extreme and opposing positions regarding psychiatric disease: (1) that psychopathology, both social and individual, is everywhere and that therapeutic intervention may be useful for all human conditions; (2) that mental illness is a myth, and therefore lies out of the purview of medicine.

Conceptual Models in Psychiatric Thinking

There are many conceptual frameworks by which psychiatrists attempt to organize their thinking about patients with mental disorders. The presence of multiple approaches, particularly when thay are not made explicit, commonly leads to misunderstanding amongst psychiatrists and between psychiatrists and other medical professionals, mental health professionals, and patients. The four conceptual models most often used are (1) the biologic; (2) psychodynamic; (3) sociocultural and (4) the behavioural.

(1) According to the biologic model, psychiatric illness is a disease like any other. Its cause will be found to be related to disorders of genetics, biochemistry, and/or the functional anatomy of the brain. Abnormal behaviours are understood as partial manifestations of a syndrome or underlying disease process. In his relationship to the patient, the biologic psychiatrist behaves like any other physician: he elicits the history through careful questioning, establishes a diagnosis and recommends a treatment plan which the patient is expected to accept. The biologic approach, after giving psychiatry its classification of mental illness in the late nineteenth century, was generally unproductive until the 1950s. From that time until the present its contributions to psychiatry have included the development of antipsychotic, antidepressant, and antimania medications; the increased understanding of the genetic transmission of some mental illness; and metabolic studies of

depressive disorders. The biologic model has been least helpful in the study of the neuroses and personality disorders.

(2) According to the psychodynamic model, it is the development deficit, fixation, regressive response to current stress, and/or conflict within the mind that leads to psychiatric symptoms. The symptom represents both an expression of an underlying conflict as well as a partial attempt to resolve it. The concept of unconscious mental processes is all important. In the relationship to the patient, the therapist assumes a nondirective posture in order to elicit meaningful associations, as well as to develop a transference reaction in which the patient reacts to the therapist as he would to other important people in his life. The psychodynamic model had its origin with Sigmund Freud in the late nineteenth and early twentieth centuries. There have been significant theoretical developments since 1950 in ego psychology, object relations theory, and self psychology. Although the psychodynamic model is a general psychology of normal and abnormal behaviour, it is most helpful in the understanding and treatment of neuroses and personality disorders.

(3) The sociocultural model focuses on the way the individual functions within his social system. Symptoms are traced not to conflicts within the mind nor to manifestations of psychiatric disease, but to disruptions or changes in the social support system. According to the sociocultural approach, symptoms, disorders, or the designation that someone is mentally ill may be seen as social phenomena: responses to breakdown or disorganization of social groupings, attempts at social communication, a cultural or ethnic expression of distress, or a message by the social group that certain behaviours are no longer acceptable. Treatment consists in helping the patient deal better with the existing social system. The sociocultural approach was reawakened in the 1950s. From that time until the present, the psychiatric ward was viewed as a social system, the relationship between social class and mental illness was established, and federal legislation was enacted to provide psychiatric care for catchment areas in the community.

(4) The behavioural model regards symptoms in their own

right as the problem. Symptoms are manifestations neither of disease, intrapsychic conflict, nor social breakdown. In order to develop a treatment strategy, the behavioural formulation takes into account conditions antecedent to and reinforcing of the pathologic behaviours. The behavioural model, like the three models previously discussed, began its period of rapid growth in the late 1950s. Behavioural therapists are hopeful of offering several possible advantages to other forms of treatment including a shorter duration of treatment and applicability to a broad range of patients.

Which conceptual approach a psychiatrist uses depends on several factors including his own training and ideology, the diagnosis of the patient, and the availability of clinical services. The use of a single approach to explain all psychopathology (including the belief that all psychopathology will ultimately be explained by biochemistry) is reductionistic. In optimal clinical practice, the psychiatrist attempts to understand the patient simultaneously by means of several conceptual approaches or frames of references, with the understanding that even the four approaches described above may not exhaust the ways in which psychopathology of people can be understood. Various attempts to integrate several conceptual frameworks have been referred to as systems theory, biopsychosocial approach, multidimensional approach, or eclecticism.

Psychiatric Treatments

Psychiatric treatments can be divided into two major categories: the biologic approaches (somatotherapy) and the psychologic or verbal therapeutic approaches. The most commonly used somatic treatments are drugs followed by electroconvulsive treatments. Other somatic treatments much less used include insulin treatment and neurosurgery. Drugs may be divided into four major groups: (1) the anti-anxiety agents; (2) antidepressant agents; (3) antimanic agents; and (4) antipsychotic agents. The anti-anxiety agents such as Librium and Valium are useful in the short-term treatment of some anxiety states. Their sedative-hypnotic effect makes them also useful for the short-term treatment of insomnia. This class of anti-anxiety agents (benzodiazepines), because of their relative safety, has rendered the barbiturates virtually obsolete. Antidepressant agents such as Tofranil and Elavil (tricyclics) and Nardil (MAO inhibiter) reverse depressive symptomatology while the antimanic agents such as Lithium Carbonate reverse symptoms of mania or hypomania while sometimes functioning as an antidepressant. The antipsychotic agents such as Haldol and Thorazine are useful in managing the excitement, delusions, hallucinations, and disorientation of various psychotic states in schizophrenia, depressive psychoses, and organic psychoses. With prolonged use, the antipsychotic agents can cause tardive dyskinesia, a permanent involuntary movement disorder involving primarily the tongue, neck, and facial muscles. Electroconvulsive therapy, the passage of electrical current through the brain, is used primarily for depressed patients for whom drug therapy has failed, has or will produce serious side effects, or will take too long before exerting a therapeutic effect.

There are hundreds of psychologic treatments. They may be classified according to theoretical approach, structure of the treatment, and duration. In terms of ideology the psychodynamic approach, based on the principles of psychoanalytic theory, is the most widely used. Behaviour therapies which include the specific techniques of relaxation, cognitive restructuring, and flooding have made major inroads in clinical practice during the past twenty-five years. In addition, there are various interpersonal, existential, Jungian, Adlerian, and other therapies. To what degree specific dimensions of each ideological approach are uniquely therapeutic and to what degree there are common therapeutic dimensions of many approaches is a subject of considerable interest. As to structure, the therapist may treat the patient alone, with a spouse, as part of a family, together with a broader social network, or with a group of other patients. When therapy is provided to a couple or to a family, then the couple or family, not the individual, may be regarded as the patient. Most therapies take place once a week but may occasionally be as infrequent as once a month or as frequent as four or five times per week as in psychoanalysis. Depending on the goals of treatment, the sessions may range from one visit (evaluation), eight to twelve visits (brief or short-term therapy), one to four years (long-term therapy), or three to seven years (psychoanalysis). Treatment may take place in a private office, in a mental health centre, or in a psychiatric inpatient unit.

The therapeutic efficacy of the somatic treatments is well established. The efficacy of particular psychological treatments for designated symptoms or disorders has been receiving increasing confirmation during the past ten years. For certain depressive and schizophrenic disorders, it has been established that a combination of drug and psychological or social treatments is more effective than either used alone. Psychiatric treatment has also been shown to diminish patients' use of medical facilities.

Psychiatry – Past and Future
Psychiatric illness is not new to modern society. In the Hippocratic writings (400 B.C.) there are clear descriptions of the major psychiatric disorders. Throughout the centuries psychopathology was described, explained, and classified by the great physicians of the time. The degree of sophistication, or lack thereof, paralleled that for medicine in general. There was no autonomous discipline of psychiatry.

The historian George Mora divides modern scientific psychiatry into three overlapping periods: (1) From 1800 to 1860, the mental hospital, or asylum, was the centre of psychiatric activity. It was staffed by a new type of physician, the alienist, totally devoted to the care of the mentally ill. The major accomplishments of this period were the practice of 'moral therapy', the description and classification of mental disorders, and the study of brain anatomy. Famous names associated with this period are Esquirol, Morel, Kahlbaum, Tuke, Rush, and Ray. (2) From 1860 to 1920, the centre of psychiatry moved from the hospital to the university which could simultaneously treat patients, teach, and do research. The important names of this era include Griesinger, Meynert, Forel, Bleuler, Charcot, Jackson, Kraepelin, A. Meyer, and S. Freud. It was Kraepelin who provided a classification of mental disorders that is the intellectual precursor of DSM-III. Meyer developed the psychobiologic approach, trained a whole generation of leaders in American psychiatry and provided the fertile ground for the growth of psychoanalysis in this country. (3) The period from 1920 to the present has been referred to as the 'psychiatric explosion'. As described earlier, the greatest expansion of knowledge in psychodynamic, sociocultural, biologic, and behavioural approaches began in the 1950s.

It is anticipated that within the next one to two decades there will be important new developments in psychiatry. These will include: (1) greater sophistication in nosology with improved validity for certain diagnostic categories; at the same time there will be philosophical and empirical sophistication in understanding the limitations of the diagnostic or categorical approach to other mental disturbances; (2) significant advances in understanding the biology of mental processes in general and of the depressive and schizophrenic disorders in particular; (3) significant advances in the evaluation of psychologic therapies so that more effective matches can be made between disorder and treatment; (4) significant advances in the integration of biologic, psychodynamic, behavioural, and social approaches to the diagnosis and treatment of mental disorders; (5) advances in the integrative efforts between psychiatry and other medical disciplines such as neurology, medicine, and paediatrics.

The advances described above will further define psychiatry both as a mental health profession and as a medical speciality.

Aaron Lazare
Massachusetts General Hospital

Further Reading

American Psychiatric Association (1980), *Diagnostic and Statistical Manual of Mental Disorders (DSM-III)*, 3rd edn, New York.

Baldessarini, R. (1983), *Biomedical Aspects of Depression and Its Treatment*, Washington, DC.

Brenner, C. (1982), *The Mind in Conflict*, New York.

Gedo, J. E. and Goldberg, A. (1973), *Models of the Mind: A Psychoanalytic Theory*, Chicago.

Greenhill, M. and Gralnick, A. (1983), *Psychopharmacology and Psychotherapy*, New York.

Lazare, A. (1973), 'Hidden conceptual models in clinical psychiatry', *New England Journal of Medicine*, 288.

Lazare, A. (1979), 'Hypothesis testing in the clinical interview', *in Outpatient Psychiatry: Diagnosis and Treatment*, Baltimore.

Lishman, W. (1978), *Organic Psychiatry: The Psychological Consequences of Cerebral Disorder*, Oxford.

Papajohn, I. (1982), *Intensive Behavior Therapy: The Behavioral Treatment of Complex Emotional Disorders*, New York.

Rutter, M. and Hersov, L. (eds) (1984), *Child Psychiatry – Modern Approaches*, 2nd edn, Oxford.

See also: *biological psychiatry; DSM-111; mental disorders; mental health; psychoanalysis; psychopharmacology.*

Psychoanalysis

Psychoanalysis is a procedure for the treatment of mental and emotional disturbances. Sigmund Freud originated and developed psychoanalysis as a result of his individual researches into the causes of hysteria, one of the common forms of mental illness in Europe in the latter part of the nineteenth century (see Jones, 1953).

The unique characteristic of psychoanalysis as a therapy derives from its theory of psychopathology. The central finding of psychoanalysis is that mental and emotional disturbances result from unconscious mental life. Treatment therefore depends upon the ability of the patient, with the help of the analyst, to reveal unconscious thoughts and feelings. The formula that propelled the psychoanalytic method from its inception ('what is unconscious shall be made conscious') remains vitally significant today. The changes that have occurred in the formula have resulted from a broadened and deepened understanding of the nature of unconscious mental life and how it functions developmentally in relation to consciousness and to the environment.

According to Freud's first conception of symptom formation, morbid thought patterns occurred during a dissociated state and were prevented from normal discharge because of the altered states of consciousness. The undischarged tensions produced symptoms. The cure required some method of discharge – an abreaction or mental catharsis. By applying hypnosis, the noxious material could be brought to the surface and discharged through verbal association. This chain of inference, formulated first in collaboration with Joseph Breuer (1842–1925) who described his clinical experience in treating a female patient he named Anna O. (Freud, 1955, Vol. II) was dependent upon a quantitative hypothesis concerning unconscious mental life and its relation to conscious states. In this prepsychoanalytic period of research, excessive excitation and the blockage of discharge were thought to produce pathological effects.

A major shift occurred both in research and in the explanatory theory toward the turn of the century. Freud recognized, largely through his self-analysis but also through careful attention to what his patients told him, that a qualitative factor was as important as the quantitative in the pathological process. The unconscious thoughts and feelings contained sexual content and meaning which was linked to arousal, or in earlier language, the quantity of excitation.

The introduction of the qualitative factor altered the theory of neurosis and the therapeutic procedure and, indeed, the method of research. Instead of managing a procedure designed to discharge quantities of noxious excitation stored within the psyche, the problem shifted to uncovering the meaning of the symptoms, and, through association, their roots in the unconscious. Hypnosis no longer served the purpose, since it was imperative that the entire treatment procedure elicit the full participation of the patient. Freud asked his patients to recline on the couch and to say whatever came to mind. This method, called 'free association', created a contradiction in terms. Freud discovered that it was difficult for the patient to carry out his request. Difficulty in associating did not seem to be a random effect, but along with the symptoms could be understood as an inherent aspect of the patient's manner of thinking and feeling and the particular form and content of the presenting symptoms. Freud visualized the difficulties of free association as *resistance* and as part and parcel of the problem of unconscious content, attempting to break through the barriers that guarded conscious mental life.

The research and treatment method, called psychoanalysis, replicated the individual's intrapsychic struggle with the unconscious. Freud's model of neurotic suffering combined both the quantitative and qualitative ideas in the concept of intrapsychic conflict. Symptoms, those alien and debilitating conditions, appear as a result of conflict within the psyche.

According to this model, the terms of neurotic conflict begin with desire; the aim is gratification. The impulse to act, to seek direct gratification of desire, is inhibited by restrictive forces within the psyche. The most familiar type of restriction arises from the individual's moral standards, which render unacceptable the direct gratification of desire. This opposition of the forces of desire and morality produces the debilitating symptoms but in forms that will allow a measure of gratification of desire, however small and costly. Symptoms, resulting from intrapsychic conflict, are the individual's best effort at compromise.

However, as Freud discovered, symptom formation, since it utilizes compromises, follows principles of mental function which apply across a broad spectrum of activity. Therefore, the dynamics of intrapsychic conflict go beyond the pathological and enter into the realm of a general psychology. Normal mental activity such as dreaming, to cite one illustration, follows the same principle as the activity that leads to symptom formation (Freud, 1955, Vols IV and V). A dream is a symptom of mental conflict since it represents a compromise among forces in the unconscious that simultaneously push toward gratification of desire while inhibiting this tendency. The symbolic content of the dream disguises the conflict but also expresses all the terms of the conflict – both desire and prohibition.

This model of intrapsychic conflict underwent a variety of modifications throughout Freud's lifetime. For example, the idea of desire shifted from a dual instinct theory of sex and self-preservation to a dual instinct theory of sex and aggression. Closer attention to the object of desire (in contrast to the aim of discharge) revealed that while its normal pathway was outward toward objects and the environment, it could turn inward, particularly during stressful episodes in the individual's life. But even where desire turned inward, the object remained important in the psychoanalytic theory of conflict because of the observation that the individual retained an internalized image of the object, while seemingly relinquishing it in its real form. Even in the case of the most severe psychological disturbances – psychoses – the individual may appear uninterested in the object world, but the internal conflict evolves around the representations of these objects both in their beneficent and malevolent forms.

The formalization of the model of conflict led to the structural hypothesis which postulates three parts of the psychic structure: id, super-ego, and ego. The id is the part of the mind which generates desire, both sexual and aggressive impulses. The super-ego is the agency that involves the conscience (the imperatives of 'thou shalt not') and the ideals (the imperatives that one must achieve in order to feel loved and to experience self-esteem). The ego is the executive apparatus that consists of a variety of functions which together mediate the terms of the conflict between id, super-ego and, finally, reality.

Several problems arise in the application of the structural hypothesis, indeed, in working with all of these superordinate hypotheses in psychoanalytic theory. The hypothesis, called the metapsychology of psychoanalysis, poses a number of problems in application, both in strict scientific research as well as in clinical work. Some of these problems can be dismissed readily, such as the use of the structural hypothesis as though it referred to 'real' agencies of the mind. The id, super-ego, and ego are abstract concepts, an attempt to organize a theory of conflict. They are not anatomical entities, nor are they especially valuable as a guide to the phenomenology of conflict. But the structural hypothesis and the concepts of id, super-ego and ego serve a number of intellectual purposes in the theory of psychoanalysis. One example is the concept of resistance, or what prevents unconscious content from direct appearance in conscious images and thoughts. The work of psychoanalysis indicates that the derivatives of unconscious mental life are omnipresent in consciousness, but in such indirect and disguised forms (except in the case of delusional thinking and hallucinations) as to stretch credulity about the idea of unconscious derivatives affecting conscious thinking and activity. The structural hypothesis organizes Freud's observations and conclusions about resistance as a part of unconscious mental life: he posited the need to broaden the term of resistance (from barriers to consciousness) to defence as an unconscious function of the ego to limit the danger that occurs when the pressure to act on impulses becomes great (Freud, 1955, Vol. XX).

Another problem with the structural hypothesis of psychoanalysis derives from the logical consequences of using this hypothesis to distinguish among and explain the forms and functions of various pathologies. Psychological conflict implies that a psychic structure exists within the individual, so that, for example, moral imperatives no longer depend upon the parents for their force. The individual has a conscience which inflicts some measure of painful anxiety and guilt when unconscious desire seeks gratification.

The classical theory of psychoanalysis presumes that psychic conflict and structure become established during the last stages of infantile development, which is called the Oedipal stage (Freud, 1955, Vol. VII). In relinquishing incestuous desire, the child of approximately age five identifies with the objects and consequently emerges from infancy with a reasonably self-contained psychic structure. The pathologies linked to conflict in psychic structure, the transference neuroses, include hysteria, obsessional neuroses and related character neuroses. These pathologies are called transference neuroses because they do not impair the patient's ability, despite pain and suffering, to establish attachments to objects. However, the attachments are neurotically based in that the patient shifts the incestuous struggle from parents to other people. In the transference neuroses, the relationship to objects is not totally determined by the persistence of neurotic disturbance. For example, a person may be able to function reasonably well with other people except that he is incapable of sexual intimacy as a result of neurotic inhibition.

Psychoanalytic investigation, especially of the post-World War II period, has given rise to doubt about some of the formulations of the structural hypothesis and some of its derivatives in the explanation of pathologies. For example, can one clearly differentiate structural conflict from earlier developmental problems which derive from the deficits of infancy? The investigation of borderline conditions (a consequence of developmental deficits) or narcissistic disturbances (the conditions of impaired self-esteem and painful self-awareness), suggest that early internalizations of objects so colour the later identifications as to minimize the effects of psychological structure (see Segal, 1964). Critics argue that to treat such patients using classical techniques will prove futile. On the more theoretical plane, the critics also dispute the distinction between transference and narcissistic disturbances because of the importance of object attachments in the latter category of disturbance. Perhaps underlying the controversies within the psychoanalytic profession are more fundamental differences than the suggestion that one or more hypotheses are open to question. After all, any scientific endeavour attempts to disprove hypotheses and to modify the theory as a result of fresh observation and experimentation.

Almost from its inception, psychoanalysis has been the centre of debate in which the contenders, more than disputing particular hypotheses, are engaged in a test of contradictory world views. As indicated earlier, a tension inherent in psychoanalytic observation and explanation pervades the field. The dialectics of quantity and quality, of mechanics and meaning, colour the evaluation and practice in the field. The tension extends into more abstract polarities: humanity between science and humanism, tragic and utopian views of humanity, and conservative versus imperialistic visions of the place of psychoanalysis in improving human relations.

Freud cautioned against abandoning points of view implicit in the quantitative and qualitative position in psychoanalysis.

While he was an artist in his observation of pathology and mental function (see, for example, Freud's exquisite narrative of an obsessional illness in his case 'The Rat Man' (Freud, 1955, Vol. (X)), Freud never abandoned the theory of instincts and its grounding in biology. From early on, the disputes in psychoanalysis have resulted from attempts to frame the theories of pathology and therapy along a single dimension, what Freud called the error of *pars pro toto*, or substituting the part for the whole. Thus, in contemporary psychoanalysis, the stress on developmental deficits over structural conflict arises in part from a humanistic perspective and leads to the use of the therapist not as an object in a transference drama that requires interpretation, but as a surrogate who will use his beneficent office to overcome the malevolence of the past, particularly of early infancy. These debates within psychoanalysis have strong intellectual, as well as cultural and philosophical, foundations. Some investigators place psychoanalysis squarely in the midst of interpretive disciplines rather than the natural sciences (Ricoeur, 1970). They link psychoanalysis to hermeneutics, linguistics and the humanities as against biology, medicine, psychiatry and the sciences. These debates also have economic and political ramifications concerning what constitutes the psychoanalytic profession and the qualifications of those who seek to enter its practice.

Psychoanalysis began as a medical discipline for the treatment of neurotic disturbances. It continues this therapeutic tradition of classical psychoanalysis in broadened application to the psychoses, borderline and narcissistic conditions through variants of psychoanalytic psychotherapy. As a result of its methods of investigation, its observations and theories, psychoanalysis has become a part of the general culture. The applications of psychoanalysis in literary criticism, history, political and social sciences, law and business are evidence of its infusion into the general culture. Writers, artists and critics, while debating the uses of psychoanalysis beyond the couch, understand the theory and experiment with its applications to the arts. Freud gave birth to a therapy and a theory and perhaps beyond his intent, to a view of the world and the human condition.

Abraham Zaleznik
Harvard University

References

Freud, S. (1953–66), *Standard Edition of the Complete Psychological Works of Sigmund Freud*, 24 vols, edited by J. Strachey, London.

Jones, E. (1953), *Sigmund Freud: Life and Work*, 3 vols, London.

Ricoeur, P. (1970), *Freud and Philosophy: An Essay on Interpretation*, New Haven.

Segal, H. (1964), *Introduction to the Work of Melanie Klein*, New York.

See also: *countertransference; defences; free association; Freud, S.; hysteria; Klein; super-ego; transference; unconscious.*

Psychology

Almost a hundred years ago, William James (1890) epitomized psychology as 'the science of mental life'. It is the discipline that gathers together all those who have a systematic interest in the mind and its workings, in people and the lives they lead. To say this, though, is to pose a puzzle, even a paradox. For what the visitor finds, when he enters a university department of psychology, opens a textbook of psychology, or dips into psychology's professional journals, seems both startling in its diversity, and, often, to have little to do either with the mind or with people. It is this puzzle that an account pf psychology must explain.

Looking back to James and his contemporaries, the founding fathers of psychology, one sees scarcely a trace of the diversity to follow, or of the retreat, real or apparent, from their conception of the psychologist's subject-matter. These men wrote about the mind and about people, and did so without embarrassment. Francis Galton, for instance, allowed his curiosity to range from hereditary studies of genius, the invention of rudimentary statistics and the first attempts to test intelligence, to discussions of the mind that sit comfortably beside those of the early psychoanalysts. While Freud was still a young man, with his life's work ahead of him, Galton (1883) wrote: 'There seems to be a presence chamber in my mind where full consciousness holds court, and where two or three ideas are at the same time in audience, and an ante-chamber full of more or less allied ideas, which is situated just beyond the full ken of consciousness. Out of this ante-chamber the ideas most nearly allied to those in the presence-chamber appear to be summoned in a mechanically logical way, and to have their turn of audience.' Beyond or below this ante-chamber, Galton also discerned 'a darker basement, a storehouse from which older and remoter ideas can with greater difficulty be called up into consciousness.' Such language and assumptions were accessible not only to Galton's academic neighbours, but also to those outside psychology; Poincaré, for example, the great French mathematician, was intrigued by the source of his own mathematical insights, which seemed to arrive unbidden (Hadamard, 1945).

Without question, Galton's imagination was circumscribed by what we now see as ugly Victorian prejudices. 'It is in the most unqualified manner,' he said (1883) 'that I object to pretensions of natural equality.' He also observed that 'The mistakes the negroes made in their own matters were so childish, stupid, and simpleton-like, as frequently to make me ashamed of my own species.' Nowadays we would expect Galton to distinguish altogether more crisply between questions of diversity, essential to our evolution as a species, and questions of value. Nevertheless, he entertained the great problems of human self-awareness, and did so with unbridled energy. Thus, one morning, he decided that he would view the world around him as though being spied upon (Burt, 1961). By the time his walk was over 'every horse on every cabstand seemed to be watching me either openly or in disguise'. These 'persecutory delusions' lasted for the rest of the day, and could be revived at will three months later.

In the years after the First World War, the intellectual freedom of men like Galton was gradually abandoned.

Psychology became the focus of a new enthusiasm: behaviourism. Under this influence, psychology, then establishing itself as an academic subject in universities, began to settle upon two of its abiding preoccupations: the first, with its status as a science, as opposed to a scholarly pursuit like history or a therapeutic one like medicine; the second, with the need to banish from the discipline all 'subjective' considerations, all mention of mental states, and to root psychology instead in the prediction of relationships between stimulus and response.

Gradually, throughout the 1930s and 1940s, the influence of behaviourism strengthened; to the extent that, by the early 1950s, the subject-matter of psychology itself had been redefined. Instead of being taught that psychology was the science of mental life, students were taught that it was the 'science of behaviour' (Skinner, 1953). The behaviour in question, their professors made plain, was not just that of human beings, but of all animal species, from octopus to man – and these creatures, not in their wild state, but in the artificial environment of the laboratory.

Behaviourism was to remain the dominant orthodoxy in university departments of psychology until the late 1960s, when doubts were voiced (for example, Kagan, 1967; Hudson, 1972). The mood, since, has grown more pluralistic. While behaviourism produced neither the centrally placed bodies of knowledge nor the intellectual mastery that pioneers like Watson and Skinner promised, its legacy is all round us, in that the activities of professional psychologists make less than complete sense if this influence is ignored. The anxiety over psychology's status as a science remains, scarcely abated; and so too does the distrust of any argument that cannot be tethered to objective evidence about what people, animals or, more recently, computers can be seen to do.

Worries about the scientific respectability of psychology have led, in turn, to a sense of hierarchy within psychology. Precisely controlled experimental research, designed to test a theory that is itself carefully formulated, is highly regarded; field research or research which is geared to the practical needs of the world at large have a lower status. As in the scientific community as a whole, the pure is elevated over the applied. The subject-matter of academic psychology has organized itself, too, around a variety of abstract themes: learning, memory, attention, motivation, intelligence, personality, creativity, and so on. Pursuing these, psychologists have sometimes seemed to execute a wilful retreat from questions of practical relevance.

In the 1950s, when this retreat was at its most pronounced, it seemed at times that psychological research enjoyed higher prestige the further removed from ordinary human concerns it became. Experimental studies, of course, were not always narrowly conceived; Gregory's (1966) work on visual illusions, for example, combined elegance with a wider sense of implication. But research on issues of pressing social concern was usually treated, in comparison, as suspect. McClelland's (1961) studies of the motives of the entrepreneur were accorded a certain respect, as was the work, inspired by Nazi Germany, on the authoritarian personality (Adorno, 1950), and the research by social psychologists like Asch (1955) and Milgram (1963) on social pressure and compliance. Even here, though, the lure of theory, and of the apparent rigour of tests and statistics, were sometimes to prove disruptively strong. Only rather exceptionally did psychologists study a pertinent slice of life without the protection of either, as Bronfenbrenner (1970) was to do in his comparison of Russian and American experiences of childhood.

Another feature of psychology at this stage in its growth, despite its optimism and energy, was its reliance on sources outside itself for new initiatives. Obvious instances are the impact on the discipline of the early information theorists and of a linguist like Chomsky. Another instance, more subtle, is that of Kelly (1955). His background was complex: first in mathematics and physics, then in educational sociology and psychology. He earned a living as an aeronautical engineer before settling on a career in psychology. Perhaps because of this grounding, half inside psychology, half out, his work on the semantics of everyday life has remained fertile, even though the area was one that more conventional psychologists like Osgood (1957) had already begun to develop. In the hands of

the orthodox, the wider implications of a good idea were sometimes buried beneath technique that was rigorous but subtly
misplaced, evidence that was copious but inconclusive. Preoccupied with questions of rigour, psychologists also allowed
academic neighbours like the sociologist Goffman (1959) to pre-
empt important parts of their own subject-matter, placing upon
it constructions in which psychological notions played only an
insignificant part.

Whatever its excesses, behaviourism helped establish a
concern for rigour over questions of method. Less directly, it
pointed to a source of uncertainty – and, hence, of diversity –
that lies at the very heart of psychology, and which refuses to
go away. For the study of the mind is based upon an unresolved,
and some would say unresolvable, tension: that between human
consciousness and the brain in which that consciousness is
housed. At the centre of psychology, there is the baffling relation
of the mind to body; of the meanings in terms of which human
beings order their lives, some crisply determinate, others
ambiguous, vague or half-hidden, and the central nervous
system without which such meanings could not exist.

In practice, psychologists leave the mind/body problem to
philosophers. The shape that their discipline takes nevertheless
reflects this point of strain. Psychologists have in the past tended
to form two camps: on the one hand, the 'soft', those concerned
with people, the relations between them, and the meanings with
which their lives are imbued; on the other, the 'hard', who are
committed to the study of the brain and how it works. The
'soft' have a natural affinity with social scientists, historians,
therapists, while the 'hard' have close links with brain chemists,
biologists, computer scientists.

This distinction between 'soft' and 'hard', although it still
enjoys wide currency, is an unfortunate one. It provides a
tempting line of fissure, and it is unrepresentative, too, of the
variety that the inhabitants of many psychology departments
nowadays display. If you walk into a psychology department,
anywhere in the Western world, and listen to what is taught,
or speak to the teachers about their research, you will probably
find as many instances that violate this simple distinction

between 'soft' and 'hard' as conform to it. In order to make sense of psychology as it now stands, another, more complex, model or metaphor is required.

Consider the members of staff in a particular department who have joined forces to teach an introductory course in psychology to first-year students (the instance is real rather than imagined). There are four of them. The first is a young woman who usually describes herself as a social psychologist. Her special concern is with stress, and her research has carried her into the clinical world, where she studies the anxieties experienced by surgical patients, especially those with breast cancer. She works in close collaboration with surgeons, and the aim of her research is in part the practical one of reducing the distress that serious illness and surgery induce.

Her teaching partner, in the first term of the course, is, superficially, of a different stamp. He was trained in a famous physiology department rather than a department of psychology, and his research is squarely scientific: it deals with the brain's ability to assimilate information reaching it from the eye, and he conducts it in a small, electrically-screened cubicle, with a high degree of experimental refinement and control. His interests in psychology range quite widely, but what he publishes is addressed to an audience that is very specialized indeed.

In the second term, another pair of lecturers take over. The first studies the relations of young mothers to their infants, the ways in which patterns of child-raising differ from one social class to another, and, more generally, the emergence of the individual's sense of identity – the ideas and commitments around which a sense of self is hung. Her partner started out in life as a mathematician. He is an expert in the study of memory and of mental imagery; and has carried out studies, for example, of the effects on memory of the kinds of head injury sustained in traffic accidents. More recently, he has become interested, too, in methods of teaching, and in the ways in which university students learn.

These four psychologists, members of a single department, plough four distinct furrows. Next year, their places on the introductory course could be taken by others. One, whose appointment is half in psychology, half in biology, specializes in animal behaviour, and is knowledgeable about the interaction of hereditary and environmental forces. He might speak to the students about the mating behaviour of red deer, or show them films of rats running in mazes. Another deals with psychoanalytic theory and feminism. Yet another does research on the chemistry of the brain, and hopes to shed light on the causes of senile dementia. A fourth is interested in the relation of Kelly's repertory grid analysis to information technology; a fifth pays systematic attention to the skill of reading.

The diversity that these academics represent is far greater than one would find in any other discipline on the university's campus. Yet they all see themselves and are seen by others as psychologists. They combine to teach the same students, and the students they teach see themselves, in turn, as becoming psychologists.

Despite their differences, a visitor might expect all these psychologists to share a belief in the same body of theories, in the sense that physicists share a belief in the theoretical edifice that Newton, Einstein, Hiesenberg and others have built. If so, he would be mistaken. There is no commonly accepted body of psychological theory. In practice, the best theorizing in psychology has been done at the local level, and attempts to create grand, overarching theories have met with little success.

This absence of a uniting theory may come as an uncomfortable surprise. Even more uncomfortable is the discovery that psychologists of different persuasions often have little to say to one another about research, and can differ with one another quite sharply about the kinds of psychology that students should be taught. They may disagree, for example, about whether a grounding in elementary statistics is essential, or whether students ahould be exposed to the ideas of Freud. Rather than exchanging views with one another, they often find it easier and more natural to talk to academic neighbours, outside psychology. The psychologist who specializes in animal behaviour may well find that he goes to conferences where he meets ethologists and geneticists, rather than psychologists whose special interests differ from his own. And his colleagues likewise.

Not only do many psychologists lack a driving interest in one another's research; it frequently happens that they cannot understand one another's publications. Thus a psychologist working on the computer simulation of short-term memory may find it hard, even impossible, to follow a paper written by a colleague who is excited by recent critiques of psychoanalytic theory, advanced by scholars on the Continent (see, for example, Bowie, 1979). And vice versa. At this point, the visitor may well protest that psychology is not a discipline at all; simply a cacophany, a muddle. To reach this conclusion is an error, however; and it is so, because it rests on an excessively simple view of what a discipline is like.

The point is best made in terms of diagrams, as Campbell (1977) suggests. The usual assumption about a discipline like chemistry is that it consists of a common core of agreed theory, and a number of subsidiary specialities or applications. In diagrammatic terms, this might be represented as a pyramid, or as a nest of concentric circles, like the layers of an onion. Pyramids and concentric circles are not the only diagrams one can draw, though. Consider this:

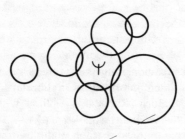

Figure 1

Psychology is represented by the centrally placed circle, marked 'Ψ'; other, related disciplines – social science, biology, computer science – by the adjacent circles. Some of the neighbouring circles overlap the 'psychological' circle, but none includes it. If the circle representing psychology is now abstracted from the rest, one sees this:

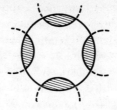

Figure 2

This diagram poses some interesting possibilities: for example, that it is in its areas of overlap with its neighbours – here, shaded – that the field of psychology is at its most exciting. It is in these zones of overlap that their interests bring the psychologist and his neighbours into contact – and, often, conflict. Thus both psychologist and computer scientist may have an interest in human memory, but very different presuppositions about how memory can best be explained. Likewise, psychologists and sociologists share an interest in crimes of violence but disagree sharply over their likely causes.

Analogous conflicts arise continually, and three or more disciplines sometimes stake a claim, as has happened in the field of sex and gender and the explanation of the psychological differences that men and women display. Those, like Kinsey, with a background in biology, have generated bodies of evidence about regularities in behaviour, although their researches, as it happened, were often informed by a libertarian, permissive system of moral values (Robinson, 1969). At the same time, evidence was drawn from anthropology, pioneers like Margaret Mead stressing the extent to which male and female patterns of behaviour were culturally rather than biologically determined (D'Andrade, 1967); and, then, from medicine and from within psychoanalytic tradition, there evolved a further body of work stressing the confusions of gender identity that can arise, and tracing these to the relation of the infant in question to the parent of the opposite sex (Stroller, 1968; Money and Ehrhardt, 1972). Into this area, there also moved endocrinologists, interested in the impact of sex hormones on behaviour; feminists, concerned with the extent to which evidence about sex differences becomes muddled with political prejudice; and those studying abnormalities of sexual behaviour – a perversion like fetishism, for instance, which seems a male preserve.

Such areas of overlap usually arise from contact between psychologists and their academic neighbours, but, from time to time, the contact is with specialists whose concerns are more immediately practical: the doctor concerned with the care of his patients, the police superintendent worried about relations between his junior officers and the Black community. Whether academic or practical, the moral pointed by the diagram is the same: intellectually, psychology is a discipline that thrives on exchange with the worlds of expertise that surround it.

Other morals flow too. If psychology is a field in which excitement characteristically arises around the edges, its heartland will consist not so much of specific theories or bodies of evidence, as of those broader concerns which have remained unchanged since psychology's beginnings as a branch of philosophy: the relation of mind to body, the origins of knowledge, the distinction between the real and the illusory. It is in their sensitivity to these centrally placed foci of conceptual unease that psychologists of quality mark themselves out from those whose contribution is more technical. It also follows that, in the shaded areas around the edge of the field, specialized languages and techniques will evolve in response to local needs. A consequence is that, considered as a whole, psychology will tend to be a polyglot, containing a number of languages rather than a single language. The risk, plainly, is that the task of translation will be skimped, and that psychology will tend to split apart as nations do. If this were to happen, professional life in the short run might be more tranquil, but the uniting commitment to the study of mental life would dissolve, and with it would be lost the chance to resolve the more complex problems that human beings pose.

Grant such a model of psychology, more complicated than the onion with its skins or the pyramid with its layers, but down-to-earth nonetheless, and what one finds inside a psychology department fits comfortably into place. The diversity and polygot nature of psychology represent not a lapse from some simple ideal, but the consequences that flow, quite properly, from the complexities of the psychologist's subject matter. This complexity, it is important to see, is not just a question of the styles that psychologists adopt, the schools of thought they form or the methods of inquiry they find it most comfortable to use. It is inherent in the problems themselves, as the work on sex and gender shows. The direction of an individual's sexual desires, his sense of his own maleness or femaleness, his presentation of himself in terms of his interests, habits and social style as typically male, typically female or more androgynous: all this will depend on physical questions – his chromosomes and sex hormones, his anatomy – but on these overlaid with the influence of parents and contemporaries and the values implicit in the wider culture. The confusions and perplexities that characterize this aspect of human experience demand patient scrutiny; and this, in its turn, may depend as much on clinical and on literary skills (see Brown, 1966; Gass, n.d.; Barthes, 1979) as it does on those of scientific research.

This point about the multifaceted nature of the psychologist's subject-matter can equally be made elsewhere. The question of mental illness, far from seeming depressing or sordid, is the focus of keen interest among laymen and psychologists alike. Insight into its causes or cure could come from a variety of quite different directions, and these could prove to be complementary. The attraction of mental illness as a research problem is precisely its many-sidedness.

The traditional view is that mental illness – or, more specifically, schizophrenia – is congenital. In support of this, there is the evidence of genetics. This shows that the closer the kinship between two people, the more likely both are to be schizophrenic, identical twins seeming to show the highest concordance of all (Kallmann, 1953). Adjacent, but separate, there is the work of the pharmacologists and brain chemists. They point to certain substances that can be recovered from the brains of schizophrenics that are not present in the same quantities in the brains of those who are not schizophrenic. Adjacent again, but again separate, there are arguments based on the analogy

with the computer: the suggestion, for instance, that the schizophrenic brain is like a computer suffering from information
overload.

Such theories and speculations can be categorized broadly as
'physical'. They have been subjected to vigorous attack over
the last twenty years or so. One onslaught (for example, Laing
and Esterson, 1964) advanced the claim that rather than going
mad, people are driven mad – and driven mad, characteristically, by parents who exert 'double binds' upon them. More
sweeping still has been the argument, often attractive to
students of social science, that schizophrenia is what results
when a society stigmatizes, isolates and humiliates its deviants,
a process in which orthodox psychiatrists are seen as playing a
malign role.

The key to the problem of schizophrenia, if there is one,
could emerge from any of four or five separate areas of research,
or from a combination of these. Along one path, a cure might
arise from better parental practices; along another, from a revolutionary new drug therapy.

At meetings between opposed camps, an air of awkwardness
often reigns, and, frequently, there are displays of mutual
incomprehension. More tellingly, though, rival camps also have
the chance to probe the logical weaknesses in each other's
positions. Thus it was quickly discovered that the genetic
evidence about identical twins was less conclusive than it
seemed, because identical twins share not only their genetic
endowment but very similar environments too (Newman, 1937).
In search of rigour, the debate was forced back from concordance in identical twins in general to concordance in those few
pairs who had been separated from birth, and whose environments had of necessity been different (Shields, 1962). Inexorably logical, this step precipitated another, however. Gradually,
research workers realized that, as they could not know in
advance which aspects of an individual's environment might
play a crucial part in causing schizophrenia, they had no means
of demonstrating that the separated twins' environments were
dissimilar in significant rather than trivial respects.

Step by step, in other words, the logical demands made upon

the competing bodies of evidence were sharpened; and, one after another, bodies of evidence which at first sight had seemed clinching were revealed as helpful but inconclusive. More generally, it was also realized that the discussion of causes was logically separate from the discussion of cures. Many participants in the debate about the causes of schizophrenia assumed that evidence from genetics must be resisted because it was evidence that schizophrenia could not be cured. Only slowly did it dawn that schizophrenia might prove to be genetically transmitted, after all, and yet that, in one form or another, perfectly satisfactory clinical or social treatments might nonetheless be established.

While the debate about the causes of schizophrenia has recently seemed to lose a little of its intensity, another topic, eclipsed for several decades, is now moving back towards the limelight: the question of why we dream. Again, this is multifaceted. A popular view, derived from Freud (Sulloway, 1979), is that we dream in order to fulfil repressed sexual wishes. This line of reasoning, which sees dreams as pregnant with hidden meaning, did not recommend itself to behaviourists, however, who professed to believe, many of them, that dreams do not exist; or, if they did, that they were purely random. The 1950s saw the establishment of laboratories for the study of sleep and dreaming. While important discoveries were made, the theorizing within these laboratories tended to be biological in inspiration. The dream, more often than not, was seen as a by-product of some physiological or chemical process in which a balance in the brain is restored (Oswald, 1980). More recently, analogies between brain and computer have led to the suggestion that the dreaming brain is akin to a computer in its 'off-line' state, during which its programmes are up-dated or 'cleaned'.

Such biological research nonetheless faced a difficulty: that of explaining the evolutionary function that sleep and dreaming must perform. The sleeping, dreaming animal is at the mercy of its predators; and any pattern of behaviour so blatantly dangerous must have a vital adaptive function if it is to survive. One task, then, is to state what this adaptive function is. Another is to explain (rather than explaining away) the widely held and carefully substantiated view that dreams, although in code, can sometimes serve as a complement to and comment upon waking thought (Rycroft, 1979); that, as Darwin (1871) observed, dreams are an involuntary kind of poetry.

Again, four or five bodies of evidence are relevant; there are four or five circles that can in principle overlap. Adopting an evolutionary frame of reference, and drawing heavily on the computer analogy, Crick and Mitchison (1983) have proposed that animals have the dreams associated with rapid eye movement sleep in order that their brains can clear themselves of 'parasitic' patterns of response; and that, without this capability, the brain would quickly become overloaded. A corollary of this argument, as the authors point out, is that we dream in order to forget; that dreams, on the whole, neither can nor should be recalled.

Such a theory is difficult if not impossible to test directly. One would have to show that the occurrence of a thought in an unrecalled dream reduces the likelihood of that thought recurring. On the other hand, it is an error to restrict psychology to the study of theories that can be directly verified or falsified; and an error, too, to assume that the issue of the dream's meaning is closed. Einstein was not alone among scientists in treating the dream as a useful source of insight, both in its own right and as part of a more general access to intuitive or imaginative modes of thought. There is no inherent reason why a theory like Crick and Mitchison's should not be modified to allow the brain to scan its own 'parasitic' products, and to glean from them ideas that it can set to good use. If this modification were adopted, dreams would be seen less as household rubbish, more as items jumbled together on a bric-a-brac stall, most virtually worthless, a few of genuine value and richly deserving rescue.

As with research on schizophrenia, there also exists the need to specify, with detachment and precision, what it is that dream theories are seeking to explain. In research on schizophrenia, there is still uncertainty about symptoms – whether 'thought disorder' is always present, and what 'thought disorders' consist of. Similarly with dreaming. The laboratory research on sleep and dreaming makes it clear that many dreams are more 'thought-like' than had previously seemed likely. This finding has implications that run in several directions. It brings to mind the possibility that this distinction between thought-like and dream-like dreams has its basis in the activities of the left and right cerebral hemispheres respectively. It raises once again the question of 'cognitive style' and the differences that individuals display in their access to the nonrational aspects of their own experience (Getzels and Jackson, 1962; Hudson, 1966); and it suggests that one might with profit look more closely at the dream-like states that occur while we are awake: not just reveries and fantasies, but at the dream-like states evoked in an altogether more disciplined and fastidious way in the verbal and visual arts (Hudson, 1982). As with schizophrenia, so with dreaming; a more scrupulous mapping of mental states could sharpen the pressures under which relatively simple-minded evolutionary and computer-based theories are at present placed.

Of course, not all debates in psychology appeal as directly to the layman as do those about schizophrenia or sleep and dreaming. Nor can all be contained relatively comfortably within frames of reference that are familiar. Sometimes, the discipline faces a challenge from outside, and one with implications that cannot be foreseen. One such is the computer.

While early computers were 'stupid', their descendants are showing signs of adaptability: the ability to learn from experience, and even to evolve their own instructions (Boden, 1977). Arguably, students of artificial intelligence can now learn from the adaptive systems that have evolved naturally: the brain and also the genetic mechanisms whereby inherited patterns of behaviour are passed from one generation to the next. It could be of real value to designers of artificial brains, for example, to know why natural brains dream. This new field – that of 'intelligent systems' – cuts across the established boundaries between computer science, biology and psychology, and it will be of interest to see how lively a part psychologists play in it.

The implications of the computer, though, are not tidily circumscribed. It opens a door onto an immediate future in which, to a wholly unprecedented degree, human beings will live in intimate contact with machines: not only the computer and word processor but the camera and television set – and these instruments not just as useful servants, but as devices that invade the individual's consciousness and alter it in both profound and superficial ways.

The tendency of psychology over the last half century, a period of massive professional growth and proliferation, has been somewhat inward-looking. It has addressed certain themes – ones that, over the years, have come to be seen as the 'classical' ones – and it has preserved from its formative stages a deep preoccupation with objectivity in judgement, correctness in method. Yet it seems unlikely that the human implications of information technology can satisfactorily be met from such a stance. Social change, both in this area and in others, will in all probability be too rapid and too radical.

Whether the question at issue is the human implication of the computer, or some other respect in which an advanced industrial society is subject to change – the impact, for example, of structural unemployment on the lives of those on whom idleness is imposed – the challenge is in principle the same. In order to make contributions of value, psychologists may have to recover some of the intellectual freedom and vitality (though not the ugly prejudices) that founding fathers like Galton and James enjoyed.

Liam Hudson
Brunel University, Uxbridge

References

Adorno, T. W. *et al.* (1950), *The Authoritarian Personality*, New York.

Asch, S. E. (1955), 'Opinions and social pressure', *Scientific American*.

Barthes, R. (1979), *A Lover's Discourse*, London.

Boden, M. (1977), *Artificial Intelligence and Natural Man*, Hassocks.

Bowie, M. (1979), 'Jacques Lacan', in J. Sturrock (ed.) *Structuralism and Since*, Oxford.

Bronfenbrenner, U. (1970), *Two Worlds of Childhood*, New York.

Brown, N. O. (1966), *Love's Body*, New York.

Burt, C. (1961), 'Galton's contribution to psychology', *Bulletin of the British Psychological Society*, 45.

Campbell, D. T. (1977), *Descriptive Epistemology*, preliminary draft of William James Lectures, Harvard University, unpublished.

Crick, F. and Mitchison, G. (1983), 'The function of dream sleep', *Nature*, 304.

D'Andrade, R. G. (1967), 'Sex differences and cultural institutions', in E. E. Maccoby (ed.), *The Development of Sex Differences*, London.

Darwin, C. (1871), *The Descent of Man*, London.

Galton, F. (1883), *Inquiries into Human Faculty*, London.

Gass, W. (no date), *On Being Blue*, Boston.

Getzels, J. W. and Jackson, P. W. (1962), *Creativity and Intelligence*, New York.

Goffman, E. (1959), *The Presentation of Self in Everyday Life*, New York.

Gregory, R. (1966), *Eye and Brain*, London.

Hadamard, J. (1945), *The Psychology of Invention in the Mathematical Field*, Princeton.

Hudson, L. (1966), *Contrary Imaginations*, London.

Hudson, L. (1972), *The Cult of the Fact*, London.

Hudson, L. (1982), *Bodies of Knowledge*, London.

James, W. (1890), *Principles of Psychology*, New York.

Kagan, J. (1967), 'On the need for relativism', *American Psychologist*, 22.

Kallmann, F. J. (1953), *Heredity in Health and Mental Disorder*, New York.

Kelly, G. A. (1955), *The Psychology of Personal Constructs*, New York.

Laing, R. D. and Esterson, A. (1964), *Sanity, Madness and the Family*, London.

McClelland, D. C. (1961), *The Achieving Society*, New York.

Milgram, S. (1963), 'Behavioral study of obedience', *Journal of Abnormal and Social Psychology*, 67.

Money, J. and Ehrhardt, A. A. (1972), *Man and Woman, Boy and Girl*, Baltimore.

Newman, H. H. *et al.* (1937), *Twins: A Study of Heredity and Environment*, Chicago.

Osgood, C. E. *et al.* (1957), *The Measurement of Meaning*, Urbana.

Oswald, I. (1980), *Sleep*, Harmondsworth.

Robinson, P. A. (1969), *The Sexual Radicals*, London.

Rycroft, C. (1979), *The Innocence of Dreams*, London.

Shields, J. (1962), *Monozygotic Twins Brought up Apart and Brought Up Together*, Oxford.

Skinner, B. F. (1953), *Science and Human Behavior*, New York.

Stoller, R. J. (1968), *Sex and Gender*, London.

Sulloway, F. J. (1979), *Freud, Biologist of the Mind*, London.

Psychopathic Personality

The condition of the psychopathic personality has been variously labelled by psychiatrists over the past two hundred years as 'hereditary moral insanity', 'constitutional psychopathic inferiority', 'psychopathic personality', 'sociopath', and more recently, 'antisocial personality disorder'. Each of these labels suggests a different aetiology. The aetiology remains debatable, and even the condition itself defies precise description.

Some psychiatrists regard this disorder as an unreliable category, as a 'wastebasket' condition which lacks the features of a genuine mental disorder. Critics of the psychopath label also decry the use of this term as obscuring what, in their view, is instead criminal, immoral or other situationally based behaviour. The supposed core of psychopathy includes egocentricity and lack of respect for the feelings and rights of others, coupled with persistent manipulative and/or antisocial behaviour – at times, of an aggressive, even violent, type. These core characteristics are manifested by certain criminals, but also by other, more outwardly successful, persons. As William McCord (1982) writes, 'The psychopath simply does not care, one way or another, about the communality of human beings known as society.'

While appearing superficially normal (because cognition is

intact and the individual does not manifest any obvious mental pathology) the psychopath's destructive pattern of activities is manifested over time, usually resulting in social and personal tragedies for himself and others.

The best-known modern criteria for psychopathic personality disorder were developed by Cleckley (1982). Cleckley's approach stresses the psychopath's persistent personality features such as untruthfulness and insincerity, poor judgement and failure to learn by experience, pathological egocentricity and incapacity for love, and inadequately motivated antisocial behaviour. Psychodynamically-oriented psychiatrists explain these features as attributable to pathological super-ego development, inner emptiness and compensatory impulsivity. Recent, more 'objective', non-aetiological diagnostic approaches recommended by the American Psychiatric Association (DSM-III) stress a constellation of long-standing antisocial behaviour dating from childhood, and poor adult work behaviour, violation of social and interpersonal norms, and impulsivity.

The prevalence of psychopathy in normal and criminal populations is unknown. Over the centuries, the aetiology has been variously attributed to genetic predisposition or other constitutional problems and, more recently, to emotional deprivation in childhood with poor, inconsistent and sadistic parenting. Biological theories are related to the psychopath's putative brain immaturity, autonomic nervous system defects which inhibit learning of social norms, or hormonal defects. In some instances, aspects of the psychopathic syndrome may appear following brain injury. However, the aetiology of psychopathy remains obscure and controversial.

Little is known about treatment. The natural history of this disorder, however, includes attrition with age of certain diagnostic features and psychopathic behaviour. After age forty, the psychopath is said to 'burn out'. Current treatment approaches (usually not successful) include milieu therapy to promote the psychopath's identification with better-adjusted, more prosocial peers. From the psychological or behavioural perspective, consistent, limit-setting treatment approaches are advocated. Individual psychotherapeutic work directed towards uncovering and resolving inner conflicts is usually not successful. The psychopath is neither a neurotic nor a psychotic. The nature and extent of past social adjustment (not the mental status) best predict the psychopath's future adjustment.

The challenge of psychopathy, including the appropriateness of categorizing mental disorders along somewhat vague socially based criteria, will probably persist for a long time.

Loren H. Roth
University of Pittsburgh

References
McCord, W. (1982), *The Psychopath and Milieu Therapy*, New York.
Cleckley, H. (1982), *The Mask of Sanity*, New York.
See also: *character disorders*.

Psychopharmacology

The last thirty years have witnessed dramatic progress in our knowledge of drugs to treat the major psychiatric disorders. Prior to the 1950s, psychiatrists possessed only a few nonspecific sedative and stimulant drugs to treat anxiety and depression. Electroconvulsive therapy (ECT) had also been found effective for patients with depressive illness, but it proved much less useful for patients with chronic schizophrenia. For many of the half-million patients in American mental hospitals in the 1950s, and hundreds of thousands more throughout the world, no effective treatment existed.

Then, in the space of only six years – from 1949 to 1955 – three pharmacological discoveries sparked a revolution in psychiatric treatment. These were: (1) antipsychotic drugs; (2) antidepressant drugs; and (3) lithium.

(1) *Antipsychotic drugs* counteract delusions (beliefs in things which are not real) and hallucinations (seeing visions, hearing voices, and the like) – symptoms common in schizophrenia and manic-depressive illness. Within a few weeks, these drugs may bring a patient from a floridly psychotic state, in which he must be confined to a locked ward of a mental hospital, to a state of

near-remission, in which he can be discharged and return to normal social and occupational life. Indeed, the introduction of antipsychotic treatment is credited with decreasing the population of American mental hospitals from 550,000 to 430,000 in the twelve years after 1955, despite a steady rise in the population.

Remarkable as their effects may seem, however, all antipsychotic drugs may have annoying side-effects: sedation, muscle stiffness, restlessness, slowed physical and mental functioning, and other problems. Perhaps as a result of these side effects, the antipsychotic drugs have often been misnamed 'major tranquillizers'. In fact, they are not tranquillizers at all; it is a serious misconception to think that they 'tranquillize' the patient into being free of his symptoms. Rather, they seem to have specific and selective effects on the psychosis itself. Any sedative or tranquillizing properties of the antipsychotic drugs appear purely accidental. In fact, if a normal person were to take even a small dose of one of the more potent antipsychotic drugs – such as fluphenazine or haloperidol – he would in all likelihood notice no tranquillization, and, indeed, might possibly experience a jumpy, restless feeling called akathisia.

Fortunately, given the wide range of available antipsychotic drugs, and the various medications developed to treat the side-effects, it is usually possible to reduce the side-effects to a tolerable level. This is important, since many patients must take the drugs for months or years to ensure protection from recurrent psychotic symptoms.

(2) *Antidepressant drugs* include the tricyclic antidepressants (such as imipramine and amitriptyline) and the monoamine oxidase inhibitors (such as phenelzine and tranylcypromine), discovered in the 1950s, together with several newer families of agents. These drugs provide relief for patients suffering from so-called major depression, or from the depressed phase of manic-depressive illness – conditions formerly responsive only to electro-convulsive therapy. The effect of antidepressants, like that of the antipsychotics, may be dramatic: a patient too depressed to eat or sleep, unable to perform even the most rudimentary tasks, and thinking constantly of suicide, may

respond so well that he is completely back to normal functioning in three or four weeks.

Like the antipsychotics, antidepressants are the subject of various misconceptions. In particular, they are not 'psycho-stimulants' or 'mood elevators'; a normal person taking them would typically notice some sedation, lightheadedness, dry mouth, and a few other side-effects, but no increased energy or euphoria. Antidepressants appear to act by correcting some underlying chemical imbalance in the brain, rather than propelling the patient into an artificial euphoria.

(3) *Lithium* is unique among psychiatric medications in that it is a simple ion, rather than a complex molecule. For reasons still poorly understood, it counteracts the manic phase of manic-depressive illness (it appears less effective in acute depression), and, taken over the long term, protects patients against relapses of mania or depression. Since it has relatively few side-effects, it may be taken for years at a time with few problems. Such long-term prophylactic use of lithium has transformed the lives of thousands of sufferers from manic-depressive illness and related disorders. Prior to lithium, many patients were accustomed to frequent psychiatric hospitalizations for the exacerbations of their illness, with severe disruption of their personal lives and their careers. Now they often enjoy partial or total protection against such occurrences.

Other Psychiatric Drugs

Other types of psychiatric drugs continue to be introduced. Benzodiazepines, such as chlordiazepoxide and diazepam, have been found safer and perhaps more effective than barbiturates for sedation in anxious patients; other benzodiazepines, such as flurazepam and temazepam, are excellent sleeping-pills. Stimulants, such as methylphenidate and magnesium pemoline, have ameliorated the symptoms of childhood hyperkinesis or minimal brain dysfunction, now called 'attention deficit disorder'. Anti-convulsant drugs, such as carbamazepine and sodium valproate, appear effective in some cases of manic-depressive illness. Even two food substances – a fat called lecithin and the amino acid L-tryptophan, which are now used primarily for research purposes – may be helpful in mania and depression, respectively. But none of these recent discoveries has matched the impact of the introduction of the antipsychotics, the antidepressants and lithium. Not only have the latter three classes of drugs greatly reduced the ravages of schizophrenia and manic-depressive illness, but they appear helpful for a number of other disorders, among them, panic disorder and agoraphobia, some forms of drug and alcohol abuse, anorexia nervosa and bulimia, certain organic mental disorders, and others.

The discovery of these medications has not only great clinical and public-health consequences, but major theoretical implications. It is an important observation that the drugs have little psychiatric effect on normal individuals, but a profound effect on patients suffering from actual psychiatric disorders. In other words, unlike the nonspecific sedative and stimulant medications, these compounds appear specifically to correct some underlying abnormality in the brain. This specificity not only suggests that there are biological abnormalities underlying many of the major psychiatric disorders, but gives clues as to what the abnormalities may be. Studies of the action of psychopharmacologic agents have given impetus to the growing field of biological psychiatry. In time, this research may greatly enhance our knowledge of the aetiology of psychosis, depression, and other symptoms – and yield even more specific and effective treatments.

Harrison G. Pope
The Mailman Research Center
Belmont, Mass.

Further Reading

Baldessarini, R. J. (1977), *Chemotherapy in Psychiatry*, Cambridge, Mass.

Davis, J. M. (1975), 'Overview: maintenance therapy in psychiatry. I: schizophrenia', *American Journal of Psychiatry*, 132.

Davis, J. M. (1976), 'Overview: maintenance therapy in

psychiatry. II: affective disorders', *American Journal of Psychiatry*, 133.

Goodwin, F. K. (ed.) (1976), 'The lithium ion: impact on treatment and research', *Archives of General Psychiatry*, 36.

Hollister, L. E. (1983), *Clinical Pharmacology of Psychotherapeutic Drugs*, 2nd edn, New York.

Jefferson, J. W. and Greist, J. H. (1977), *Primer of Lithium Therapy*, Baltimore.

Klein, D. F., Gittleman, R., Quitkin, F. and Rifkin, A. (1980), *Diagnosis and Drug Treatment of Psychiatric Disorders: Adults and Children*, 2nd edn, Baltimore.

Quitkin, F., Rifkin, A. and Klein, D. F. (1979), 'Monoamine oxidase inhibitors: a review of antidepressant effectiveness', *Archives of General Psychiatry*, 36.

See also: *biological psychiatry*.

Psychosomatic Illness

In the broadest sense of the term, all human illness is psychosomatic, since the functions of mind and body are closely interwoven. Emotional disorders are commonly accompanied by bodily symptoms, and physical illness often leads to pathological emotional responses. Clinical practice reflects this duality. Psychiatrists working in general hospitals are often called upon to evaluate and treat patients (1) whose illnesses are the response to an emotional stress, and (2) those for whom physical illness or injury is in itself a stressful precipitant of a pathological emotional reaction that, in turn, complicates the underlying physical disorder.

(1) In the first category of psychosomatic illness, emotional factors may be a major precipitator of physical illness. In many patients with a variety of chronic bodily disorders (such as peptic ulcer, hyperthyroidism, and bronchial asthma), severe emotional stress (the loss of a wife or husband, for example) appears to play a significant role in the onset and recurring episodes of the physical illness. Such patients often have major defects in their capacity to experience and express emotions aroused by stress. The arousal, barred from discharge over the psychological, emotional and behavioural channels that

normally attenuate it, is shunted directly into nervous and endocrinal pathways that control the body's organs. The resulting chronic stimulation of these organs leads to pathological changes manifested as physical illness. Modern scientific investigation of the psychosomatic process is beginning to uncover a wealth of facts that shed important light on the psychological, neuronal, endocrinal and immunological mechanisms at work in stress-induced psychosomatic illnesses. The knowledge thus gained will ultimately be translated into more effective treatment measures for a host of hitherto chronic, debilitating human diseases.

(2) In the latter category of psychosomatic illness, the individual patient's characteristic personality features help to determine the response to the stress of illness. As psychiatrists see it, these personality features often not only induce complications in the course of the illness, but create problems in the medical management of the case. Dependency needs, in particular, pose a central psychological difficulty. The incapacitation resulting from a serious illness or injury compromises the patient's autonomy, independence, and self-sufficiency, and forces him into the role of an invalid who must look to others for help and care. Individuals who are fiercely independent may find it difficult to give up their autonomy. As a consequence, they deny the seriousness of their illness and refuse to comply with the treatment programme necessary for their recovery. On the other hand, in persons with strong, overt dependency needs, the symptoms of a physical disorder provide a means of gratifying those needs. As a result, both the symptoms and the incapacitation arising from the illness are intensified and often prolonged beyond the time when physical healing has taken place.

John C. Nemiah
Beth Israel Hospital, Boston
Harvard University

Further Reading
Nemiah, J. C. (1961), 'Psychological complications of physical illness', in J. C. Nemiah (ed.), *Foundations of Psychopathology*, New York.
Weiner, H. (1977), *Psychobiology and Human Illness*, New York.
See also: *anxiety; stress.*

Reaction Times

For experimental psychologists, the study of reaction times is both a methodological preoccupation and a topic of intrinsic theoretical interest. It was launched when the Rev. Nevil Maskelyne, then British Astronomer Royal, discovered (in 1796) that he and his assistant David Kinnebrook produced estimates for timings of stellar transits which differed by as much as 0.8 secs. He dismissed Kinnebrook 'with regret', and the event was later mentioned in a history of the Royal Observatory. Twenty-four years later Friedrich Bessel read this account, and investigated individual differences between the timings made by careful observers who all used precisely the same method. He found that mean differences between all possible pairs of readings ranged from 0.044 secs to 1.021 secs. This was probably the first quantitative measurement made on the decision speed of human beings. It was also an elegant insight which had important practical and theoretical results. Thenceforward individual astronomers, however eminent, calibrated themselves to obtain 'personal constants' which might be used to adjust their observations. After this moment it became impossible to sustain the romantic belief that 'nothing in the universe is faster than the speed of thought', or to retain the more prosaic fallacy that all humans can make decisions equally rapidly if only they will try hard enough. The study of individual differences had its small beginning.

The methodological study of reaction times concerns the reliability of experimental procedures involving comparisons of times taken for different types of decisions and by different individuals. Many psychological experiments involve decisions which are so easy that people make very few, or no, mistakes in any of the tasks which are compared. In such cases we can only judge which task is slightly harder by timing, preferably in milliseconds, how long people take to make these different decisions. We then assume that decisions that take longer are more difficult for the human central nervous system to make. Thus measurements of reaction times can be used to deduce the way the nervous system works. This can be illustrated by the first, perhaps apocryphal, theoretical use of reaction times made by Helmholtz (allegedly in about 1852) in which people were given electrical shocks, either on one foot or on the cheek and, in either case, responded by rapidly clenching their teeth on a response-key. Helmholtz is said to have found that response times to foot-shock were reliably longer than to cheek-shock. Dividing the differences between mean reaction times (RTs) for foot and for cheek stimulation by the mean physical distance in metres between these locations on his subjects' bodies, he obtained an estimate, quite surprisingly accurate, of the mean speed of human nerve conduction.

Later studies by Donders and by Wundt extended the use of RTs to examine latencies for otherwise unexaminable internal processes, such as the differences between the times required to identify signals and the times required to select responses to them. These studies have been extended by S. Sternberg (1969) in attempts to compare the times taken to search the contents of short-term memory, as the number of items to be remembered increases; by R. Sternberg, to obtain differences in the times taken to solve logical problems; by Shepherd and Metzler (1971) in an attempt to examine differences in the times required to rotate mentally images of complex objects, and by Neisser (1963), Rabbitt and Vyas (1970) and others in attempts to study the strategies that people use to locate objects by visual search.

Reaction times have also been a fascinating theoretical study in themselves. This is because, superficially, they seem to offer a means of studying very elementary neural processes underlying decision making. This optimism may arise from the following, naïve consideration: if healthy young people practise at a simple task in which they have repeatedly to make the same response whenever a particular signal (such as light flash or tone) occurs, their response times to particular signals average 170 msecs to 180 msecs. We know that about 40 msecs of this time is necessary for peripheral processing of the signal in the eye or the ear. We also know that a further 40 or 50 msecs is needed by muscles and joints to execute any chosen response. Thus only 90 msecs or so seems to be required by internal decision processes in the central nervous system. We also know that since no neurone can communicate with another in less than a millisecond this means that a system of not more than 90 neurones, in series, end to end, must subserve the decision process whose latency we have measured.

A few moments thought convinces us that this line of logic, tempting to the great nineteenth-century investigators such as Donders and Wundt, is simplistic. Any organism which could only react to events as soon as they occurred would lag, perpetually, from 90 to 170 msecs behind the phenomenal present. This would make it too slow to compete successfully with other organisms who manage to develop means of anticipating future events. Thus the study of simple reaction times is, essentially, the study of the way in which humans formulate and vary their anticipations of events which have not yet taken place. The study of times taken to decide which of several different events has taken place (choice reaction times) has become the study of why humans process different kinds of information at different rates (Hick, 1952), of how humans adjust their decision speeds in order to trade off accuracy to gain speed (Schouten and Bekker, 1956; Rabbitt and Vyas, 1970) and of how humans learn to anticipate selectively which of several events, of different probabilities of occurrence, will happen next and when it will occur.

In these respects the study of reaction times is both a topic of considerable practical interest (as when we need to know how much time people need to begin to apply their car brakes in response to unexpected events on motorways, or what is the minimum time within which fighter-pilots can make any of the complex decisions required of them). It is also one of the most important methodologies we have with which to deduce how the brain interprets sensory information and successfully predicts future events by relating what is currently perceived to memories of past contingencies.

Patrick Rabbitt
University of Manchester

References

Hick, W. E. (1952), 'On the rate of gain of information', *Quarterly Journal of Experimental Psychology*, 4.

Neisser, U. (1963), 'Decision time without reaction-time: experiments in visual scanning', *American Journal of Psychology*, 76.

Rabbitt, P. M. A. and Vyas, S. M. (1970), 'An elementary preliminary taxonomy of errors in laboratory choice RT tasks', *Acta Psychologica*, 33.

Schouten, J. F. and Bekker, J. A. M. (1967), 'Reaction time and accuracy', in *Attention and Performance* 1, ed. A. F. Saunders, Amsterdam.

Shepherd, R. N. and Metzler, J. (1971), 'Mental rotation of three dimensional objects', *Science*, 171.

Sternberg, S. (1969), 'On the discovery of processing stages; some extensions of Donders's model', *Acta Psychologica*, 30.

Reich, Wilhelm (1897–1957)

There is no more audacious figure in the history of modern psychiatry than Wilhelm Reich. Born on 24 March 1897 in an eastern province of the Austro-Hungarian empire, he died sixty years later in a US penitentiary. His various accomplishments included the development of *character analysis* (or the investigation of defensive character traits) within the framework of psychoanalysis. This work, undertaken in Vienna in the 1920s, profoundly influenced the later growth of ego psychology, especially Anna Freud's *The Ego and the Mechanisms of Defense*, (1936).

Between 1927 and 1933 in Vienna and Berlin, Reich made conceptual contributions towards the integration of psychoanalysis and Marxism. His practical 'sex-political' work during this period brought sex education and counselling to large numbers of people in a way that connected emotional issues with social concerns. These activities later influenced the new left in the 1960s and the orientation of the women's movement towards 'politicizing the personal'.

Following his expulsion from the German Communist Party in 1933 for his psychodynamic emphases, and from the International Psychoanalytic Association in 1934 for his social stance, Reich moved to Oslo. There he delineated the *muscular armour*, that is, chronic muscular spasms representing the somatic anchoring of characterological rigidities. This work provided the originating impulse for such latter-day therapies as Bioenergetics, Gestalt Therapy and Primal Therapy.

In the 1940s and 1950s in America, Reich, whose work had always been radical, began to investigate *orgone energy*, an energy which, he asserted, functioned as the life energy inside the organism and in nature at large. These ideas were dismissed by almost the entire psychiatric and psychoanalytic community. Reich subsequently invented and distributed a device, the *orgone energy accumulator*, which, he believed, had therapeutic and preventive properties for a number of illnesses. When he continued to distribute the accumulator after an injunction against it was obtained by the US Food and Drug Administration, the accumulators were destroyed, most of his publications were burned, and he was imprisoned on 11 March 1957.

Reich's extraordinary and defiant journey across scientific boundaries merits serious evaluation of both its fruitfulness and its error.

Myron Sharaf
Cambridge Hospital and Harvard University

Further Reading
Higgins, M. Boyd (1960), *Wilhelm Reich: Selected Writings*, New York.
Reich, W. (1961), *Character Analysis*, New York. (Contains translations of *Charakteranalyse*, 1933, and *Psychischer Kontakt und vegetative Strömung*, 1935.)

Sharaf, M. (1983), *Fury on Earth: A Biography of Wilhelm Reich*, New York.

See also: *gestalt therapy*.

Rogers, Carl R. (1902–1987)

Founder of client-centred or non-directive psychotherapy, Carl Rogers is considered part of the 'third force' in psychotherapy, a force which is characterized in opposition to psychoanalytic approaches on the one hand and behaviourist approaches on the other. Rogers himself thinks of his therapy as a 'person-centred approach' to human relationships, which can be extended to education, marriage and family relationships, intensive groups and even international relations.

Like other members of the third force, Rogers's basic premise is that every human being has an 'actualizing tendency' towards complete growth that can be mobilized in the correct therapeutic setting. Rogers's theory and therapy emphasize the actual here and now relationship between therapist and patient or client rather than the transference. The therapist is encouraged: (1) to be genuine (congruence between his or her feelings and their expression to the client); (2) to show unconditional positive regard for the client; and (3) to demonstrate empathic understanding of the client. The goal is 'to free the client to become an independent, self-directing person'. This method is in contrast to a behaviourist approach, where the therapist selects particular reinforcement techniques to modify particular behaviours.

Beginning his studies at the Union Theological Seminary in New York City, Rogers soon crossed the street to Columbia University's Teachers College (Ph.D. 1931). His early work with children, as Director of the Society for the Prevention of Cruelty to Children in Rochester, New York, led to his 1939 book, *Clinical Treatment of the Problem Child*. Challenging the medical model of psychiatric diagnosis and psychoanalysis, he chronicled the development of his client-centred approach through several books, beginning with *Counselling and Psychotherapy* in 1942. As professor of clinical psychology at the University of Chicago, he published *Client-Centered Therapy*

(1951), a statement of his technique which included applications in education – as student-centred teaching – as well as group therapy, and play therapy for children.

On Becoming a Person (1961) brought together Rogers's writings from the 1950s, in which he emphasized that the therapist must be personally present to infuse the therapeutic relationship with an 'I-Thou' quality, a theme taken from the works of the philosopher Martin Buber. Carl Rogers's treatment method has had a profound effect on the practice of psychotherapy, particularly among nonpsychiatrists in their counselling of 'clients' without serious mental illness. Although Rogers himself spent several years attempting to treat patients with serious mental illness, this work was less successful. In the early 1970s, Rogers examined the encounter group movement and the changing institution of marriage. His 1980 collection, *A Way of Being*, highlights autobiographical material about his half-century as a 'practising psychologist'.

Louisa B. Tarullo
Harvard University

Further Reading
Rogers, C. R. (1967), 'C. R. Rogers', in E. Boring and G. Lindzey (eds), *A History of Psychology in Autobiography*, vol. 5, New York.
See also: *group therapy*.

Schizophrenia

The technical term for madness, psychosis, refers to a mental state in which a person perceives, thinks, and/or behaves in strange ways. Thus, the psychotic person may hear voices that other people do not perceive (auditory hallucinations), have beliefs that others would consider irrational (delusions), behave in strange ways, such as carrying around a bag with small bits of paper, or have difficulties in thinking clearly, such as having thoughts follow each other in a disorganized fashion.

Schizophrenia is one form of madness or psychosis. It is the disorder marked by a psychotic state or states and identified especially by certain characteristic symptoms. These symptoms include particular kinds of auditory hallucinations and certain delusions, such as feeling controlled by an outside force. Bizarre behaviour and formal thought disorder are also common. However, since these symptoms can also be found in other types of psychosis, the diagnosis of schizophrenia is frequently one of exclusion – having a psychosis in which affective symptoms (depression or elation) are not predominant, and where no organic origin has been identified. Another criterion often included for diagnosing schizophrenia is that the condition continue for at least several months.

Perhaps because it is such a terrifying disorder, there are many existing beliefs about schizophrenia that far outdistance the available information. Thus, for example, people who are not mental health professionals often believe that schizophrenia means a split personality, or that it involves only people who are totally 'out of touch with reality'. Such views are either incorrect and/or oversimplifications, and thus neither do justice to the complexities of the disorder nor to the basic humanity of the people afflicted with it.

Other common but distorted beliefs about schizophrenia are that it is entirely hereditary, that patients never recover, and that people who have it are totally incapacitated. Although research suggests that there may be a genetic component in the causation of schizophrenia, it is likely that those genetic characteristics make a person vulnerable to developing schizophrenia rather than causing the disorder as such. In fact, schizophrenia appears to be caused by a wide range of biological factors and life experiences, probably acting together in ways that are not currently understood.

It has often been believed that people with schizophrenia do not recover, but a group of longitudinal studies has now demonstrated the inaccuracy of this notion. While many patients have the disorder over a long period of time, about 60 per cent of people diagnosed as schizophrenic recover completely or have only limited residual impairment.

Finally, although many people with schizophrenic disorders are impaired severely, at least for periods of time, with treatment and rehabilitation it is often possible for such persons to return to the community and function effectively.

Certain hallucinations, delusions, bizarre behaviour, and 'formal' thought disorder are indicative of schizophrenia, but it is important to note that this condition is not totally different from more normal human experience. There are, for example, degrees of intermediate states between florid schizophrenia and normal behaviour, and many of these states are considered normal. The existence of these intermediate states suggests that many manifestations of schizophrenia and other psychoses may be extremes on continua of functioning, functioning that may be found in people who are normal and not psychotic. Thus, the person who has been paged by name all day on a loud-speaker system may hear his name being called at night after leaving the building where the system operates. Sometimes people believe that someone in their organization is out to ruin them when there is little evidence for this. There are particular types of religious beliefs that may or may not be based in reality. Some behaviours which appear strange may nevertheless have a purpose. A person who has just heard some shocking news or encounters some other kind of highly unusual situation may be disorganized in his thinking for a brief period.

Treatments of schizophrenia focus both on direct control of symptoms and on countering the underlying causes, although it is not certain that treatments supposedly directed at the causes do in fact operate in that way. Antipsychotic medications are pre-eminent among the treatments focused more directly on symptom reduction or elimination. These do not merely 'tranquillize' or sedate the person generally, but appear to have a more specific action tending to reduce the psychotic symptoms themselves, at least in some patients. Although the development of these medications has been an important advance in the treatment of schizophrenia, there is a growing opinion that they do not resolve the basic processes of the disorder. There has also been increasing concern about the side effects of these medications. Some of these effects, such as abnormal involuntary movements of the face and other parts of the body, may not appear until after a prolonged use and then may be irreversible.

There is evidence to suggest that certain kinds of personal or social treatments are also helpful for schizophrenia. Thus, hospitalization that temporarily provides an environment with reduced stimulation, and the more reality-oriented forms of group and individual psychotherapy appear to be helpful. The acquisition of insight and interpersonal and occupational skills may help reduce the person's vulnerability to recurrence of psychosis. If a particular stressful event or situation appears to have contributed to a recurrence of the psychotic state, it may also be helpful to assist the person to understand and/or change that circumstance.

Schizophrenia is a shocking and striking condition, causing much agony for the individual, as well as for family, friends, and co-workers. Because schizophrenia relates to the human condition more generally in so many ways, it also has much to teach us about biology, psychology and social attachments. Considerable progress has been made in understanding and treating this condition, but much remains to be learned.

John S. Strauss
Yale University

Further Reading
Kaplan, H., Freedman, A. and Sadock, B. (1980), *Comprehensive Textbook of Psychiatry*, 3rd edn, Baltimore.
Strauss, J. S. and Carpenter, W. T. Jr (1982), *Schizophrenia*, New York.
See also: *genetic aspects of mental illness; psychiatry; psychopharmacology*.

Self-Concept

The self-concept has had a diversity of meanings, due in part to its multidisciplinary heritage. Philosophy and theology have emphasized the self as the locus of moral choices and responsibility. Clinical and humanistic psychologies have stressed the self as the basis of individual uniqueness and neurosis. Within sociology the self-concept has acquired an indelibly social character, with the emphasis on language and social interaction as the matrix for the emergence and maintenance of the self. The current popularity of self-concept within experimental social psychology places greater emphasis on its cognitive and motivational aspects, such as the self-concept as a source of motivation, as a performance aimed at managing impressions, and as a source of perceptual and cognitive organization.

At its core, the idea of self-concept or self-conception is based on the human capacity for reflexivity, frequently considered the quintessential feature of the human condition. Reflexivity or self-awareness, the ability of human beings to be both subjects and objects to themselves, can be conceptualized as the dialogue between the 'I' (for example, the self-as-knower) and the 'me' (the self-as-known), an internal conversation, which emerges (at both the ontogenetic and the phylogenetic levels) with the emergence of language – an argument extensively developed by G. H. Mead (1934). Language requires us to take the role of the other with whom we are communicating, and in the process enables us to see ourselves from the other's perspective.

Properly speaking, this process of reflexivity refers to the concept of self. The self-concept, on the other hand, is the *product* of this reflexive activity. It is the conception the individual has of himself as a physical, social, moral and existential being. The self-concept is the sum total of the individual's thoughts and feelings about himself as an object (Rosenberg, 1979). It involves a sense of spatial and temporal continuity of personal identity, a distinction of essential self from mere appearance and behaviour, and is composed of the various attitudes, beliefs, values, and experiences, along with their evaluative and affective components (such as self-evaluation or self-esteem), in terms of which individuals define themselves. In many respects the self-concept is synonymous with the concept of ego (see Sherif, 1968), although psychologists have preferred the latter term and sociologists the former. The various aspects of the self-concept can be grouped into two broad categories: (1) identities and (2) self-evaluations.

(1) The concept of identity focuses on the meanings constituting the self as an object, gives structure and content to the self-concept, and anchors the self to social systems. 'Identity'

has had its own interesting and complex history in the social sciences. In general, it refers to who or what one is, to the varius meanings attached to oneself by self and others. Within sociology, identity refers both to the structural features of group membership which individuals internalize and to which they become committed, for example, various social roles, memberships, and categories, and to the various character traits that an individual displays and that others attribute to an actor on the basis of his conduct in particular social settings. The structure of the self-concept can be viewed as the hierarchical organization of a person's identities, reflecting in large part the social and cultural systems within which it exists (Stryker, 1980).

(2) Self-evaluation (or self-esteem) can occur with regard to specific identities which an individual holds, or with regard to an overall evaluation of self. People tend to make self-evaluations on the basis of two broad criteria: their sense of competence or efficacy, and their sense of virtue or moral worth (Wells and Marwell, 1976; Gecas and Schwalbe, 1983).

Several processes have been identified as important to the development of self-concepts: reflected appraisals, social comparisons, self-attributions and role-playing. The most popular of these in sociology is reflected appraisals. Based on Cooley's (1902) influential concept of the 'looking-glass self' and Mead's theory (1934) of role-taking as a product of symbolic interaction, reflected appraisals emphasize the essentially social character of the self-concept, such as the idea that our self-conceptions reflect the appraisals and perceptions of others, especially significant others, in our environments. The process of reflected appraisals is the basis of the 'labelling theory' of deviance in sociology, and of self-fulfilling processes in social psychology.

Social comparison is the process by which individuals assess their own abilities and virtues by comparing them to those of others. Local reference groups or persons are most likely to be used as a frame of reference for these comparisons, especially under conditions of competition, such as athletic contests or classroom performance. Self-attributions refer to the tendency to make inferences about ourselves from direct observation of our behaviour. Bem's (1972) 'self-perception theory' proposes that individuals determine what they are feeling and thinking by making inferences based on observing their own overt behaviour. Role-playing as a process of self-concept formation is most evident in studies of socialization. It emphasizes the development of self-concepts through the learning and internalizing of various social roles (for example, age and sex roles, family roles, occupation roles).

The self-concept is both a product of social forces and, to a large extent, an agent of its own creation. Along with the capacity for self-reflexivity discussed earlier, the agentive aspect of the self-concept is most evident in discussions of self-motives (that is, the self-concept as a source of motivation). Three self-motives have been prominent in the social psychological literature: (1) self-enhancement or self-esteem motive; (2) self-efficacy motive; and (3) self-consistency motive.

(1) The self-esteem motive refers to the motivation of individuals to maintain or to enhance their self-esteem. It is manifest in the general tendency of persons to distort reality in the service of maintaining a positive self-conception, through such strategies as selective perception, reconstruction of memory, and some of the classic ego-defensive mechanisms.

(2) The self-efficacy motive refers to the importance of *experiencing* the self as a causal agent, that is, to the motivation to perceive and experience oneself as being efficacious, competent and consequential. The suppression or inhibition of this motive has been associated with such negative consequences as alienation, 'learned helplessness', and the tendency to view oneself as a pawn or victim of circumstances (see Gecas and Schwalbe, 1983).

(3) The self-consistency motive is perhaps the weakest of the three, yet it continues to have its advocates. Lecky (1945), an early advocate, viewed the maintenance of a unified conceptual system as the overriding need of the individual. Those theorists who view the self-concept primarily as an organization of knowledge, or as a configuration of cognitive generalizations, are most likely to emphasize the self-consistency motive. The self-concept as an organization of *identities* also provides a motivational basis

for consistency, in that individuals are motivated to act in accordance with the values and norms implied by the identities to which they become committed.

In the past, the bulk of research on the self-concept has focused on self-esteem (see Wells and Maxwell, 1976; Wylie, 1979), that is, on the antecedents of self-esteem, the consequences of self-esteem, and the relationships between self-esteem and almost every other aspect of personality and behaviour. Much of this research focus continues to be evident. But there are noticeable trends in other directions as well. The most evident are: the dynamics of self-presentation and impression management in naturalistic and experimental settings; the development and the consequences of commitment to specific identities (especially gender, ethnic group, deviant, and age-specific); historical and social structural influences on self-conceptions (such as wars, depressions, cultural changes, and organizational complexity); and, increasingly, we find a focus on the effect of self-concept on social structure and social circumstances. The self-concept is rapidly becoming the dominant concern within social psychology (both the sociological and the psychological varieties), as part of the general intellectual shift from behavioural to cognitive and phenomenological orientations in these disciplines.

Viktor Gecas
Washington State University

References

Bem, D. J. (1972), 'Self-perception theory', in L. Berkowitz (ed.), *Advances in Experimental Social Psychology*, vol. 6, New York.

Cooley, C. H. (1902), *Human Nature and the Social Order*, New York.

Gecas, V. and Schwalbe, M. L. (1983), 'Beyond the looking-glass self: social structure and efficacy-based self-esteem', *Social Psychological Quarterly*, 46.

Lecky, P. (1945), *Self-Consistency: A Theory of Personality*, New York.

Mead, G. H. (1934), *Mind, Self and Society*, Chicago.

Rosenberg, M. (1979), *Conceiving the Self*, New York.

Sherif, M. (1968), 'Self-concept', in D. K. Sills (ed.), *International Encyclopedia of the Social Sciences*, vol. 14, New York.

Stryker, S. (1980), *Symbolic Interactionism: A Social Structural Version*, Menlo Park, Calif.

Wells, L. E. and Marwell, G. (1976), *Self-Esteem: Its Conceptualization and Measurement*, Beverly Hills, Calif.

Wylie, R. C. (1979), *The Self-Concept*, Lincoln, Neb.

Further Reading.

Gecas, V. (1982), 'The self-concept', *Annual Review of Sociology*, 8.

Rosenberg, M. (1979), *Conceiving the Self*, New York.

Semantic Differential

The semantic differential was developed by Charles Osgood and his colleagues at the University of Illinois during the 1950s as an objective method for the measurement of the connotative meaning of concepts. The aim was to produce a scaling instrument which gave representation to the major dimensions along which meaningful reactions or judgements vary, and which would allow any concept to be described in terms of those dimensions.

The method of investigation required informants to describe various concepts (for example, Psychology) on a series of scales, consisting of pairs of polar adjectives such as successful-unsuccessful, difficult-easy, or serious-humorous. This method is based on the proposition that many of these scales are essentially equivalent and represent a single dimension of meaning, and that only a limited number of dimensions are needed to define a semantic space within which the connotative meaning of any concept can be specified.

The empirical problem was to identify this limited set of dimensions, and then to demonstrate repeatedly, using different samples of concepts, descriptive scales and subjects, and different methods of data collection and analysis, that essentially the same set of dimensions appears, and appears with the dimensions having the same relationships to one another.

In the original empirical test of these propositions (Osgood and Suci, 1955) fifty-seven-step scales were used by 100 subjects to describe twenty different concepts. The ratings of each scale, averaged over both subjects and concepts, were then subjected to factor analysis to summarize the pattern of correlations of scales with scales.

The analysis produced three factors which were termed:

Evaluation (such as good-bad, beautiful-ugly, clean-dirty)
Potency (such as large-small, strong-weak, heavy-light) and
Activity (such as fast-slow, active-passive, sharp-dull).

In numerous subsequent studies, these same three factors repeatedly emerge, indicating the stability of the underlying dimensions of semantic judgement. They regularly account for some 50 per cent of the total variance, with Evaluation the major factor, accounting for double the variance of either the Potency or Activity factors. In each study the variance which remains is taken up by a number of minor factors, which are specific to particular concept areas.

Thus a semantic differential could be constructed, consisting of only a small number of scales (typically ten–twelve) chosen to represent the three principal dimensions, and yielding, when used to describe a concept, three scores describing it with respect to a three-dimensional semantic space.

Osgood, Suci and Tannenbaum (1957) reported studies of the connotative meaning of many different concept areas, including studies of attitude structure and change, the changing semantic space of a patient during psychotherapy, the description of a case of multiple personality, a study of the structure of aesthetic judgements, and investigations of the effects of the mass media. Since these original studies, an enormous number and variety of studies of affective meaning have been conducted (a selection of which are reprinted in Snider and Osgood, 1969), and variations on the procedure have become standard techniques used by social scientists in many different disciplines.

In addition, a major cross-cultural research effort has established the generality of these dimensions across thirty grossly different language-culture communities (Osgood, May and Miron, 1975) and provided an Atlas of affective meanings of over 600 diversified concepts. These results suggest that the structure of meaning may be a human universal irrespective of linguistic and cultural differences.

Guy Fielding
Sheffield City Polytechnic

References

Osgood, C. E., May, W. H. and Miron, M. J. (1975), *Cross-Cultural Universals of Affective Meaning*, Urbana, Ill.

Osgood, C. E. and Suci, G. J. (1955), 'Factor analysis of meaning', *Journal of Experimental Psychology*, 50.

Osgood, C. E., Suci, G. J. and Tannenbaum, P. H. (1957), *The Measurement of Meaning*, Urbana, Ill.

Snider, J. G. and Osgood, C. E. (1969), *Semantic Differential Technique: A Sourcebook*, Chicago.

Sensation and Perception

Sensation and perception refer to the mechanisms by means of which we are aware of and process information about the external world. Aristotle classified the senses into the five categories of seeing (vision), hearing (audition), smelling (olfaction), tasting (gustation), and the skin senses. It is now commonplace to subdivide further the skin senses into separate categories of pain, touch, warmth, cold, and organic sensations. In addition, two senses of which we are not normally aware are also included – kinesthesis, or the sense of position of our limbs, and the vestibular sense which provides information regarding movement and position of the head.

Early theorists often regarded sensation as more elementary and less complex than perception, but the distinction has not proven to be useful. Physical energies such as light, sound waves, acceleration, are *transduced* by the sensory end organs so as to activate nerves which carry the signals to the central nervous system. The properties of the sense organs determine the acceptable range of physical stimuli. For example, the human ear responds to vibrations of the air only between 20 and 20,000 cycles per second. The minimum physical energy required to activate the sensory end organs is referred to as the *absolute threshold*. Thresholds for hearing depend systematically on the frequency of the vibrations, being minimal in the intermediate frequency range which involves speech sounds, and progressively higher for both lower and higher frequencies. Similarly, within the range of wave lengths which activate the eye, the visual system is most sensitive to yellow and yellow-green, and less sensitive to red and blue. Wave lengths outside of this range do not activate the visual system although infra-red radiation may be perceived as heat.

The quality of sensation – whether it is perceived as light, sound, pain, smell and so on – is not determined directly by the nature of the physical stimulus but rather by the nervous pathways being activated. Under normal conditions, light energy will typically stimulate visual pathways because the light threshold for the eyes is much lower than for any other form of physical energy. Pressure on the eyeball, however, will elicit a light sensation. Similarly, all the sense organs have the lowest thresholds for the appropriate forms of stimulus energy. The relationship between the quality of sensory experience and the specific nervous pathways activated is referred to as Mueller's doctrine of *specific nerve energies*. This concept was important in the early history of psychology because it focused attention on the role of the nervous system in mediating experience. We do not perceive the external world directly, but rather are aware of the activity of the nerves. Since awareness and knowledge depend on nervous activity, the study of the nervous system is fundamental to the science of psychology.

The intensity of sensation is not predictable from the absolute energy in the stimulus but is rather related to some multiple of stimulus energy. For example, the energy required for a light to appear just noticeably brighter than another light is closely predicted by the *ratio* of energies. An increment of a light unit which is just noticeable when viewed on a 10 light unit background will not be visible when viewed on a 100 light unit background. The just noticeable difference is closely predicted by the ratio of energies. The *differential threshold* for the 100 unit background would, in this case, be 10. To a first approximation, the ratio of the just noticeable difference to the background, historically known as *Weber's law*, is a constant. In the last century, the physicist Fechner argued, on the basis of Weber's law, that the subjective magnitude of sensation is determined by the logarithm of the stimulus energy. This relationship was viewed by Fechner as representing a quantification of the mind and the solution of the mind-body problem. The procedures devised to study sensory functions, known as *psychophysics*, provided an important methodology in support of the founding of experimental psychology as an independent laboratory science in the late nineteenth century.

Information from the senses is combined with past experience, either consciously or unconsciously, to construct our awareness of the external world and to guide our motor responses. For the most part, these perceptions are accurate, but there are instances in which they are in error. Incorrect perceptions are referred to as *illusions* which may result when normal mechanisms are inappropriately activated. When viewing two-dimensional photographs or drawings, distortions of size, shape and direction may occur because of the misapplication of sensory and perceptual mechanisms which normally subserve three-dimensional vision. Illusions should be differentiated from hallucinations, which refer to perceptions which have no basis in the external world. Hallucinations are typically associated with psychopathology, drugs, or pathology of the nervous system.

The theoretical importance of sensation and perception derives from the empirical point of view in philosophy which maintains that knowledge is mediated by the senses. In this context, limitations of sensory systems, illusions, and distortions by past experience or bias relating to motivational factors play a central role, because they determine the content of the mind. The predominance of the empirical view was responsible for the emphasis on the study of sensation and perception during the early history of experimental psychology.

Sensory systems can act independently or in conjunction with other senses. The 'taste' of food results from the combination of inputs from olfaction, gustation, the skin senses, and kinesthesis. This can be demonstrated by comparing the taste of foods when the nasal passages are blocked. In this case, taste is reduced to a less complex combination of the four basic gustatory qualities of salt, bitter, sour and sweet. The wide variety of food qualities is made possible in large part by olfactory cues. The appearance of food, its temperature, and resistance to chewing also contribute to these complex sensations.

Spatial orientation depends on the integration of visual, vestibular and proprioceptive information, all of which contribute to the maintenance of erect posture and location. The interactive nature of the sensory systems subserving spatial orientation is responsible for the fact that overactivation of the vestibular sense can lead to the illusory sensation that the visual world is moving. Similarly, if a large area of the visual environment is moved, an objectively stationary observer will experience a compelling illusory sensation of body motion (vection).

The correspondence between the physical pattern of stimulation and our corresponding perception of the world has remained a problem of major interest in perception. If two adjacent stationary lights are alternately flashed, the observer will report apparent movement between them. This phenomenon was cited by the *Gestalt* psychologists in support of their position that perception consists of more than the elements of stimulation. It is also the basis for the perceived movement in motion pictures and television. The contribution of the observer to perceptual experience is emphasized in numerous theoretical analyses of perception. In the case of *Gestalt* psychology, the organization is provided by inherent properties of the nervous system. Within the context of theories which stress the role of attention or motivation, the observer 'selects' only certain aspects of the environment for processing, in other words, we tend to see and hear what we want to see and hear and actively exclude information which is potentially embarrassing or unpleasant. The phenomenon of selective perception is illustrated by the reaction to painful stimuli which may be mini-mized or ignored if associated with an otherwise pleasant event such as victory in an athletic contest, but may be reported as very painful under unpleasant circumstances. Since the study of human perception frequently depends on the verbal report of an observer, it can not be evaluated directly and is therefore subject to modification by motivational states.

The active contribution of the observer to perception is also illustrated by the phenomenon of perceptual constancy. The first stage of sensing or perceiving visual stimuli is the formation of an optical image in the eye. This image is determined by geometric principles so that its size will be inversely proportional to the distance from the observer. In spite of wide variation in retinal image size, the perceived sizes of objects tend to remain constant and to correspond to their true dimen-sions. The tendency to perceive the veridical sizes of objects in spite of the continually changing pattern of the retinal image is referred to as perceptual 'constancy'. Other perceptual attri-butes also demonstrate constancy effect. The foreshortening of the retinal image resulting from oblique viewing is not perceived. Circular objects appear round even though the retinal image is elliptical, for example, shape constancy. When we move our eyes, the retinal image also moves but the percep-tion of the environment remains stationary, for example, space constancy. A white object appears 'white' and a dark object appears 'dark' even under wide ranges of ambient illumination, for example, brightness constancy. Similarly, the colours of objects tend to remain the same even though the spectral quality of the light reflected from them varies as they are illuminated by the different wavelengths provided by natural and artificial illumination, for example, colour constancy. Perceptual constancies are essential in biological adjustment because they permit the organism to be aware of and to respond to the biologically relevant, permanent physical characteristics of objects in the environment. The eye has been likened to a camera, and they are similar, as both have an optical system for focusing an image on a light sensitive surface. However, whereas the camera is passive, the eye, as well as other sensory systems, is connected to the brain so that the final perception is a result of the active combination of physical stimuli with information from the observer's past experience, motivation and emotions.

Sensation and perception have been of interest, not only because of their central role in the acquisition of knowledge and in mediating awareness, but also because they play an essential role in many aspects of human and animal behaviour. Pain is an essential protective mechanism which is normally activated whenever the integrity of the organism is in danger. Olfaction provides warning against ingestion of poisons. Serious threats to health are a consequence of the fact that no information is provided by our sensory systems for some dangers, for example, ionizing radiation, carbon monoxide, early stages of some diseases.

Knowledge of sensation and perception is important in performance evaluation and prediction and in medical diagnosis. Many tasks in modern society place unusual demands on the individual's sensory capacities as, for example, in aviation. Consequently sophisticated batteries of tests have been developed to identify those individuals with the superior visual and perceptual capacities necessary to operate high-performance aircraft. In a technologically-oriented society, the ability to acquire information from reading is indispensable and has led to the development of an extensive visual health-care system. The systematic changes in vision, balance and hearing which occur as a consequence of ageing are relevant to the design of safe environments and the successful adjustment of the elderly. Visual tests are sensitive to pathology and are used to evaluate the consequences of disease, in diagnosis, and in the evaluation of therapy.

Perceptual tests provide a methodology for evaluating group dynamics and personality. If a single stationary point of light is viewed in an otherwise dark room, it will appear to move. The extent of this reported *autokinetic* movement has been shown by Sherif to depend on the magnitude of apparent movement reported by other observers and their social status. The extent to which one's reports are influenced by others is taken as a measure of social pressure and conformity. Ambiguous stimuli are also used to evaluate personality. In the Rorschach test, subjects are asked to describe what they see in patterns formed by inkblots. It is assumed that the reports will be a reflection of the individual's personality dynamics which are attributed or 'projected' unconsciously into the ambiguous stimulus.

Herschel W. Leibowitz
Pennsylvania State University

Further Reading

Boring, E. G. (1942), *Sensation and Perception in the History of Experimental Psychology*, New York.

Boring, E. G. (1950), *A History of Experimental Psychology*, 2nd edn, New York.

Carterette, E. C. and Friedman, M. P. (eds), *Handbook of Perception*, New York (1974); Vol. I, *Historical and Philosophical Roots of Perception*; (1973), Vol. III, *Biology of Perceptual Systems*; Vol. IV, (1978), *Hearing*; (1975), Vol. V, *Seeing*; (1978), Vol. VIA, *Tasting and Smelling*; (1978), Vol. VIB, *Feeling and Hurting*; (1978), Vol. VIII, *Perceptive Coding*; (1978), Vol. IX, *Perceptual Processing*.

Held, R. H., Leibowitz, H. W. and Teuber, H. L. (1978), *Handbook of Sensory Physiology, Vol. VIII, Perception*, Heidelberg.

Kling, J. W. and Riggs, L. (eds) (1971), *Woodworth and Schlosberg's Experimental Psychology*, 3rd edn, New York.

Pastore, N. (1971), *Selective Theories of Visual Perception: 1650–1950*, London.

See also: *nervous system; sensory and motor development; vision.*

Sensory and Motor Development

In describing the stages of intellectual growth from birth to maturity, Piaget (1953) emphasized the initial and continuing importance of motor activity. In his view, the basis for later cognitive growth is constructed in the first two years by the production of physical rather than mental transformation of reality. Since this activity depends on sensory information about objects and events, the capacity to detect, discriminate, classify and integrate input from the different senses is basic to an understanding of behavioural development. Despite the motor and linguistic incompetence of the young infant, ingenious advances in technology permit a reassessment of the origins of sensori-motor activity, the role of experience, and the manner in which information from one sensory modality is related to that of another.

Behavioural and physiological measures are used to index responsiveness to sensory stimulation. Fundamental to all aspects of pattern perception is the resolution of visual detail when contrast is varied from low to high. This capacity improves rapidly during the early months, probably as a consequence of neuronal maturation. There are, as well, changes in the structure of the eye, improvement in the control of extra-ocular muscles and in visual accommodation. From birth, there is a preference to look at patterned rather than plain surfaces. An early ability to discriminate differences in brightness and colour is combined with a tendency to classify the colours of the spectrum in much the same fashion as adult humans. Colours from the one hue (for example, blue) are perceived as more similar than colours from different hue categories (for example, blue and green) although the physical difference between them is similar (Bornstein, 1981). In the auditory domain, early discrimination and classification of stimulation can also be observed. Perhaps the most striking example is the sensitivity to the acoustic properties that differentiate the phonetic segments of speech sounds (Jusczyk, 1981). This ability is not confined to sounds that are phonemic in the parental language. The discrimination and classification of consonants and vowels clearly precede and facilitate language acquisition.

Most research on sensory development has been concerned with the visual and auditory modalities. Recent findings on intermodal perception suggest that the haptic, kinaesthetic and proprioceptive senses also may not be as primitive as had previously been assumed. Although interpretation of these findings is controversial, there is a view that young infants are predisposed to recognize equivalence in the information derived from different modalities. Thus, for example, they detect the correspondence between the appearance of a speaker articulating a speech sound and the auditory characteristics of that sound, and they can match the visual appearance of an object with haptic information obtained from its oral exploration (Meltzoff, 1981). The age at which imitation first occurs is not yet clear. Nevertheless the reproduction of the facial expression of another person implies the translation of visual input into structurally similar but unseen proprioceptive output. It is clear that all these intermodal perceptions do not originate from a long period of gradual associations between the separate senses, as Piaget argues. It is equally clear that they are not the product of tuition of other senses by a primary touch sense, as classical theories maintain.

The study of early sensory and motor development has revealed a competence that was previously unsuspected. The exciting aspect of this research lies not so much in the demonstration of precocity as in the challenge to specify the nature of the relevant stimulus characteristics and the mechanisms that detect them. Recent findings have theoretical implications for normal development and clinical implications for those with sensory disabilities.

B. E. McKenzie
La Trobe University, Australia

References

Bornstein, M. H. (1981), 'Psychological studies of color perception in human infants: habituation, discrimination and categorization, recognition, and conceptualization', in L. P. Lipsitt (ed.), *Advances in Infancy Research*, Vol. 1, Norwood, NJ.

Jusczyk, P. (1981), 'Infant speech perception: a critical appraisal', in P. D. Eimas and J. L. Miller (eds), *Perspectives on the Study of Speech*, Hillsdale, NJ.

Meltzoff, A. N. (1981), 'Imitation, intermodal coordination

SEPARATION AND LOSS 397

and representation in early infancy', in G. Butterworth
(ed.), *Infancy and Epistemology*, Brighton.
Piaget, J. (1953), *The Origins of Intelligence in the Child*, London.

Further Reading
Lipsitt, L. P. (ed.) (1982), *Advances in Infancy Research*, Vol. 2,
Norwood, NJ.
See also: *developmental psychology; Piaget; sensation and perception.*

Separation and Loss

Separation and loss are central life events which impinge on all
individuals throughout the life cycle. The significance of these
common human experiences, particularly in early childhood,
are viewed quite differently by psychoanalysts, learning theorists and critical period theorists. Psychoanalysts emphasize the
potential for fixation and regression, with the possibility of
permanent limitations in emotional vitality as a response to
losses in infancy. Learning theorists suggest that, given the
appropriate environmental stimulation, humans are plastic and
can transfer their attachments and recover from periods of
loss or deprivation. Critical period theorists believe that phase-
specific development requires adequate environmental
conditions and that the absence of such (for example, maternal
contact) at a critical period can result in permanent developmental arrests.

Psychiatric research after the Second World War, which left
many European children without parents, attempted to trace
the long-term effects of orphanhood on the children. Early
research relied on dubious methods and reported a wide spectrum of pathological results, the common finding being a loss
of affectivity in personal relations. Since that time, there have
been attempts to obtain more exact information about infants
and children who have been separated from their primary caretakers through death, parental hospitalization and adoption.
Rene Spitz (1946) and John Bowlby (1969; 1973) are central
figures in the pioneering investigations of early childhood
response to maternal separations.

Spitz is best known for his description of depressive reactions in six-to-nine-month-old infants deprived of their mothers' presence for a duration of three to five months. He called this reaction – characterized by listlessness, immobility, setbacks in psychomotor development, and profound weight loss – anaclitic depression, postulating that the loss of the love object left the dependent infant with no outlet for his aggressive and libidinal drives. But since his subjects were not provided with substitute caretakers, his research describes the results of loss of mothering rather than, as he seems to suggest, the loss of the love object.

Bowlby described separation anxiety and grief reactions in infants six months and older. He characterized the mourning process in three stages: (1) a protest stage, viewed as an angry and anxious attempt to regain the object and protest the abandonment; (2) the despair stage; and (3) the detachment or readjustment stage. This same behaviour pattern had been noted by observers of young primates separated from their mothers.

Separations and losses have also been addressed at other phases in the life cycle. Reactive stages to the knowledge that one is dying, responses to marital separations and divorce, as well as reactions to the death of a loved one in later life have also been detailed. Bowlby's triad of rage, despair and readjustment often figure prominently in clinical descriptions of response to loss.

Grief reactions are regarded as both normal and adaptive responses to separation and loss. Mourning is only viewed as pathological when the individual becomes fixated over time in the early stages of rage and despair and is unable to detach and re-acclimate. Separation responses are pathological when the individual becomes excessively anxious, fearful and unable to initiate autonomous activity.

The impact of loss and separation from the caring parent continues to be a subject of great interest to psychotherapists. It would be fair to say that it now rivals the Oedipus complex in its psychotherapeutic significance as a critical developmental event. These are questions of great political significance as well, because they bear on the advisability of day care centres and the entry of women into the work force.

Karen Stone
Belmont, Massachusetts

References
Bowlby, J. (1969; 1973), *Attachment and Loss*, Vols I and II, London.
Spitz, R. (1946), 'Anaclitic depression', *Psychoanalytic Study of the Child*, 2.
See also: *attachment; bereavement; Bowlby.*

Skinner, Burrhus F. (1904–   )

A behaviourist and the most prominent figure in contemporary American psychology, Skinner has devoted most of his professional career to studying the effects of the consequences of behaviour on behaviour. He received his Ph.D. from Harvard in 1931, and from 1948 to 1975 was a professor there. His approach is descriptive and inductive; he is unconcerned with the physiological, mental, or affective processes taking place within organisms (see *The Behavior of Organisms*, 1938). The prototypic environment for Skinnerian (operant) conditioning is the Skinner Box, a chamber designed to give the animal being conditioned little room to move around in; it is equipped with a lever or other manipulandum which when activated produces a specific consequence (for example, food, water, avoidance of electric shock) according to a predetermined schedule. A consequence which, over trials, leads to an increase in the frequency of the response producing the consequence is referred to as a reinforcing stimulus. One of Skinner's major contributions has been to demonstrate that various schedules of reinforcement are characterized by unique response-frequency patterns. The ability to generate predictable response patterns has, in turn, found useful application in almost all areas of psychological research. Operant conditioning techniques also comprise the primary procedural foundation of behaviour modi- fication, a set of intervention strategies which have been effectively employed in all major institutional settings, particularly in schools, mental hospitals, and care facilities for the psychologically retarded. Skinner was one of the pioneers of programmed learning. As a social critic, he has throughout his professional life advocated the reorganization of societies so that positive reinforcement (rewarding desired behaviours) rather than punishment or the threat of punishment be used to control human actions. His philosophy is detailed in two widely read books, *Walden Two* (1948), a novel about an entire society being controlled by operant techniques, and *Beyond Freedom and Dignity* (1971). Skinner's most important general contribution to the social and behavioural sciences may be to inspire methodological precision and accountability.

Albert R. Gilgen
University of Northern Iowa

Further Reading
Gilgen, A. R. (1982), *American Psychology since World War II: A Profile of the Discipline*, Westport, Connecticut.
See also: *behaviourism; conditioning, classical and operant; learning*.

Sleep

Sleep is an area of human behaviour which occupies a third of the total life span and occurs thoughout all societies and all of history. Despite its pervasiveness it has been largely ignored by social scientists until recently. As laboratory-based studies began in earnest in the early 1950s to describe the nature and dimensions of sleep as a regularly recurring behaviour (Aserinsky and Kleitman, 1953; Dement and Kleitman, 1957), it became clear that this period was far from a passive state of quiescence or non-behaviour. By recording the electroencephalogram (EEG), electro-oculogram (EOG) and electromyogram (EMG) continuously throughout the time period from waking into sleep until the final reawakening, it was found that there were regular cyclic changes within sleep itself. The discovery that sleep consists of two distinct types, Rapid Eye Movement (REM) sleep and Non-Rapid Eye Movement (NREM) sleep, which differed as much from each other as each did from wakefulness, led to a series of studies detailing the properties of these two states and their interactions within the context of the whole circadian (sleep-wake) rhythm. Each hour and a half the shift from a synchronized, physiologically quiescent, NREM sleep in which motor activity is intact, to the desynchronized, physiologically active, REM state accompanied by motor paralysis, became known as the ultradian rhythm. Within NREM sleep, variations in EEG pattern were further differentiated by convention into numerical sleep stages 1, 2, 3, 4. This laid the basis for the descriptive mapping of a night's sleep by the number of minutes spent in each sleep stage across the hours of the night and by the length of the ultradian cycle. This plot is referred to as sleep architecture. Once these conventions were established (Rechtschaffen and Kales, 1968) age norms for these sleep characteristics were also established (Williams, Karacan and Hursch, 1974). Study of these developmental changes provided insight into sleep-wake relations. Individual differences in sleep parameters were also explored and related to variations in intelligence, personality and life-style. For example, although it is still a matter of some debate, long sleepers (those sleeping in excess of nine hours per night) were found to differ reliably from short sleepers (who sleep less than six hours per night) in psychological makeup, with long sleepers being more introverted, with lower energy and aggressive drive than short sleepers. It is clear that there is a selective difference in the type of sleep that is increased for these people. Long and short sleepers have the same amount of stages 3 and 4, but long sleepers have twice the amount of REM sleep and their REM sleep has increased eye movement density. Thus it is in the area of REM function that the need of long sleepers for more sleep must be explored. Other variations also occur, for example, in depth of sleep. These have been studied using the degree of auditory stimulation needed to produce an arousal as the measurement. This procedure has established that all sleep stages become progressively lighter with age, making sleep more fragile in the elderly.

Beyond the descriptive and correlational studies there has

been the continuing challenge concerning the question of sleep function. This question has been approached most often by looking into the effects on waking behaviour of sleep deprivation, either total or selective. Until recently these studies have been hampered by the limits to which human subjects could be subjected. Short studies of sleep loss have produced only small and equivocal results. These have been summed up ironically as: the effects of sleep deprivation are to make one more sleepy. However, the effects on subsequent sleep are clear. After total sleep loss, sleep architecture is changed. REM sleep is postponed in favour of a prolonged period of stages 3 and 4 sleep. It appears that this synchronized sleep is preemptive and is recouped first. In fact, if the degree of sleep loss has been more than a night or two, the first night of recovery sleep may contain no REM sleep at all. This may not reappear until a second recovery night. The opposite is true of the recovery following a period of selective REM sleep deprivation. On the first night of ad-lib sleep, REM sleep appears earlier in the architectural plot and the total amount may be increased above the usual proportion when total sleep time is controlled. In other words, both NREM stages 3 and 4 and REM sleep act as if they have the properties of needs requiring they be kept in homostatic balance. Recently, a long-term sleep deprivation study using rats and employing yoked non-sleep-deprived animals as controls has established that extreme sleep loss results in debilitative organic changes and death (Rechtschaffen *et al.*, 1983). This is the first study to establish that sleep is necessary to sustain life. How much sleep of what kind is necessary at the human level to ensure well-being will probably be determined not from experimental studies, but may come from the many clinical studies currently being carried out of patients suffering from various disorders of sleep and of sleep-wake relations.

Against the background knowledge of normative sleep architecture, for each sex across the whole life span, significant deviations in amount and type of sleep can now be identified as well as differences in the distribution of sleep across the circadian cycle. Studies that have sought to relate waking psychopathology to sleep pathology have been most productive in the area of depression. Although it has been well known that most persons suffering from affective disorders also suffer from insufficient and poor quality sleep, the detailed laboratory monitoring has revealed the nature of this dysfunction to be specific to REM sleep. This is found to be significantly displaced in the overall architecture. The first REM sleep occurs too soon, at half the normal cycle length, is often abnormally prolonged on first occurrence, from a norm of ten to as much as forty minutes, and with an increase in the density of eye movements within this time period and a change in total time distribution. Instead of REM being predominant in the second half night, as in normal individuals, in the depressed the distribution in the first and second halves of the night is equal (Kupfer et al., 1983). Since REM deprivation is known to increase waking appetite and sexual activity in cats and depression is associated with reduction of these behaviours, the finding of a specific REM dysfunction in these patients hints that this sleep stage is implicated in the regulation of appetitive behaviours.

Studies of sleep under time-free conditions have established that the normal human circadian rhythm is not twenty-four hours but slightly greater than twenty-five. This finding suggest that social learning has played a part in entraining sleep to a twenty-four hour cycle. Loss of these social cues or *zeitgebers* during vacation time or when unemployed, for example, often leads to later sleep onset time and longer sleep periods leading to later arousal hours. Most normal individuals have little trouble becoming re-entrained. However, some individuals with withdrawn schizoid personalities, or perhaps some neurological deficit, have no established sleep-wake rhythm. These people suffer from an inabililty to function in regular occupations due to the unpredictabililty of their time periods for active prosocial behaviours.

Nocturnal sleep studies of persons whose waking life is interruped by uncontrollable episodes of sleep have revealed several different types of sleep disturbance that are responsible for these intrusions, including narcolepsy and sleep apnoea syndromes.

The study of sleep and its interaction with waking behaviour has enlarged the capacity of the social and behavioural scientist to account for some aspects of human behaviour previously poorly understood and has changed the time frame of observation to one including the full circadian cycle.

Rosalind D. Cartwright
Rush-Presbyterian-St Luke's Medical Center, Chicago

References

Aserinsky, E. and Kleitman, N. (1953), 'Regularly occurring periods of eye motility and concomitant phenomena during sleep', *Science*, 118.

Dement, W. and Kleitman, N. (1957), 'Cyclic variations in EEG during sleep and their relation to eye movements, body motility and dreaming', *Electroencephalography and Clinical Neurophysiology*, 9.

Kupfer, D., Spiker, D., Rossi, A., Coble, P., Ulrich, R. and Shaw, D. (1983), 'Recent diagnostic treatment advances in REM sleep and depression', in P. J. Clayton and J. E. Barretts (eds), *Treatment of Depression: Old Controversies and New Approaches*, New York.

Rechtschaffen, A., Gilliland, M., Bergmann, B. and Winter, J. (1983), 'Physiological correlates of prolonged sleep deprivation in rats', *Science*, 221.

Rechtschaffen, A. and Kales, A. (eds) (1968), *A Manual of Standardized Terminology, Techniques and Scoring System for Sleep Stages of Human Subjects*, Los Angeles.

Williams, R., Karacan, I. and Hursch, C. (1974), *Electroencephalography (EEG) of Human Sleep: Clinical Applications*, New York.

Further Reading

Cartwright, R. (1978), *A Primer on Sleep and Dreaming*, Reading, Mass.

Dement, W. (1972), *Some Must Watch While Some Must Sleep*, San Francisco.

Hartmann, E. (1973), *The Functions of Sleep*, New Haven.

Webb, W. (1975), *Sleep, the Gentle Tyrant*, Englewood Cliffs, NJ.
See also: *dreams*.

Social Identity

In its most general sense, social identity refers to a person's self-definition in relation to others. Within social psychology, however, it usually has a more specific connotation – namely, a self-definition in terms of one's membership of various social groups. This sense of the term owes much to G. H. Mead, who emphasized a social conception of the self, arguing that individuals experience themselves 'from the standpoint of the social group as a whole' to which they belong (Mead, 1977). It is important to distinguish this public (or *social*) aspect of identity from the more private (or *personal*) aspects. Indeed, Mead himself, in stressing the importance of the group, can be seen as contrasting his approach from the more individualistic psychodynamic formulations. Thus, it has become common to refer to social identity in the manner above, and to personal identity as reflecting those parts of one's self-definition which have to do with personality traits, physical attributes, interpersonal styles and the like. More recently, Brown and Turner (1981) have argued that this is not merely an abstract theoretical distinction but one which, following Tajfel (1978), may have important behavioural implications: according to whether 'personal' or 'social' identities are psychologically uppermost in any situation may determine whether people exhibit sporadic and idiosyncratic 'interpersonal' behaviours, *or* organized and socially uniform 'intergroup' behaviours.

Historically, the concept of social identity has occupied a central place in both social-psychological and sociological theorizing. For instance, Lewin (1948), whose field theory inspired a whole generation of post-war social psychologists, wrote and researched extensively on the psychological significance of group affiliations, especially for minority and marginal groups. Within a more psychoanalytic tradition, the work of Erikson (1960) on identity conflicts and identity diffusion in the individual's life cycle has had important clinical applications. Within sociology, too, social identity has not gone unnoticed. For example, in Parson's General Theory of Action it is defined as a subsystem of personality and assigned a major role in determining a person's participation in the social system (see, for example, Parsons, 1968).

Reflecting these theoretical concerns, much empirical research has attempted to measure different components of identity. The bulk of this work has concentrated on aspects of personal identity focusing on such topics as self-esteem, locus of control, and level of aspiration. These methodologies have been comprehensively reviewed by Wylie (1974). In contrast, very few attempts have been made to measure social identity. One of the earliest, and still widely used, techniques is the Twenty Statements Test devised by Kuhn and McPartland (1954). This simply involves a respondent giving up to twenty responses to the question 'Who am I?' These responses may then be analysed to reveal the nature of that person's social and personal identity referents, the evaluative quality of the terms used, and the importance attributed to different elements. A typical finding is that social identity referents emerge earliest in response protocols, the most commonly mentioned categories being sex and occupational role. Zavalloni (1971) has proposed a technique for investigating a person's social identity idiographically. This method allows the respondent to differentiate between different subgroups within a larger category, some-times attaching very different valence and meaning to those subgroup identifications. However, both of these techniques yield essentially qualitative data and, in the latter case, are time-consuming to administer and analyse. A simpler and more practicable instrument is suggested by Driedger (1976). This consists of a short scale in which the respondent is permitted to affirm or deny, in varying degrees of strength, different aspects of ingroup membership. Although designed to measure ethnic identity, there is no reason why the technique could not be extended to measure the strength of other group identifi-cations also.

Despite these methodological difficulties, the concept of social identity continues to excite considerable research interest.

Much of this has been stimulated by Tajfel's Social Identity Theory (for example, Tajfel, 1978), which proposes a causal link between social identity needs and various forms of intergroup behaviour. Central to this theory is the hypothesis that people's social identities are sustained primarily through social comparisons, which differentiate the ingroup from relevant outgroups. From this simple idea it has proved possible to explain the prevalence of intergroup discrimination, even in the absence of real conflicts of interest, and to provide persuasive analyses of the plight of minority groups, industrial conflicts over pay differentials, and linguistic differentiation between ethnic groups.

Rupert Brown
University of Kent

References

Brown, R. J. and Turner, J. C. (1981), 'Interpersonal and intergroup behaviour', in J. C. Turner and H. Giles (eds), *Intergroup Behaviour*, Oxford.

Driedger, L. (1976), 'Ethnic self-identity: a comparison of ingroup evaluations', *Sociometry*, 39.

Erikson, E. H. (1960), 'The problem of ego identity', in M. R. Stein, A. J. Vidich and D. M. White (eds), *Identity and Anxiety*, New York.

Kuhn, M. H. and McPartland, T. S. (1954), 'An empirical investigation of self attitudes', *American Sociological Review*, 19.

Lewin, K. (1948), *Resolving Social Conflicts*, New York.

Mead, G. H. (1977), *On Social Psychology*, revised edn, A. Strauss, Chicago.

Parsons, T. (1968), 'The position of identity in the General Theory of Action', in C. Gordon and K. J. Gergen (eds), *The Self in Social Interaction*, New York.

Tajfel, H. (1978), *Differentiation between Social Groups: Studies in the Social Psychology of Intergoup Relations*, London.

Wylie, R. C. (1974), *The Self Concept*, London.

Zavalloni, M. (1971), 'Cognitive processes and social identity through focussed introspection', *European Journal of Social Psychology* 1.

Further Reading
Gordon, C. and Gergen, K. J. (1968), *The Self in Social Interaction*, New York.
Tajfel, H. (1982), *Social Identity and Intergroup Relations*, London.
See also: *self-concept*.

Socialization

Socialization has been defined as 'the process whereby the individual is converted into the person'. The study of this process forms large areas of psychology, anthropology and sociology; and it is interesting that the emergence of socialization as a field of study occurred almost simultaneously, in the late 1930s, in all three disciplines. One early school of thought, perhaps best known as the 'culture-personality' school, attempted to draw together the approaches of different disciplines by applying psychoanalytic theory to anthropological data. Abram Kardiner led a series of seminars in New York in the 1930s whose aim was to determine the personality characteristics associated with different cultural groups, and to establish their antecedents in child-rearing practices. The effort failed, probably because of the overwhelming scale and interdisciplinary nature of the task; and current studies of socialization tend to be intra- rather than interdisciplinary. Sociologists concentrate on the effects of social institutions such as the family, the school, or the media; and psychologists work on the individual level by investigating topics such as parent-child interaction, sex-role identity, play, moral thinking, and the development of the self-concept. This last topic probably has more potential for fruitful collaboration between psychologists and sociologists than any other – cognitive-developmental theory and symbolic interactionism have a good deal in common, for example – though few attempts have been made to develop the link.

In psychology, the term 'socialization' was originally used by a group of American theorists to connote a particular view of the nature of human development, a view which derived from 'behaviourism' or 'reinforcement theory'. In its purest form this tries to explain human behaviour as conditioned responses to environmental stimuli, learnt by association with different rewards and punishments. These 'neobehaviourists', including Robert Sears, Neal Miller, John Dollard and Albert Bandura, were concerned to explain development in a manner that was objective, neutral, value-free and thoroughly susceptible to scientific investigation. Whereas 'education' implies some deliberate guidance of, or intervention into, development, with a predetermined end-state or goal in view, 'socialization' was intended to convey a detached, dispassionate approach to the study of the influence of society upon the individual.

This early psychological approach ran into severe problems. It was clearly not possible to explain the full complexity of human behaviour in terms of simple learning processes. In investigating phenomena such as children's imitation of aggressive behaviour and the effects of parental discipline, for example, it became necessary to introduce concepts like *internalization* and *identification*. These are essentially cognitive, or 'internal', concepts, that is, they cannot be pinned down in terms of identifiable 'pieces' of behaviour. The less rigorous form of reinforcement theory that resulted from this kind of modification became known as 'social learning theory'.

The last twenty years has seen a radical shift away from this kind of explanation. Indeed, the changing view of the nature of socialization has transformed developmental psychology from a quiet backwater of the discipline into one of its most vigorous and active areas. Three broad characteristics of the new view can be distinguished:

(1) The reciprocal, interactive nature of the relationship between the child and its environment is stressed. The environment is not seen to condition, or 'shape', the passive child any more than the child is seen to 'shape' its own environment; rather, the two form an active, symbiotic system in which any change in one has immediate effects upon the other. This is very different from what Danziger (1971) has called the 'social problem' approach to the study of child-rearing, which is closely related to social learning theory. This approach, now largely

abandoned, sought correlations between ratings of parental behaviour on dimensions such as 'punitiveness' and 'permissiveness', and of children's behaviour on dimensions such as 'dependency' and 'aggressiveness' – the best-known study being that of Sears, Maccoby and Levin (1957). The difficulties of establishing direction of causality, as well as the uncertain status of the dimensions of behaviour employed, contributed to its eventual abandonment. One alternative strategy is to carry out longitudinal studies, in which the development of a selected subject group is systematically assessed at a series of points in time. Several famous investigations of the long-term stability of different aspects of behaviour have been carried out using this technique (for example, Thomas, Chess and Birch, 1968).

(2) The second major characteristic of the new view of socialization is a shift towards what might be called a 'cognitive' approach. The revival of interest in Piaget's cognitive-developmental theory has provided considerable impetus in this respect. Piaget emphazises the active part played by the child in imposing meaning upon its world; and these constructions of meaning are 'negotiated' with others, notably, of course, the parents in the first instance. The extremely complex patterns of mother-infant interaction being investigated in the 1970s and 1980s are seen as a developing series of 'conversations', in which the mother's interpretations of her child's intentions are reflected in the child's responses to her. The newly-coined term 'intersubjectivity' summarizes this aspect of the interaction, now regarded as a key feature of early socialization.

(3) There is a new emphasis on an 'ecological' approach. Early research took an extremely stereotyped view of family relationships, such that the mother-infant bond was studied more or less to the exclusion of all others. In recent years father-child relationships are being studied more, as well as relationships with siblings. The ecological approach argues that no single relationship (such as between mother and child) can be studied adequately without taking into account the significant others in what is a highly complex network of relationships. These others include other members of the immediate family; they may also include grandparents, babysitters, childminders

and so on. Such changes in research emphasis may well relate to other changes in society, such as the greatly increased proportion of working mothers in the population, and the correspondingly greater degree of involvement of fathers in child care. There can be no doubt, when seen in this light, that socialization research has important practical as well as theoretical implications.

David J. Hargreaves
University of Leicester

References
Danziger, K. (1971), *Socialization*, Harmondsworth.
Sears, R. R., Maccoby, E. E. and Levin, H. (1957), *Patterns of Child Rearing*, Evanston, Ill.
Thomas, A. S., Chess, S. and Birch, H. G. (1968), *Temperament and Behavior Disorders in Children*, New York.

Further Reading
Cairns, R. B. (1979), *Social Development*, San Francisco.
McGurk, H. (ed.) (1978), *Issues in Childhood Social Development*, London.
See also: *culture and personality; developmental psychology; Piaget.*

Social Psychology

Many textbook authors have attempted to define the field of social psychology in a few succinct words. Their definitions focus on social influence processes as they affect the individual, or responses to so-called 'social stimuli', or on the variables that affect interactions between persons. Most would agree that social psychology is the biochemistry of the social sciences, a field lying between the study of customs and social norms on the one hand, and the study of individual personalities on the other. Although the field is in this sense interstitial, this should not demean its significance as a major social-science discipline. In its theories and research, social psychology provides vital information concerning how personalities are shaped and how cultural norms and values are translated into individual thoughts and actions.

Though there remain a number of highly resonant pockets of similar interest in sociology, most of the research literature and the recent texts in social psychology have been written by psychologists. It is also the case that social psychology, at least until recently, has been dominated by theories and research generated in America. Many of the seminal figures behind this array of contributions did, however, emigrate from Europe in the 1930s: Brunswik, Heider, Katona, Lazarsfeld and Lewin. In addition, under the stimulus of the European Association of Experimental Social Psychology (founded in 1967), there has been considerable recent momentum toward redressing the imbalance represented by America's pre-eminence.

The field of social psychology grew out of the recognition of human diversity within cultural uniformity. Essentially the field focuses on choices and behavioural decisions among the competing options that confront us all in complex contemporary societies. It has become a field that, more than any other, deals with the psychology of everyday life: the psychology of conversations, of self-presentations, of conformity, of persuasion, of winning and losing, helping and hurting, liking and avoiding.

Recent History

Gordon Allport argued three decades ago (1954) that most of the major problems of concern to contemporary social psychologists were recognized as problems by social philosophers long before psychological questions were joined to scientific methodology. Perhaps the most fundamental question was that posed by Comte: How can man be simultaneously the cause and consequence of society? But the discipline of social psychology has a more recent history than its flavouring ideas and concerns. Although many conveniently mark its birth in 1908 with the publication of influential early texts by McDougall and Ross, in a very real sense the field began to cohere and develop its own identity only in the mid-1930s and did not really take on momentum until after World War II. This coherence and subsequent momentum depended largely on the development of indigenous theories and methods, usually associated with the contributions of Kurt Lewin in the late 1930s and early 1940s. Partly through sustained advocacy and partly through example, Lewin championed the possibilities of experimentation in social psychology. His experimental studies of autocratic, democratic, and *laissez-faire* leadership atmospheres (with Lippitt and White in 1939) showed how complex situational variables could be manipulated, validated, and shown to produce distinctive but orderly consequences. Lewin hoped to solve the problems of generalizing from the laboratory to the 'real world' by advocating (a) the linkage of experimentation to theory and (b) the parallel conduct of laboratory and field experimentation on conceptually cognate problems.

Though there would be wide agreement that Kurt Lewin deserves the title of the father of *experimental* social psychology, there were many other influences gathering under the social psychology umbrella during the 1920s and 1930s in America. These included the sustained series of empirical studies on group problem solving, the ingenious attitude measurement methodologies of Thurstone (1929) and Likert (1932), and the development of respondent sampling and survey research techniques.

But the central identity of social psychology was to remain anchored in the experimental approach. One of Lewin's students, Leon Festinger, exemplified Lewin's emphasis on going back and forth between the laboratory and the field, and showed in particular how experimentation made sense only if it were wedded to theory. During the two post-war decades when he was active as a social psychologist, Festinger (1954; 1957) developed two theories that had a profound impact on the field. The first of these was a theory of social comparison processes, a detailed set of postulates and propositions concerning the consequences for social interaction of man's need for the kinds of information about himself and the outer world that only other people could provide. The second was a theory of cognitive dissonance, which portrayed the various mental and behavioural manœuvres by which people attempt to restore cognitive consistency. The power of this theory was greatly enhanced by Festinger's recognition that some cognitions are more resistant to change than others, and that behavioural commitment is a potent source of such resistance. This recognition permitted rather precise predictions concerning the form that dissonance reduction would take in different situations. In particular, changes would be observed in the least resistant cognition. The ideas informing both of these theories remain important in much of current social-psychological thinking and have become a part of our cultural wisdom. Equally important, perhaps, the voluminous research generated by the theory of cognitive dissonance provided a clear example of coherent progress through experimental research in social science, research yielding cumulative insights that helped to refine and amplify the theory inspiring it.

A very different kind of theoretical orientation became prominent in the late 1960s, just as the enthusiasm for investigating dissonance phenomena began to wane. This was the attributional approach to social behaviour, an approach associated with Fritz Heider and identified with his seminal treatment of the *Psychology of Interpersonal Relations* (1958). The basic premise of the attributional approach is that people are motivated to understand behaviour, and readily do so by viewing it within a meaningful causal context. Our response to others, in other words, is a function of the causes we attribute to explain their behaviour. Though initially the focus of attribution theory was almost entirely on the perception of other persons, Kelley (1967) and Bem (1967) extended the attributional orientation to include self-perception. The perception of our own inner dispositions and emotions is mediated by our causal evaluations of our own behaviours, taking into account relevant features of the situational context.

As the attributional orientation flourished in the early 1970s, it fed and was fed by a broad revival of interest in social cognition. Though social psychology (at least since the subjectivism championed by W.I. Thomas) has always emphasized the cognitized social world, an emphasis on detailed analyses of information processing and social memory has become more

dominant over the past five years. The heritage of the attributional approach is largely reflected in a concern with attributional biases and errors in the application of inference strategies (Nisbet and Ross, 1980), though there remains a strong
current of interest in attribution of responsibility, attributional
approaches to self-presentation, and attributional analyses of
self-fulfilling prophecies.

While these developments in social cognition were occurring
within the 'mainstream' of experimental social psychology,
some social psychologists continued to concentrate on the
traditional problems of social influence and group processes.
Asch's (1956) classic studies of conformity and Milgram's
(1974) research on obedience have become standard textbook
entries. In different ways, their findings showed the remarkable
sensitivity of normal adults to social influence pressures. The
nature of group processes was especially informed by Thibaut
and Kelley's (1959) analysis of outcome exchanges in dyads
and larger groups. This analysis capitalized on the contingency
matrices of game theory, as well as building on both reinforcement and social comparison theories within psychology. It
provided a rich and provocative framework for dealing with
power relations, roles, and the development of norms. Many
publications in the 1960s and 1970s dealt with complex interpersonal conflict situations that might be resolved through
bargaining and negotiation. Throughout this period, also, a
steady stream of articles appeared shedding light on such social
phenomena as aggression, helping behaviour, attitude change,
jury decision making, crowding, social discrimination, sex-role
stereotypes, the impact of television, and a variety of other
applied topics. More comprehensive historical overviews – both
general and within specific content areas – may be found in the
Handbook of Social Psychology (Lindzey and Aronson, 1984).

Current Status of the Field
Any brief characterization of such a complex discipline must
be arbitrary and selective in many respects. Nevertheless, it is
possible to venture a few generalizations on the current state
of the field that would probably recruit a sizeable consensus.

The emphasis on experimentation has been buffeted by critical winds from several directions. Some critics have concluded that the problem of generalizing from laboratories (and sopho-mores!) is insurmountable. There is no way to extrapolate meaningfully from the historical and contextual particularities of any given experiment. Other critics have been concerned with the ethics of those deceptive cover stories which most social psychology experiments seem to require. Still others are bothered by the treatment of subjects as manipulable objects rather than collaborators with whom one negotiates appropriate explanations for behaviour. Finally, there are those who feel that experimentation implies a highly restrictive form of linear causation, misrepresenting the normal processes of situation selection and movement through complex feedback loops in which the behaviour of actors is both causal and caused. Though many of these criticisms raise vital concerns, neither singly nor in combination are they likely to relegate the exper-imental approach to a secondary position in the armamenta-rium of social psychology. The viability of the experimental approach may be even more assured as its practitioners more clearly realize its particular strengths and its limitations. Even if the generalization problem seems insurmountable, on occasion, the design of experiments may be extremely important in facilitating and disciplining conceptual thought.

The current flowering of cognitive social psychology seems to be producing new intellectual alliances and breaking down old boundaries between general experimental and social psychology. Certainly social psychologists are borrowing para-digms from the traditions of general research on thought and memory; cognitive psychologists in turn are showing greater sensitivity to the variables of social context. In a similar fashion, social psychological theory has shed light on such clinical phenomena as depression, alcohol abuse, obesity and a range of problems associated with symptom labelling. Though social psychology may in some respects play the role of a gadfly within the social sciences, borrowing here and lending there, it is not likely to lose its special identity as the one field especially concerned with the details of interpersonal influence. At present, the pendulum seems to have swung away from a concern with social interdependence and group phenomena toward a concern with individual information processing. Here there seems to be some divergence between the more 'individualistic' Americans and the more 'groupy' Europeans. It would be interesting if the more blatantly *social* psychology of the Europeans influenced an American revival of interest in groups. This seems to be an old story in social psychology: the study of individuals must be informed by a clear understanding of the matrices of social interdependence within which they function; the study of groups must comprehend the cognitive and motivational processes of group members. The tension between these two foci, in the long run, may be what keeps the field on its relatively straight track – in spite of temporary deviations in course.

Edward E. Jones
Princeton University

References

Allport, G. W. (1954), 'The historical background of modern social psychology', in G. E. Lindzey (ed.), *Handbook of Social Psychology, Vol. I*, Cambridge, Mass.

Asch, S. E. (1956), 'Studies of independence and conformity: a minority of one against a unanimous majority', *Psychological Monographs*, 70.

Bem, D. J. (1967), 'Self-perception: an alternative interpretation of cognitive dissonance phenomena', *Psychological Review*, 74.

Festinger, L. (1954), 'A theory of social comparison processes', *Human Relations*, 7.

Festinger, L. (1957), *A Theory of Cognitive Dissonance*, Evanston, Ill.

Heider, F. (1958), *The Psychology of Interpersonal Relations*, New York.

Kelley, H. H. (1967), 'Attribution theory in social psychology', *Nebraska Symposium on Motivation*, 14.

Lewin, K., Lippitt, R. and White, R. K. (1939), 'Patterns of aggressive behavior in experimentally created "social climates" ', *Journal of Social Psychology*, 10.

Likert, R. (1932), 'A technique for the measurement of attitudes', *Archives of Psychology*, 140.

Lindzey, G. E. and Aronson, E. (1984), *Handbook of Social Psychology* (3rd edn), Cambridge, Mass.

McDougall, W. (1908), *An Introduction to Social Psychology*, London.

Milgram, S. (1974), *Obedience to Authority*, New York.

Nisbet, R. E. and Ross, L. (1980), *Human Inference: Strategies and Shortcomings of Social Judgment*, Englewood Cliffs, NJ.

Ross, E. A. (1908), *Social Psychology: An Outline and a Source Book*, New York.

Thibaut, J. W. and Kelley, H. H. (1959), *The Social Psychology of Groups*, New York.

Thurstone, L. L. and Chave, E. J. (1929), *The Measurement of Attitude*, Chicago.

See also: *attitudes; attribution theory; cognitive dissonance; conflict resolution; conformity; culture and personality; environmental psychology; prejudice; social identity; socialization; stereotypes; stigma.*

Social Skills

The Meaning and Assessment of Social Competence

A socially competent person is someone who possesses the necessary social skills to produce the desired effects on other people in social situations. These may be the professional skills of teaching, selling, interviewing, and so on, or the everyday skills of communicating effectively, being persuasive, and maintaining social relationships. Social competence can be assessed by objective measures of success, for example, in selling, or self-rating scales, for example, for assertiveness, or the amount of difficulty experienced in different situations. Interviews can find out more details about areas of social difficulty. Role-playing in laboratory or clinic can provide information about specific areas of deficit. In the case of clients for social skills training (SST), the particular goals of treatment can then be decided upon.

Social inadequacy of different degrees is widespread. Among children, some are isolated, others aggressive. Over 50 per cent of students say they often feel lonely, 15–20 per cent seriously so, and 40 per cent of students say that they are shy. Between 7–10 per cent of adults are handicapped by an inability to establish or sustain normal relationships or cope with common social situations. Among outpatient neurotics the corresponding figure is 25–30 per cent, while for hospitalized psychotics it is probably 100 per cent. Failures of social competence can lead to rejection and social isolation, and ultimately to the development of anxiety, depression and other symptoms of mental disorder.

For any particular professional social skill, such as selling, teaching, or supervising working groups, some people are far less effective than others. Some salespersons may sell 25 per cent of what the better ones sell, poor supervisors may generate four times as much absenteeism and labour turnover, and much less output than better supervisors. Among people who go to work abroad, for example, for those going to parts of the Middle or Far East for commercial firms or the Peace Corps, as many as 60 per cent may fail, and return home early.

Methods of Social Skills Training

(1) *Role-playing* is now the most widely used method. An area of skill is briefly described, such as how to combine a principle with an example (teaching), how to make someone talk more (interviewing). This is followed by a demonstration, live or on film ('modelling'). The contents of this teaching depend on the results of research into the most effective way of performing the skill, for example, which teaching methods get the best results. A trainee then role-plays in front of video cameras for 5–10 minutes, with another trainee, or with a prepared stooge. Finally there is a feedback – consisting of playback of video-tape, and comments from the trainer. Between sessions trainees are encouraged to try out the new skills ('homework'), and report back on how they got on.

(2) *Supplementary exercises* for special aspects of social skills can also be used. These include training to send and receive

nonverbal communications from face and voice, in the conduct of conversations, in appearance and other aspects of self-presentation, and the handling of particular situations and relationships. These specialized methods make use of research into, for example, nonverbal communication and conversational analysis.

(3) *Educational methods* are a valuable addition to, but not a substitute for, more active methods of training. The 'Culture Assimilator' for intercultural skills consists of instruction on the situations which have been found to cause most difficulty in the other culture. Training for situation and relations can include instructions on the rules and other basic features, and can correct common misunderstandings.

The Current Extent of Social Skills Training

SST is being increasingly used for neurotics, disturbed adolescents, depressives, alcoholics, drug addicts and prisoners, usually as part of a larger treatment package. Training usually consists of role-played sessions, once or twice a week, for one to one-and-a-half hours, in groups of four to ten with two trainers, sometimes combined with individual treatment.

Teaching skills are often taught by 'microteaching', a form of role-playing, using short practice lessons to small groups of children. Similar methods are used for industrial supervisors, managers, doctors, social workers, police and other professional groups.

Training for everyday social skills is less readily available. However, in North America there is widespread assertiveness training, mainly for women, occasional training in heterosexual skills for students with 'minimal dating' problems, and training for making friends for young people who are lonely. While Americans are very interested in assertiveness, British clients for SST are more interested in making friends.

Intercultural skills training is being increasingly widely given for people who are going to work abroad – export salesmen, diplomats, military personnel, Peace Corps members and others. A variety of methods are used, including education in the different customs of the other culture and meeting members of the culture and recently returned expatriates.

Marital therapy of various kinds is widely available, but has not prevented one marriage in three failing. American Behavioral Marital Therapy is based on increasing rewardingness, and contracts in which each partner agrees to a concession, such as to go dancing together once a week in exchange for going to football once a week. Other methods of marital therapy consist of role-playing focused on interaction between the couple, or of group therapy for two.

The Effectiveness of SST

Does it work? For socially inadequate neurotics, SST does a little better than behaviour therapy aimed to reduce anxiety: SST improves the skills, and may later reduce the anxiety. The worse the patients are, the more sessions are needed. Mental patients of all kinds can be helped by SST, preferably as part of a larger package.

Professional social skills, and intercultural skills, can be trained in quite a short course of role-playing – typically six sessions. Marital problems can be somewhat alleviated by existing forms of therapy.

However, it should be emphasized that most follow-up studies have been carried out on earlier and fairly simple versions of SST. Research has now made possible much more sophisticated training, such as that embodied in the various supplementary exercises listed earlier.

Michael Argyle
University of Oxford

Further Reading

Argyle, M. (ed.) (1981), *Social Skills and Health*, London.

Argyle, M. (ed.) (1981), *Social Skills and Work*, London.

Argyle, M. (1983), *The Psychology of Interpersonal Behaviour* (4th edn), Harmondsworth.

Argyle, M. (1985), 'Some new developments in social skills training', *Bulletin of the British Psychological Society*, 37.

Bellack, A. S. and Hersen, M. (1979), *Research and Practice in Social Skills Training*, New York.

Singleton, W. T., Spurgeon, P. and Stammer, R. B. (eds) (1980), *The Analysis of Social Skill*, New York.

Spence, S. and Shepherd, G. (1983), *Developments in Social Skills Training*, London.

See also: *group therapy*.

Stereotypes

Stereotypes are usually defined as oversimplified, and often biased, conceptions of reality that are resistant to change. The term is primarily used with reference to conceptions of particular categories of people, conceptions that are often negative in tone and linked to prejudiced attitudes and behavioural discrimination. The term derives from the Greek *stereos*, meaning solid, and *typos*, meaning the mark of a blow, impression, or model. A stereotype was originally a method of duplicate printing, but the word was adapted for its present usage by Walter Lippmann in his classic book, *Public Opinion* (1922). Lippmann stressed the important function of stereotypes as cognitive preconceptions that are essential for the management of a reality that would otherwise overwhelm us with its complexity.

The phenomena of stereotyping have become standard topics in sociology and social psychology. Early empirical studies (for example, Katz and Braly, 1933) stressed the degree of consensus in the stereotypes depicting different ethnic groups. Labelling theorists in sociology have emphasized the power of stereotypes in generating invidious emotional responses to deviant or minority persons. Frustration-aggression theory in psychology also stimulated interest in the dynamics of prejudice and emphasized the motivated nature of many of our stereotypes (Dollard *et al.*, 1939).

Two important developments in social psychology shortly after World War II accelerated interest in the processes of stereotyping. One was the general atmospheric interest in the role of motivation and past experience as determinants of our perceptions. A capstone of this development was a paper by

J. S. Bruner (1957) linking perception to the concept of pre-established cognitive categories. Bruner explicitly stressed the assimilation of incoming information to the 'typical instance' of a category, thus providing a fruitful context for the discussion of stereotyping. Another influence was *The Authoritarian Personality* (Adorno *et al.*, 1950). This represented an attempt to illuminate some of the hidden dynamics of anti-Semitism and of more general predispositions toward the over-simplified thinking associated with Fascistic belief systems. Thus, stereotypic thinking was found to characterize high scorers on the various authoritarianism scales.

Gordon Allport's analysis of prejudice and stereotypy in 1954 began a general movement toward treating stereotypes as a consequence of normal cognitive functioning rather than looking at them as a by-product of frustration or pathological defensiveness. In this, and subsequent treatments, stereotypes have been viewed as the often unfortunate end-products of inevitable and even necessary strategies of information processing.

As the field of social psychology has become explicitly more cognitive, there has been renewed interest in stereotypes and the experiences and settings that contribute to them. Edited volumes by Hamilton (1981) and Miller (1982) summarize much of the recent research in the stereotyping area. Although it is still generally acknowledged that stereotypes may at times be motivated and serve as a justification for hostile or prejudiced attitudes, more stress is currently being placed on the contention that processes of prejudgement and categorization are built into every act of perception or information processing. Thus stereotypes are nothing more than cognitive categories that often satisfy emotional needs, prove quite resistant to disconfirming information, and operate as powerful cognitive magnets to which such information is assimilated. Though stereotypes are generally viewed as the maladaptive extreme of the cognitive processing continuum, and serve to perpetuate social conflict and discrimination, there is also much evidence that group stereotypes may be readily discarded when judging individual group members. Thus it appears that individuals are quite capable of having strong and rather rigid views of typical group members, but these views do not necessarily influence how a particular member is perceived or evaluated.

Edward E. Jones
Princeton University

References

Adorno, T. W., Frenkel-Brunswik, E., Levinson, D. J. and Sanford, R. N. (1950), *The Authoritarian Personality*, New York.

Allport, G. W. (1954), *The Nature of Prejudice*, Cambridge, Mass.

Bruner, J. S. (1957), 'On perceptual readiness', *Psychological Review*, 64.

Dollard, J., Doob, L. W., Miller, N. E., Mowrer, O. H. and Sears, R. L. (1939), *Frustration and Aggression*, New Haven.

Hamilton, D. L. (ed.) (1981), *Cognitive Processes in Stereotyping and Intergroup Behavior*, Hillsdale, N.J.

Katz, D. and Braly, K. (1933), 'Racial stereotypes in 100 college students', *Journal of Abnormal Social Psychology*, 28.

Lippmann, W. (1922), *Public Opinion*, New York.

Miller, A. G. (ed.) (1982), *In the Eye of the Beholder: Contemporary Issues in Stereotyping*, New York.

See also: *prejudice; stigma.*

Stigma

The sociologist Erving Goffman is usually credited with introducing the term 'stigma' into the social sciences. He begins his influential essay (*Stigma: Notes on the Management of Spoiled Identity*) with a brief etymological summary.

The Greeks . . . originated the term *stigma* to refer to bodily signs designed to expose something unusual and bad about the moral status of the signifier. The signs were cut or burnt into the body and advertised that the bearer was a slave, a criminal, or a traitor – a blemished person, ritually polluted, to be avoided, especially in public places. Today the term

. . . is applied more to the disgrace itself than to the bodily influence of it. (Goffman, 1963)

The concern with stigma fits well into a broader and older concern with deviance and its labelling. The labelling perspective favoured by many sociologists of deviance (especially those who share the orientation of 'symbolic interactionism') emphasizes the social construction of boundaries separating the 'normal' from the 'deviant'. These boundaries serve an important symbolic function of affirming in-group values and are relevant in several different domains. Goffman distinguishes between blemishes of character (for example, mental illness, homosexuality, criminal behaviour), abominations of the body (physical deformities of various kinds), and the tribal stigma of race, nation and religion. Though it is important to note that stigma can emerge in each of these domains, it should also be recognized that the tendency to avoid disabled or deviant persons may stem from the awkwardness of not knowing how to act in their presence, rather than being a reflection of the drastic discredit usually associated with the term stigma.

Cutting across the content domains of potential stigma, a number of dimensions may be identified that affect the degree of discredit likely to result from the process. One such dimension is *concealability*. Those conditions that can be concealed under normal conditions give rise to decisions about 'passing', about whether or when to disclose the condition. Another dimension is *origin*: how did the condition come about and to what extent was the person responsible? People tend to attribute greater responsibility for alcoholism and obesity than for mental retardation or the paraplegia of a combat veteran. Other dimensions of variation include *aesthetic* concerns, the extent to which the condition actually or symbolically *imperils* others, and to which it may *disrupt* normal social interaction. Deafness, for example, is typically more disruptive than blindness, though particular interaction contexts may make blindness more salient as a disability.

In spite of these sources of variation and their important differential consequences, the stigmatizing process has a number of features that transcend the particularities of any single deviant condition. Associated with a crucial act of categorizing or labelling the deviant person, there is an arousal of emotions typically featuring a mixture of revulsion and sympathy. Recent discussions of stigma (Katz, 1981; Jones *et al.*, 1984) have made much of the ambivalence involved in stigma. The act of labelling often sets in motion a process of devastating cognitive reconstruction that gives innocent behavioural data an ominous, tell-tale meaning. Thus there are strong tendencies for stigmatizing reactions to move in the direction of stereotypes that rationalize or explain the negative affect involved. Many sigmatizing reactions, however, are initially characterized by vague discomfort and unjustified 'primitive' affect.

Edward E. Jones
Princeton University

References

Goffman, E. (1963), *Stigma: Notes on the Management of Spoiled Identity*, Englewood Cliffs, NJ.

Jones, E. E., Farina, A., Hastorf, A. Marcus, H., Miller, D. and Scott, R. A. (1984), *Social Stigma: The Psychology of Marked Relationships*, New York.

Katz, I. (1981), *Stigma: A Social Psychological Analysis*, Hillsdale, NJ.

See also: *stereotypes*.

Stress

The breadth of the topic of stress is reflected both in the diversity of fields of research with which it is associated and in the difficulty of finding an adequate definition. Some stresses such as noise, heat or pain might best be considered as properties of the environment which represent departure from optimum and which differ only in intensity from levels which are normally tolerable. Thus, stress could be seen as a stimulus characteristic, perhaps best defined as an 'intense level of everyday life'. In contrast, it is possible to envisage stress as a pattern of responses associated with autonomic arousal. Initial impetus for this approach was provided by Selye (1956), who proposed that stress is the nonspecific response of the body to any demand made upon it. Physiologically committed, it assumed that the stress response was not influenced by the nature of the stressful event, but was part of a universal pattern of defence termed the 'General Adaptation Syndrome'. Selye demonstrated a temporal pattern in cases of prolonged stress. There were three identifiable phases: alarm, resistance and exhaustion. The capacity of the organism to survive was assumed to be a function of exposure time; resistance to further stress was lowered in the alarm phase, raised in the subsequent resistance phase and further lowered in the exhaustion phase.

Neither stimulus-based nor response-based definitions cope well with varied and complex stresses such as taking an examination, parachute jumping, surgical operations and public speaking. The problem that 'one man's stress is another man's challenge', is partly solved by a definition which presupposes that stress is the result of imbalance between demand and capacity, and, more importantly, by the *perception* that there is imbalance. The factors which create ambition and translate into intentions are as important in determining stress levels as those which affect capacity.

A number of models have been proposed which assume that the conditions for stress are met when demands tax or exceed adjustive resources (Lazarus, 1966, 1976; Cox and Mackay, 1978). In particular, Lazarus has proposed that several appraisal processes are involved in the assessment of threat. The intensity of threat depends on stimulus features, but also on the perceived ability to cope. In turn, coping may take the form of direct action or avoidance and may involve anticipatory preparation against harm, or the use of cognitive defence strategies.

Fisher (1984) has proposed that mental activity in the perception and response to stress forms the essential basis of worry and preoccupation, and is likely to be concerned with the assessment and establishment of control. The perception of personal control is not only a likely determinant of psychological response, but has been shown to determine hormone pattern. For example, applied and laboratory studies have suggested that control over the work pace dictates the pattern of noradrenaline and adrenaline balance, and may determine the degree of experienced anxiety.

Working conditions and events in life history together form an important source of potential stress and may have a pervasive influence on mental state and physical health in the long term. Stress at work is no longer thought to be the prerogative of white-collar and professional workers. Repetitive manual work is associated with high adrenaline levels; paced assembly line workers have been found to be very anxious, and computer operators who spend more than 90 per cent of their time working at the interface may be tense for 'unwind periods' after work. Depression is likely when personal discretion is reduced, when there is lack of social support, or when social communication is impaired, as in conditions of high machine noise.

A significant additional feature of life history is the adjustment required by change. Two important consequences of change are interruption of previously established activity and the introduction of uncertainty about future control. Studies of homesickness in university students have suggested the importance of worry and preoccupation as features of adjustment to change. Grieving for the previous life style is as much a feature as concern about the new, and in some individuals this may be an important prerequisite for the establishment of control (Fisher, 1984; Fisher et al., 1985).

Competence is a necessary condition of the exercise of personal control, but it may be difficult to maintain in stressful circumstance. Studies of the effects of environmental stress on attention and memory have indicated changes in function in relatively mild conditions of stress. Although the changes may not always be detrimental in mildly stressful conditions, at high levels of stress, behavioural disorganization and consequent loss of control are characteristic. It has been found that performance is related to arousal level in the form of an inverted 'U' curve. Mild stresses, by increasing arousal, are likely to improve performance, whereas severe stresses are more likely to cause deterioration. However, the assumption of a single dimension of arousal has been undermined by physiological evidence suggesting that there are arousal patterns which may be stimulus or response specific. The concept of compatibility between concurrent and stress-produced arousal levels is proposed by Fisher (1984) as part of a composite model of the relationship between stress and performance. The model also takes into account the influence of worry and mental preoccupation associated with stress and the establishment of control as joint determinants of performance change.

In both occupational and life-stress conditions, the pattern of behaviour – and hence the accompanying hormone balance which features in a particular stress problem – may result from decision making about control. A critical decision concerns whether a person is helpless or able to exercise control. The mental processes involved in control assessment may involve detecting and summarizing the relationship between actions and consequences over a period of time. In dogs, prior treatment by inescapable shock was shown to produce inappropriate helplessness in later avoidance learning (Seligman, 1975), which led to the hypothesis that depression and helplessness are closely associated, and may be transmitted as expectancies about loss of control. The question 'Why are we not all helpless?' is appropriate, given the high probability that most people experience helplessness on occasions in their lives; it has been partly answered by research which suggests that normal subjects resist helplessness and depression by overestimating control when rewards are forthcoming (Alloy and Abramson, 1979). Equally, they may put more effort into a task, or find other evidence suggesting that control is possible, thus raising self-esteem (Fisher, 1984). By contrast, those already depressed assess control levels accurately, but are more likely to blame themselves for circumstances which indicate that there is no control. Therefore, lack of optimistic bias and lack of objectivity in attributing the cause of failure distinguishes the depressed from the non-depressed person.

The above considerations suggest that analysis of decisions about control in different stressful circumstances may provide the key to understanding the risks attached to long-term health changes in an individual. A person who is too readily helpless may be depressed and may incur the punishment produced by control failure. He thus experiences distress. A person who struggles against the odds of success incurs the penalty of high effort. A person who practises control by avoidance may need to be constantly vigilant, and to evolve elaborate techniques for avoidance and, if successful, will never receive the information which indicates control is effective.

The outcome of decision making about control could have implications for physical health because of the mediating role of stress hormones. Repeated high levels of catecholamines may, because of functional abuse of physical systems, increase the risk of chronic illness such as heart disease. High levels of corticoid hormones may change the levels of antibody response, thus changing the risk associated with virus and bacterial born illness, as well as diseases such as cancer (Totman, 1979; Cox and Mackay, 1982).

S. Fisher
University of Dundee

References

Alloy, L. B. and Abramson, L. Y. (1979), 'Judgements of contingency in depressed or non-depressed students: sadder but wiser?', *Journal of Experimental Psychology (General)*, 108.

Cox, T. and Mackay, C. (1982), 'Psychosocial factors and psychophysiological mechanisms in the aetiology and development of cancers', *Society of Science and Medicine*, 16.

Fisher, S. A. (1984), *Stress and the Perception of Control*, Hillsdale, NJ.

Fisher, S., Murray, K. and Frazer, N. (1985), 'Homesickness, health and efficiency in first year students', *Journal of Environmental Psychology*, 5.

Lazarus, R. (1966), *Psychological Stress and the Coping Process*, New York.

Lazarus, R. (1976), *Patterns of Adjustment*, Tokyo.

Seligman, M. E. P. (1975), *Helplessness: On Depression Development and Death*, San Francisco.

Selye, H. (1956), *The Stress of Life*, New York.

Totman, R. (1979), *The Social Causes of Illness*, London.

See also: *activation and arousal; bereavement; pain; psychosomatic illness; separation and loss.*

Sullivan, Harry Stack (1892–1949)

Harry Stack Sullivan was born in Norwich, New York on 21 February 1892 and died on 14 January 1949 in Paris. Helen Swick Perry's excellent biography of Sullivan records in detail the events of his life, certain aspects of which profoundly influenced his highly original and creative contributions to psychiatry.

The first and foremost is the effect upon Sullivan's view of the world of his rural, Irish, Roman-Catholic background, and growing up socially isolated because of the then current religious prejudices, as virulent as racial prejudice. It is the fact of his having been a Roman Catholic, rather than his practising the religion itself, that is of central importance in understanding some of his points of view.

The second important biographical fact is that his formal education was limited to one semester at Cornell in 1908 and his receiving his medical degree from the Chicago School of Medicine and Surgery in 1917, a school which Sullivan himself described as 'a diploma mill'. His formal academic work in both institutions can only be described at best as marginal, at worst abysmal. Obviously Sullivan, who in his prime was an intellectual of the highest versatility, was largely self-educated.

Between 1918 and 1922, the years before he began work at Sheppard-Pratt Hospital, Sullivan served in various capacities in the Army Medical Corps and in a number of federal agencies dealing with veterans' matters. This experience in the army gave structure to his life and probably saved him from a mental breakdown. But more importantly, it gave him the chance clinically, in his various roles, to become certified by the government as a neuropsychiatrist. Thus, the loose ends of his cursory medical education were brought into synthesis. He finally had clear and formal medical status in psychiatry.

These themes of social isolation stemming from his Roman-Catholic background, his avid interest in self-education and innovation, and his profound sense not only of American patriotism but of world patriotism marked his life's work.

Sullivan began to formulate his own theoretical ideas, which were stimulated and elaborated by two close friendships: with Clara Thompson, whom he met in 1923, and Edward Sapir, whom he met in 1926. To Thompson he owed the debt of being exposed to psychoanalysis in a formal sense and to Sapir, the anthropologist, he owed support for his convictions about the importance of the interaction between individuals and their cultural and family environments. Although there is no doubt that Sapir was a brilliant intellectual foil to Sullivan through their mutual interest in culture and personality, there was a common bond which probably intensified their friendship: Sullivan as a Roman Catholic and Sapir as a Jew had both suffered religious and ethnic prejudice.

It is interesting that in formulating his theoretical propositions concerning the human condition, be it normal or pathological, Sullivan never abandoned the original intellectual stance he had hoped to realize as a student at Cornell, where he had intended to become either a mathematician or a physicist. To a degree that is equalled by no other psychiatrist before or since, Sullivan was extremely aware of when he was speaking as a scientist, profoundly influenced by the operationalism of Percy Bridgeman and other scientific thinkers and philosophers, and when he was speaking as an artist in the domain of interpersonal relationships. In his own language, Sullivan, depending on the particular situation, was the 'personification' of the natural scientist, the interpersonal artist, or the poetic, imaginative, Irish, lyric thinker. It was his ability to speak in different tongues that gave Sullivan credence in academic circles as well as in the medical domain of science. Given this basic tenet of the operational, to Sullivan what went on between people was the only data admissible to psychiatry. He largely ignored dreams and what he called reverie processes, because they could not be observed. They could create behaviour which could be observed and was thus admissible as clinical data.

A second aspect of Sullivan's theory is that it is *species specific*: human beings are not part of an evolutionary chain as seen by Freud, but are to be seen in their own right. Their primate heritage gives them a capacity no other species possesses: a symbol system and a capacity to interchange symbol systems. This conceptualization was no doubt profoundly reinforced by his friendship with Sapir, whose expertise in anthropology was linguistic relativity. Thus, as Perry has remarked, the capacity to communicate or the inability to communicate is the key to the human condition. Closely related to this idea is Sullivan's assertion that our particular primate status requires us to be in interpersonal contact at all times with significant others. If that contact cannot be maintained, deterioration and mental illness are inevitable.

Corollary to these two basic ideas was Sullivan's postulation that anxiety early in life was induced by the anxious mother and thus anxiety as what he called a 'dysjunctive state' was an inevitable part of the human condition. Sullivan can thus be seen not only as an interpersonal theorist, but as an extremely provocative expositor of the place of anxiety in human affairs. Possibly one of the most interesting aspects of Sullivan's work – given the realities of his personal history – are his highly sophisticated and value-free essays on human sexuality.

One of his most important clinical contributions was the development of milieu therapy in the treatment of schizophrenics. A natural outgrowth of his emphasis on the interpersonal, it is a standard approach in modern psychiatry.

Sullivan's theoretical creativity, for practical purposes, stopped with the onset of World War II, where he became engaged, once again, in various capacities with the military. He was one of the first to see the implications of Hiroshima and, having full knowledge that to undertake a crusade on behalf of peace was to cost him his life, with implacable will he forged ahead. His attempt to set up various foundations bridging psychiatry and the social sciences, his enlisting psychiatrists and social scientists in the cause of peace, all marked the turbulent last years of his life. It can be said that he died serving the cause of humanity.

George W. Goethals
Harvard University

Further Reading
Sullivan, H. S. (1953), *The Interpersonal Theory of Psychiatry*, London.

Super-Ego

The concept super-ego is, roughly, the psychoanalytic equivalent to the more commonly-used word, conscience. It stands for the internalized value-concerns a person learns mostly in childhood, that affect the way one is accepted, approved of, and loved. They stem from the perceptions (carried out by the 'ego') about what kind of behaviour and attitudes will gain approval from the persons who provide nurturance and care, especially during the early years of life, and who will withhold such benefits when those values are not followed. They are the product of 'instrumental learning' which is to say, trial-and-error experimentation in everyday living: what gets love and approval 'works' and is therefore replicated, remembered, and for purposes of efficiency, ultimately automated (and becomes a part of the 'dynamic unconscious').

Such childhood super-ego values are not at first reasoned out or understood beyond the fact that they work to gain approval with all of its consequences. They are life-preservative. Since so many of the values become unconcious (and automated), if inquiry were made about them and why they existed, the answer would be no more profound than, 'Just because', or 'Mummy/Daddy says I should'. Punishments for breaches are by the Talion Principle: 'An eye for an eye, a tooth for a tooth, a hand for a hand'.

With growth and development, and as the child begins to wonder 'Why?', these values are explored and re-evaluated. 'Thou shalt not kill' loses its status as a categorical imperative, and reasons why this rule is needed to achieve social equilibrium are substituted for the blindly accepted dogma of the immature super-ego. The aura of God-given (parent-given) truth is progressively eroded away under the assault of more complex, social reality-based reasoning and experience. The less absolute but more reliable and flexible reality-testing process develops and becomes a manifestation and a function of the mature psyche and its super-ego. Although some residual fragments of the childhood super-ego may remain to stir restlessness throughout life, under most circumstances the considered evaluation of goals, consequences, and other people's interests and concerns will prevail and allow effective interpersonal interactions and intrapsychic satisfaction.

In order for this process to occur, it is important for the growing child to be reared in a fairly consistent and substantially constant environment. This means that both parents (as well as most members of the child-rearing surroundings) should agree upon and communicate the values they wish the child to internalize. They must all *say* the same things and then *behave* (model) the same behaviour. A failure to do so leaves images and values in confusion and can cause subsequent emotional conflict. When the child moves out into the broader world away from his immediate family, there will ideally be a continuity of values so that he does not have to make a choice between them (when they do, home usually wins). The fact that many children nowadays are reared in mobile families means that they may be forced to adapt to several highly varied environments, and thus multiple value systems, during their formative years; this can present substantial problems.

While psychiatrists (and many others long before them) have noted that the first five years of life are crucial to the formation of the super-ego, later development may also have powerful effects upon the whole or upon specific values within it. Some values are subject to little conflict and, therefore, are relatively easy to maintain. Others are more fragile and vulnerable and need some or much reinforcement throughout life.

Andrew S. Watson
University of Michigan

See also: *Freud, S.; psychoanalysis.*

Therapeutic Community

The use of community social processes for the treatment of mentally ill and personality disordered patients has been labelled 'therapeutic community'. Factors which have led to this approach include a growing dissatisfaction with the results of individual psychotherapy, the recognition of some harmful effects of institutionalization itself, and the realization of the importance of social experiences in learning and, therefore, in therapy.

The impetus for the therapeutic community came during and after World War II with the development of therapeutic units for soldiers suffering combat fatigue. In these army centres every aspect of the soldiers' hospital life was designed to counteract the socialization experience involved in being defined as mentally ill. The success of these units in returning soldiers to full activity was in sharp contrast with previous experience, and led to efforts at their replication in the civilian community.

Procedures in therapeutic communities derive from three sources: (1) group therapy, in which patients receive continuous feedback on their behaviour as seen by others and their maladaptive use of defence mechanisms; (2) democratic traditions of self-government, including a sharing of facilities, the use of first names, and frank expressions of thoughts and feelings between patients and staff; and (3) the importance of being part of a social unit to counteract alienation and promote rehabilitation. The power of peer group pressure has long been used in self-help groups, such as Alcoholics Anonymous.

The tone of the therapeutic community is often set by a daily meeting where all patients, ward staff, and doctors openly discuss problems and psychopathology.

Problems of the therapeutic community include the blurring of roles which makes it possible for staff to evade responsibility and authority. Also, the community approach may become a vehicle for the patient's rationalizing hostility towards authority or leadership in any form.

Despite difficulties, the concept has added to the effectiveness and humanity of the psychiatric unit. Those therapeutic communities which have achieved stability have incorporated professional control while permitting patients an active voice in their own care.

Bernard S. Levy
Harvard University

Further Reading
Almond, R. (1974), *The Healing Community*, New York.
Caudill, W. (1958), *The Psychiatric Hospital as a Small Society*, Cambridge, Mass.
Cumming, J. and Cumming, E. (1962), *Ego and Milieu*, New York.
Jones, M. (1953), *The Therapeutic Community*, New York.
See also: *group therapy*.

Thinking – Cognitive Organization and Processes
The term thinking is one of those most difficult to encapsulate in a simple definition. We learn the word long before we encounter psychological research, and our ideas about thinking are strongly influenced by commonsensical notions which may not map neatly onto the concepts which psychologists have found necessary to develop when studying cognition. We may be puzzled, for example, when psychologists argue that we are not consciously aware of much of our thinking, or that it is not really sensible to draw boundaries between thinking and perceiving, understanding and remembering. In psychology the word 'cognition' (from the Latin *cognosco*, to know) has come to be used in a wide sense, encompassing perceiving, comprehending and remembering, as well as thinking, in part because psychologists are aware of the interrelationships between all these processes.

Within philosophy, from Aristotle onwards, there was a strong tradition that thought involved a chain of associations of conscious images. This view underpinned the initial founding of experimental psychology in the late nineteenth century as the scientific study of consciousness. One of the major disputes in the early 1900s followed the frequent failure of subjects at

Würzburg, when introspecting on their thought processes, to report imagery. It is easy to verify for oneself that one can think of the superordinate category of 'cat' or an example of a flower without any intervening imagery. William James had already commented that thought was like the perches and flights of a bird (1890). During the flights, we are not aware of the components which lead to the next conclusion. Subsequently, there has been general agreement that much of the processing that underlies thinking, as well as the other cognitive processes, is not available to consciousness. (Morris and Hampson (1983) discuss those processes which are not open to introspection.)

The problems which the 'imageless thought' controversy raised for the early introspective psychology encouraged the growth of behaviourism. For the founder of this school, J. B. Watson, thought was 'nothing but talking to ourselves' and since 'any and every bodily response may become a word substitute' it became difficult to separate thinking from behaviour in general; in the US the study of thinking was submerged in the rush to investigate animal learning.

In Germany, however, the reaction to the introspective psychology took another form. Gestalt psychologists argued that the mind could not be analysed into simple sensations, but actually functioned towards forming good, whole patterns. Problems arose when there was imbalance in the mental field, conceived as akin to an electromagnetic field, so that problem solutions reflected a sudden rearrangement of the field in a way analogous to the reversal of the Necker cube in perception. This change in the field corresponded to insight into the problem. One Gestalt psychologist, Kohler, produced a famous monograph on *The Mentality of Apes* (1925) claiming insight into their problem solving, which challenged many behaviourist assumptions. Others, such as Duncker and Maier, examined the conditions which aided or impeded human insight. They showed, for example, how 'functional fixity' in the way in which we think of a pair of pliers will inhibit insight into their potential use as a pendulum bob in a given problem. In a related way, the repeated use of, say, a particular order of filling and emptying jugs in successfully solving a series of problems requiring the measurement of an amount of water, will 'set' the solver to try to use this solution when a far easier one is available.

With the decline of behaviourism and the development of computer science and cognitive psychology in the 1950s and 1960s, thinking became an important research topic. The need to design computers to solve problems stimulated research on how problems were solved by humans.

It became obvious to researchers on artificial intelligence (AI) that problem solving required both a massive base of stored knowledge and suitable operators to manipulate that knowledge. Newall and Simon (1972) studied the thought processes of experts and novices while playing chess and solving other problems. By getting their subjects to 'think aloud' they produced protocols of the steps in solving their problems. They were able to show that the subjects broke the problems down into sub-goals which they tackled with various strategies until the final solution. They developed a computer program called the General Problem Solver (GPS) which was able to solve a wide range of problems. It began by identifying the initial stage, goal state, and legal operators, and broke the problem down into manageable sub-goals using the principle of means-ends analysis. This involves reducing the difference between the present state and the desired sub-goal by selecting suitable operators.

Means-ends analysis represents one way of choosing strategies. The study of AI soon showed that both computers and people need rules of thumb, known as heuristics, which they can apply to situations as a good gamble that they will lead to successful solutions. Such heuristics must often function adequately; but much of the study of thinking by psychologists has deliberately chosen problems where the normal steps to a solution will fail. By so doing, more complex problem solving can be studied and the heuristics themselves clarified.

One aspect of thinking where heuristics have been especially explored is in decision making. Tversky and Kahneman (1974) have argued that some of our decisions will be biased by the failure of the heuristics we use to estimate the probability of events occurring. They identify two common heuristics, availability and representativeness. When using the availability heuristic, we assess the likelihood of something happening, say, our having a heart attack, by recalling instances of such events happening to people of our age. If we can think of many cases, we judge a heart attack as likely. This heuristic will work well so long as the sample that we recall is not biased by the properties of our memories. Tversky and Kahneman were able to demonstrate major errors in estimates of probability, which appear to result from instances being recalled disproportionately to their real occurrence.

The representativeness heuristic appears in the gambler's fallacy. It is commonly and erroneously believed that because the red and black of a roulette wheel have equal probabilities in the long term, a run of several red wins increases the probability that the next win will be black. People expect small samples to be representative of the long-term frequency pattern and ignore the fact that each spin has the same probability of red and black. Tversky and Kahneman, and Nisbett and Ross (1980) have documented the influence of such faulty heuristics of decision making in many problems.

Attempts to make computers solve problems revealed the need for the computer already to possess a rich knowledge of the world. Schank and Abelson (1977) found it necessary to equip their computer with expectations about what should happen, for example, when using a restaurant. They called the knowledge of such events 'scripts'. The use of prior knowledge is essential not only in problem solving or question answering, but in our comprehending and making sense of our minute-by-minute experience of the world. In so far as thinking can be defined as going beyond the information given, this is common to perceiving, comprehending and remembering as well as to thinking. As the research of, for example, Bransford (1979) has shown, we are constantly going beyond the given information to construct a plausible account of, and draw deductions from, our experience. For this reason it is hard to draw distinctions among the various aspects of cognition.

There have been several attempts to model the knowledge

base used in comprehension and thought. Network models (Anderson, 1976) have been the most popular. These represent the stored knowledge as nodes (or knots) representing concepts which are joined by specified relationships such as 'is the cause of', 'is an example of', to other nodes. According to such models, thinking, at least in part, involves the activating of nodes and the tracing and evaluating of the routes that are joined between them.

Another popular way of modelling the representation of knowledge has been by production systems. A production is a rule linking defined conditions to specified actions, so that if the conditions are met the actions will be carried out. It is assumed by advocates of the production system (for example, Anderson, 1980; Allport, 1979) that our knowledge and skills are represented by a vast collection of these rules which can be activated by appropriate conditions, and can modify and transform the currently active information in the cognitive system in a very flexible way.

Psychologists have long been interested in individual differences in thinking, and have recognized that being good at solving problems is an important skill, which is closely involved in the construction of intelligence tests. Since Binet was asked in 1905 to devise the first intelligence test, their use and interpretation has been controversial. Nevertheless the standard intelligence tests clearly measure individual differences in ability, even if it can be argued that these abilities are selected and limited by cultural factors.

In recent years cognitive psychologists have tried to specify what actual cognitive skills underlie the factors, such as verbal and spatial ability, which consistently emerge from psychometric studies. Hunt (1978) and Sternberg (1977) have tried to analyse in detail the sort of tasks used in intelligence tests, and to determine how individual differences in skills and strategies may contribute to the overall IQ score.

A fundamental issue in the study of thinking which divides many current researchers is the extent to which rational thought is based upon logic. Cohen (1977) argues that human thought is logical, and that apparently illogical arguments result either from ignorance or misunderstandings, or the use of less familiar theories of probability. Many others (for example, Johnson-Laird, 1982; Evans, 1980) see the basis of thinking as being often alogical and not based upon the formal principles familiar to logicians. One theme of recent research has been to show that familiarity with real-world uses of particular rules means that subjects can easily solve reasoning problems, even though they fail with abstract problems based on the same logical structure (Cox and Griggs, 1982). Such research suggests that, whatever the fundamental rationality of human thinking, the reality of the quality of thinking and problem solving in the everyday world depends as much upon memory as logic. This illustrates the point made initially, that it is a mistake to try to separate thinking too much from the rest of cognition.

Peter E. Morris
University of Lancaster

References

Allport, D. A. (1979), 'Conscious and unconscious cognition: a computational metaphor for the mechanism of attention and integration', in L. G. Nilsson (ed.), *Perspectives on Memory Research*, Hillsdale, NJ.

Anderson, J. R. (1976), *Language, Memory and Thought*, Hillsdale, NJ.

Anderson, J. R. (1980), *Cognitive Psychology and its Implications*, San Francisco.

Bransford, J. D. (1979), *Human Cognition: Learning, Understanding and Remembering*, Belmont, Calif.

Cohen, L. J. (1977), *The Probable and the Provable*, Oxford.

Cox, J. R. and Griggs, R. A. (1982), 'The effects of experience on performance in Wason's selection task', *Memory and Cognition*, 10.

Evans, J. St B. T. (1980), 'Thinking: experimental and information processing approaches', in G. Claxton (ed.), *Cognitive Psychology: New Directions*, London.

Hunt, E. (1978), 'The mechanisms of verbal ability', *Psychological Review*, 85.

James, W. (1890), *The Principles of Psychology*, New York.

Johnson-Laird, P. N. (1982), 'Thinking as a skill', *Quarterly Journal of Experimental Psychology*, 34a.

Kohler, W. (1925), *The Mentality of Apes*, New York.

Morris, P. E. and Hampson, P. J. (1983), *Imagery and Consciousness*, New York.

Newell, A. and Simon, H. A. (1972), *Human Problem Solving*, Englewood Cliffs, NJ.

Nisbett, R. E. and Ross, L. (1980), *Human Inference: Strategies and Shortcomings of Social Judgement*, Englewood Cliffs, NJ.

Schank, R. C. and Abelson, R. P. (1977), *Scripts, Plans, Goals and Understanding*, Hillsdale, NJ.

Sternberg, R. J. (1977), *Intelligence, Information Processing and Analogical Reasoning*, Hillsdale, NJ.

Tversky, A. and Kahneman, D. (1974), 'Judgment under uncertainty: heuristics and biases', *Science*, 125.

See also: *artificial intelligence; cognitive science; intelligence; memory; problem solving*.

Time

Like philosophers and natural scientists, psychologists have been intrigued by questions about time. How, in the apparent absence of a special sense organ, can we experience time? Is time an intuitive mode of perception, as Kant suggested, or a cognitive construction? Psychological approaches over the past century have yielded a number of important insights, not the least of which is the multiplicity of time experience.

The oldest and best developed approach is the study of time perception (Block, 1980; Michon, 1978). When deprived of clocks and other measuring devices, humans can still make remarkably accurate judgements about duration and order. Yet duration judgements can also be distorted in principled ways depending upon the properties of the stimuli and the activities of the perceiver. Experiments using discrete pairs of tones or light flashes show that separations as brief as 25–90 milliseconds still allow the detection of two separate events. However, when the separation is less than about one-fifth of a second, there is a strong tendency to perceive the events as dynamically related, an impression underlying the effectiveness of 'moving' marquee lights. A number of studies indicate that humans are most accurate in judging durations of about one-half of a second. But there is virtually no progressive under- or overestimation as durations increase up to times of several minutes. Given the considerable accuracy of duration judgements, it is not surprising that some theorists have posited the existence of an internal 'biological clock'. Yet none of the candidate physiological processes (for example, heart rate, cortical alpha rhythm) seem to be responsible for time perception. In addition, the biological clock model seems inconsistent with a number of systematic distortions of subjective time estimates.

Distortions of time estimates. like other perceptual illusions, provide clues to the processes responsible for normal experience. One time illusion, noted by William James in 1890, is that interesting experiences are subjectively shortened while they occur but are overestimated in retrospect. Conversely, empty intervals seem long as they are experienced but short when they are later remembered. Several explanations have been offered for these effects including the notion that when engaged in an engrossing task, one has little attention left over to monitor the passage of time or extraneous changes in the environment. By one account of the retrospective stretching or shrinking of experiences, the 'storage space' of the corresponding memory is used as a cue to the length of the experience. Thus, simply coded events seem briefer than elaborately coded events.

The relationship between time and memory is also central in some of the more cognitive approaches to the study of time. When thinking about past events, we often have a compelling feeling that one event was more recent than another. Laboratory studies indicate that judgements of recency are better when two events are meaningfully related (Tzeng and Cotton, 1980). One intepretation is that for related pairs (for instance two plays with the same leading actor) the first event is remembered at the time that the second is experienced. This leads to the establishment of an order code. Other studies of real world memory show that personal 'temporal landmarks' often play a key role in judging the date of past events.

The structure of memory provides information about the time of past events, but how do we know the present time? Several studies of temporal orientation show that the current day of the week can be identified more rapidly just before or after a weekend than in midweek (Koriat, Fischhoff and Razel, 1976). Apparently, current or recent activities and thoughts are tested against stored associations of different days of the week. The relative indistinctness of midweek days seems to be responsible for the delay in orienting on these days.

Relatively little attention has been given to human understanding of natural periodicities and conventional time systems. But recent studies indicate that several distinct kinds of representations or processes underlie part of this knowledge. When asked to make judgements about the order of months, subjects appear to recite covertly the names of months in some tasks and to use spatial-like images in other tasks (Friedman, 1983).

Another perspective comes from developmental research (Friedman, 1982). The ability to distinguish temporal patterns is well developed by infancy. This finding is not surprising when one considers the exquisite sensitivity to order necessary for speech production and comprehension. Other abilities show a more gradual development. Adults can infer the relative durations of two events given simultaneous starts and successive finishes. Five-year-olds under some circumstances can make similar judgements but they are easily perturbed by a variety of perceptual factors including distance and end point in the case of moving objects. Other abilities show a gradual onset, including awareness of the past-present-future trichotomy and knowledge of conventional time systems. Perhaps better than other approaches, developmental studies point to the multifaceted nature of time experience.

William J. Friedman
Oberlin College, Ohio

References

Block, R. A. (1980), 'Time and consciousness', in G. Underwood and R. G. Stevens (eds), *Aspects of Consciousness*, Vol. I, London.

Friedman, W. (ed.) (1982), *The Developmental Psychology of Time*, New York.

Friedman, W. (1983), 'Image and verbal processes in reasoning about the months of the year', *Journal of Experimental Psychology: Learning, Memory and Cognition*, 9.

Koriat, A., Fischhoff, B. and Razel, O. (1976), 'An inquiry into the process of temporal orientation', *Acta Psychologica*, 40.

Michon, J. A. (1978), 'The making of the present: a tutorial review', in J. Requin (ed.), *Attention and Performance, VII*, Hillsdale, NJ.

Tzeng, O. and Cotton, B. (1980), 'A study-phase retrieval model of temporal coding', *Journal of Experimental Psychology: Human Learning and Memory*, 6.

See also: *memory*.

Traits

Traits describe individual differences in personality, ability, and temperament. They refer to stable and consistent behaviour patterns and thus provide both economical descriptions of the way one person differs from another and are the basis for predicting how a person may be expected to behave.

A trait description (for example, 'She is intelligent', or 'He is kind') gives information about the standing of the individual on that characteristic relative to others, because traits are regarded as dimensions (like physical dimensions such as height or weight) along which people can be ordered. But, unlike physical characteristics, traits can never be observed directly; they are rather inferred from behavioural signs, and in this sense their existence is always hypothetical.

Traits have been studied extensively in the mapping of individual differences in personality. Trait theorists disagree about the definition of traits and about the precise number and form of traits they consider necessary for an adequate description of personality. An early personality theorist to study traits was Gordon Allport (1937), who defined them as enduring tendencies within the individual to behave in certain ways. This is a broad definition, and it raises the question of what distinguishes a trait from other kinds of inferred constructs used to describe individuals. One particularly problematic distinction is that between trait and attitude. Allport proposed a distinction which is still generally accepted: attitudes, unlike traits, have a well-defined object of reference, are often specific as opposed to general, and typically involve an evaluation of the object.

One of Allport's views which was less well received was that individuals are characterized by their own unique traits. A more commonly accepted notion is to treat traits as dimensions, which are applicable to most, if not all people, and which are able to capture the uniqueness of each individual according to their particular combinations and relative strengths. Two contemporary advocates of this approach to personality are Cattell and H. J. Eysenck. Cattell (1973) concludes that over twenty traits are needed to capture the breadth and diversity of personality, whereas Eysenck (1969) argues for a simpler picture with only three traits; extraversion, neuroticism, and psychopathy.

One important aspect in the study of traits is trait measurement, based on the assumption that a small but carefully selected sample of behaviour will indicate an individual's score on a trait, and this score may then be used to predict how that person will behave in a wide variety of contexts. Traits are inferred from three behavioural indicators: self-report questionnaires, behaviour ratings made by observers, and behavioural responses to situations created by the tester. The questionnaire is the most convenient and widely used.

The measurement of personality traits is currently in decline, because evidence of the last two decades suggests that behaviour patterns are less consistent than one would predict on the basis of traits. A person's questionnaire score for a personality trait such as extraversion is not a particularly good predictor of how that person will actually behave in another situation (Mischel,

1968). However, test scores for traits of ability and cognitive style yield more reliable behavioural predictions. Mischel's book, *Personality and Assessment*, had a major impact on trait research, causing many to abandon the use of the trait concept in personality, but it also led others to renewed efforts to discover the circumstances in which behaviour is consistent. As a result, it is now generally accepted that, while many behaviours do remain stable when they are compared across different points in time, they do not necessarily demonstrate the same degree of cross-situational stability (Mischel and Peake, 1982).

Despite psychologists' misgivings about the value of the trait concept, trait terminology constitutes at least 5 per cent of the English language, which suggests that traits must have some predictive and descriptive value. Some psychologists believe that this wealth of trait terminology is a useful source of insights into personality (Goldberg, 1982). Recent reconceptualizations go some way towards resolving the contradiction between these opposing views of the value of personality traits.

Currently, the trait concept is experiencing a reprieve, due to a transfusion of ideas from cognitive psychology. These new conceptualizations (for example, Buss and Craik, 1983; Hampson, 1982), while differing in details, share the same basic assumption: that traits are categorizing concepts which group together diverse behaviours performed in different situations and at different times. What these behaviours have in common is a family resemblance to a prototype behaviour for that trait. The major difference between this remodelled trait concept and the traditional view, such as Allport's, is that a trait is no longer regarded as being a mental structure existing within the individual. Instead, the trait is seen as a cognitive category that helps us interpret behavioural acts.

Sarah E. Hampson
Oregon Research Institute

References

Allport, G. W. (1937), *Personality: A Psychological Interpretation*, New York.

Buss, D. M. and Craik, K. H. (1983), 'The act frequency approach to personality', *Psychological Review*, 90.

Cattell, R. B. (1973), *Personality and Mood by Questionnaire*, San Francisco.

Eysenck, H. J. and Eysenck, S. B. G. (1969), *Personality Structure and Measurement*, London.

Goldberg, L. R. (1982), 'From ace to zombie: some explorations in the language of personality', in C. D. Spielberger and J. N. Butcher (eds), *Advances in Personality and Assessment*, vol. 1, Hillsdale, NJ.

Hampson, S. E. (1982), 'Person memory: a semantic category model of personality traits', *British Journal of Psychology*, 73.

Mischel, W. (1968), *Personality and Assessment*, New York.

Mischel, W. and Peake, R. K. (1982), 'Beyond *déjà vu* in the search for cross-situational consistency', *Psychological Review*, 89.

Further Reading

Hampson, S. E. (1982), *The Construction of Personality: An Introduction*, London.

Rorer, L. G. and Widiger, T. A. (1983), 'Personality structure and assessment', *Annual Review of Psychology*, 34.

See also: *attitudes; personality*.

Transactional Analysis

Transactional Analysis (TA), the creation of Eric Berne, is a personality theory and method of treatment which dates back to the mid-1950s. It has grown in popularity and today its concepts are applied in education, management, and other fields of human relations. It is popular partly because of its clear simple language and cleverly-turned phrases; yet research has developed increasingly complex and detailed theory and it has been employed with the most difficult psychiatric problems.

Among the fundamental concepts of TA is the *ego state*, a recurrent pattern of behaviour, feelings and thoughts. Drawing upon his psychoanalytic background, Berne identifies three basic states: *child*, the archaic qualities fixed in early childhood; *adult*, the objective qualities based on rational appraisals of reality; and *parent*, derived from qualities of parental figures.

A *transaction* is a two-person interaction in which the *ego state* of one person stimulates a corresponding state from another. Transactions are called *complementary* if they are parallel, that is, both parties behave objectively in an adult transaction; *crossed*, when ego states do not correspond; and *ulterior* when there are simultaneous manifest and latent levels of transaction.

The psychological *game* is a predictable, stereotyped pattern of behaviour, frequently complex, destructive and motivated by hidden desires. Some popular examples are 'courtroom', 'kick me', 'confession', 'yes, but . . ', 'try and catch me', and 'poor me'. As these colourful names imply, the purpose of a game is not straightforward, but designed to engage another within an intrapsychic conflict. Berne's formula for the game is

$$CON + GIMMICK =$$
$$RESPONSE \rightarrow SWITCH \rightarrow PAYOFF.$$

The term *stroke* is used for the reinforcers of behaviour provided by people – the words, glances and other symbolic recognitions that motivate. A *life script* – conformity with some important early transaction – may be destructive in its later effects, for example, when one attempts to play out an unrealistic life plan. *Contracts* are the basic agreements of acceptable behaviour explicitly or implictly agreed upon between people. The treatment contract in TA is considered essential to effective psychotherapy, and should include the patient's goals and how he or she will know when these have been achieved.

The terms and theory, easily learned and shared, become a useful shorthand for analysis of otherwise confusing and compli-cated experiences. Catchy phrases invite a dimension of playful-ness in otherwise ponderous analysis in a way that enhances the working alliance. Although the process is initially intellectual, powerful affects are soon liberated.

TA has been especially valuable in the clarification of communication problems. It provides a readily grasped group of tools for the analysis and treatment of communication problems between people, in groups, and between intrapsychic parts of a person.

Arnold R. Beisser
University of California, Los Angeles
Gestalt Therapy Institute

Further Reading
Berne, E. (1961), *Transactional Analysis and Psychotherapy*, New York.
Berne, E. (1964), *Games People Play*, New York.

Transference

The concept of transference was formally brought into psychiatry by Sigmund Freud, who discovered empirically that his patient's perceptions of him during analysis were coloured, distorted, and even completely fabricated in relation to the patient's early feelings toward important figures in his own past: parents, siblings, caretakers and the like.

These early, often infantile, feelings were transferred to the analyst *unconsciously*; the patient initially believed that these essentially internal perceptions were valid reflections of the therapist himself. At times, they were recognized as internal and inappropriate to the real situation; for example, a patient might say: 'This is strange, but I seem to feel toward you as I did toward my mother.'

At first it seemed to Freud that transference feelings were an obstacle and impediment to the rational progress of the analysis. However, he came to recognize that the transference was a repetition of earlier conflicts and feelings, and thus the analysis of the transference became the central task of the analyst. Modern psychoanalysts consider the transference even more important for therapeutic exploration and treatment.

Such transference feelings were later discovered to play a part in almost all human relationships, at least to some degree. A common example is a person's tendency to see various authority figures in parental terms and to experience feelings for them which are derived from childhood. To take an extreme case, love at first sight is a phenomenon almost entirely composed of transference feelings; since this sort of attachment owes nothing to the *real* aspects of the loved one, the feelings must originate from elsewhere, in the past.

A number of dynamic psychiatrists hold the view that, for operational purposes, everything that occurs within the analytic or therapeutic session may be viewed as a manifestation of transference feelings by one or the other parties. More recently, two areas relevant to this issue have become the focus of attention. The first is the so-called 'real' relationship, that is, those elements of the therapeutic relationship that are transference-free (or relatively so). The second is the idea that certain psychological entities may best be diagnosed by noting the specific types of transference formed during therapy itself (for example, narcissistic personality disorders).

The usual form of transference in therapy (and life in general) might be described as 'neurotic transference', in the sense that the feelings transferred derive from the original neurotic conflicts of the individual. One characteristic of this sort of transference is that it is 'testable'; the patient can correct his own misperception once attention is called to the nature and form of the error. Thus, a patient might say in such a situation, 'I see that I was automatically expecting you to reject me as my father once did.' On occasion, however, the transference perception is *not* testable, and resists reality testing. Such a fixed transference is called a psychotic transference, in which the patient is unalterably convinced of the reality of the transference perception: thus the patient might say, 'You *are* rejecting, there is no doubt about it; my father's nature is irrelevant to the matter.' These psychotic transferences are quite common among patients with the borderline syndrome, and contribute to the difficulty of therapeutic work with them.

It may be a safe generalization that the major source of difficulty with all parts of therapy, especially the therapeutic alliance, is the feelings that derive from the transference. This problem is balanced by the fact that the ability to work successfully with transference material is often the hallmark of the successful therapist.

Thomas G. Gutheil
Harvard University
Program in Law and Psychiatry, Boston

Further Reading
Freud, S. (1958), *The Dynamics of Transference*, London.
Greenacre, P. (1954), 'The role of transference', *Journal of the American Psychoanalytic Association*, 2.
Greenman, R. R. (1965), 'The working alliance and the transference neurosis', *Psychoanalytic Quarterly*, 34.
Orr, D. (1954), 'Transference and countertransference: an historical survey', *Journal of the American Psychoanalytic Association*, 2.
See also: *countertransference; psychoanalysis*.

Unconscious

Perhaps the single most important idea in Freud's theory is that human beings are influenced by ideas, feelings, tendencies and ways of thinking of which they are not conscious. Freud's original 'topography' of the mind had three divisions: the conscious, the preconscious, and the unconscious. His theory can be pictured as follows: the mind is like a darkened theatre, with a single spotlight to illuminate the actors on the stage. Consciousness is equivalent to the actor in the spotlight at any moment. All of the other actors who can be illuminated as the spotlight moves across the stage are equivalent to the preconscious. To complete Freud's picture we must imagine that there are many actors who are off-stage, in the unconscious. Unless they make the transition to the stage, the light of consciousness cannot illuminate them. Seen or unseen, on-stage or off, all the actors take part in the play of psychic life. The barrier between off-stage and on-stage is removed or weakened in dreams, and by free association, which is the basic technique of psychoanalysis.

Freud understood the unconscious as dynamic. Unconscious

impulses were thought to be constantly active, influencing the preconscious and conscious – sometimes in discernible ways. Freud's explanation for slips of the tongue (now commonly called Freudian errors) is the substitution of an unconscious thought for what was consciously intended. By considering these unconscious influences, Freud found meaning in what others saw as trivial mistakes – for example, when a man calls his wife by his mother's name. Freud's theory of humour is similarly based on the dynamic interaction between conscious and unconscious. The joke allows the pleasurable release of some repressed idea or feeling; aggressive sexual jokes are thus a classic example.

Freud's theory of the unconscious became more complex in the course of his writings. At first he assumed that everything which was unconscious had once been conscious and had been repressed. The paradigmatic example was the subject who under hypnosis could be given some post-hypnotic suggestion, such as to open an umbrella indoors, but told to *forget* that he had been given that instruction. When the trance was ended, the subject would comply with the suggestions and open the umbrella indoors, but be unable to explain why he had done such a silly thing. Thus his behaviour was influenced by an idea about which he had no conscious awareness. Freud believed that his patients, like hypnotic subjects, were capable of splitting off from consciousness certain ideas and feelings by a defensive process he called repression. These repressed unconscious ideas could influence the patient's behaviour, producing neurotic symptoms without his awareness.

Freud's clinical work demonstrated that the most significant repressed ideas led back to childhood experiences. The content of the unconscious seemed to be ideas and tendencies, mainly sexual and aggressive – which he thought of as instinctual and biological – which were repressed under the moral influence of the environment. But the repressed remained active in the unconscious and continued in dynamic interaction with the conscious. Thus Freud's conception of the unconscious emphasized the continuing and irrational influence of the past on the present.

The idea of the splitting of consciousness was not original to Freud, nor was that of an instinctive unconscious. These ideas in some form go back at least as far as Plato. The German philosophers of the nineteenth century, Schopenhauer and Nietzsche, had a view of human nature which, in many ways, anticipated Freud. Freud's theory of the unconscious nonetheless met with intense philosophical criticism, even ridicule. The idea that what was mental was not identical with consciousness and that the mental might be a mystery to consciousness was problematic for certain philosophical notions. Descartes had said, 'I think therefore I exist.' He used this introspective claim as the basis of a theory of knowledge. Freud's concept of the unconscious challenged the certitude of all such introspective claims about the certainty of self-knowledge. The idea of unconscious influences also called into question the notion of free will. Perhaps because Freud emphasized the sexual aspects of the unconscious, his views were easy for philosophers to ridicule. The philosopher Sartre, who was in many ways more sympathetic than most contemporary philosophers to Freud's emphasis on the importance of sex, still found it necessary to reject Freud's fundamental concept of the unconscious. He interpreted repression as self-deception; asserting that it is impossible to lie to oneself, he described repression as 'bad faith.'

Freud's concept of the unconscious derived from his study of dreaming. He viewed the unconscious (associated with the infantile, the primitive, and the instinctual) as striving toward immediate discharge of tension. Dreaming and unconscious thinking are described as primary process thought, that is, they are unreflective, concrete, symbolic, egocentric, associative, timeless, visual, physiognomic and animistic, with memory organized about the imperative drive, in which wishes are equivalent to deeds and there is a radical departure from norms of logic – for example, contradictory ideas exist side by side. Primary process thought is contrasted with the modulated and adaptive discharge of tension in secondary process. By contrast, conscious thinking is reflective or directed, abstract, specific and particular, situation oriented, logical, chronological, auditory, verbal and explanatory. Memory is organized around the conscious focus of attention; thought and actions are clearly distinguished; thinking is rational and logically oriented. Freud's view was that although the child advances from primary process to secondary process thinking, primary process does not disappear, but remains active in the unconscious. It can be revealed in dreams, in psychotic thinking, and in other regressed mental states. Preconscious thinking was characterized as intermediate between these two types. The distinction between primary and secondary process is a key development in Lacan's linguistic reinterpretation of Freud.

Carl Jung, probably the greatest figure in psychoanalysis next to Freud, was an early advocate of what he called the collective unconscious. He assumed that in addition to repressed content, there was an inherited component to the unconscious shared by the human race. He based this conception on the evidence that certain symbols and complexes endlessly recur in the history of civilization. The Oedipus myth of the Greeks is the Oedipal dream of modern times. Freud and Jung took these ideas quite literally, believing that the individual was born not just with instinctual tendencies, but with inherited complexes and symbols – for example, the serpent as a phallic symbol. Despite his eventual break with Jung, Freud maintained his own version of a collective unconscious, which also included the idea that certain moral concepts such as taboos had been inherited.

Freud subsequently reconceptualized his ideas about the unconscious in terms of the ego, the super-ego and the id. The id and the unconscious are now often used interchangeably in the psychiatric and psychoanalytic literature. While the theory of the unconscious remains controversial even today, the intuition that consciousness does not fully grasp the deeper mystery of our mental life continues to play an important role in twentieth-century thought.

Alan A. Stone
Harvard University

Further Reading

Freud, S. (1953 [1900]), *The Interpretation of Dreams*, The Standard Edition of the Complete Psychological Works of Sigmund Freud, Vol. IV, New York.

Ellenberger, H. F. (1970), *The Discovery of the Unconscious: The History and Evolution of Dynamic Psychiatry*, New York.

See also: *Freud, S.; Jung; psychoanalysis.*

Vision

The principal advantages of the visual system over other senses are two in number: (1) The individual can respond to stimuli at distances that are very large as compared with his size: this makes for safety and can have competitive advantages. (2) The large ratio between the objects giving rise to visual stimuli and the wavelengths of the radiations whereby information is transmitted optimizes the quantity and quality of the information that arrives at the eye.

The description of the stimulus can be rationalized by a presentation in terms of a five-dimensional continuum. One dimension scales the spectral wavelengths of the radiation, partnered by dimension No. 2, namely stimulus intensity. No. 3 gives the size of the stimulus in angular measure: a Fourier transform (Campbell and Robson, 1968) can be shown to have parallels with the radiational spectrum, large objects being characterized by long spatial waves and vice versa. No. 4 measures contrast: a high intensity cannot make an object visible unless it can be made to stand out from its visual surround. And No. 5 represents the dimension of time.

It is feasible to view the whole of the visual system, beginning with the cornea and terminating with the locus of sensory perception, as a series of filters which operate on the five-dimensional input so as to maximize the wanted-signal/noise ratio. The use of the word 'wanted' is used advisedly because the response to a stimulus can be modified by earlier stimuli and responses, memory, and so on. Although the filters act independently they affect dimensions other than their own. For example, a change in intensity may modify apparent duration, contrast, and even spectral appearance.

Since the eye has evolved in response to sunlight its reaction to electro-magnetic radiations – the 'visible' spectrum – is easy to understand. The intensity of sunlight is maximal approximately in the spectral range to which the photo-sensors in the retina are mainly sensitive. The band seen is a window between the absorptive walls of the cornea and lens which protect the retina from noxious effects of ultra-violet light on the one hand, and the absorption of vitreous, that is, water, which fails to transmit infra-red radiations, on the other. The optics of the eye – made up essentially of cornea, contractile pupil and accommodative lens – serve to form a high contrast image on the retina where radiation triggers chemical events in the photo-receptors. These initiate an electric response that ultimately reaches the cortex and more central sensory areas. The pupil is a spatial filter providing a short-wavelength limit to the spatial spectrum transmitted by the eye. It is a characteristic of the resolving power of the retina that, in its central region called the fovea, it accurately matches the relation between contrast transmission and spatial wavelength of the ocular optics. This is more economical than is true of the spectral response of the retinal rods and cones which does not quite match the spectral distribution of natural light reaching them: the result is energy waste.

The size of the pupil is under reflex control and varies homeo-statically not only with stimulus intensity but also so as to maximize retinal contrast, for example, when the ocular axes converge to a nearby visual target. This pupillary near-response is evoked alternatively by the lenticular mechanism of accommodation, another reflex that ensures that a high-contrast retinal image is formed independently of object distance.

Both the iris tissue, which determines the pupillary area, and the crystalline lens, which can accommodate its optical power as just noted, are subject to significant changes due to senescence. The pupil aperture is controlled by the interplay of the dilator and the sphincter under sympathetic and parasympathetic control respectively. Of the two smooth muscles, the former atrophies faster with age so that the pupil constricts in the old, admitting less light to the retina. A number of senescent changes occur in and around the lens which interfere with its power to accommodate. The result is presbyopia and the need for reading-glasses if a high-contrast retinal image of close objects is to materialize.

Given high contrast, the visual system can resolve normally visual angles of the order of 1 minute of arc. This high performance, inexplicable in terms of evolutionary pressures that have existed within the recent biologically significant time-scale, depends not only on optical normalcy, but also on good illumination (Davson, 1976). It tends to fall off – as in blue light – probably because contrast sensitivity is poor in this part of the spectrum.

The transduction of radiation into a nervous response takes place in the rods and cones; the former mediate vision in darkness, the latter in light. The latter also are associated with colour vision and high contrast sensitivity. Hence, if they are absent, as happens in certain diseases, vision is severely handicapped (Ripps, 1982). Rod and cone mechanisms also differ as regards temporal responses, the former being more sluggish and having the longer latent period of the two.

Considerable contrast, spatial, and temporal analysis takes place in the retina as it would be uneconomical to propagate redundancy to the cortex. It would also be difficult since the visual pathways converge onto a relatively tight optic nerve only to diverge again at the level of the optic radiation (past the lateral geniculate body) and, of course, in the cortex. At the level of the lateral geniculate body there occurs a confluence of the messages from the two eyes, but binocular cell-responses can be recorded only from inner cortical areas. Current evidence suggests that the visual field is not dissected cell by cell, but that there is provision for multiple projections specializing in different types of analysis, for example, colour, disparity (for space perception), and so on. It is unknown how the ultimate synthesis, if any, occurs.

Some attention has recently been given to the possibility that there exist significant sex differences in the sphere of vision. There is evidence that women are a little short-sighted in comparison with men, which may be due to the fact that their crystalline lenses have a higher optical power than those of men (Weale, 1983). Moreover, senescence appears to affect the two sexes differently in most of the ectodermal tissues that have been studied. Women apparently become presbyopic some five years earlier than do men (the lens, like the retina, the skin, hair, is derived from ectoderm). The visual acuity of older women is poorer than that of men by a small, but statistically significant, amount. Recent observations on squirrel monkeys show that chromatic responses recorded from the lateral geniculate body reveal highly significant sex-differences apparently related to their colour vision. Defects in the latter have, of course, been long known to be inherited on a sex-linked basis.

These observations are sufficiently weighty to point to the need to keep visual performance and related data separate for the two sexes, unless they have been shown not to differ on a statistically significant basis. Only some of the differences may be explicable in terms of different hormonal environments. However, this is unlikely to be the only explanation as the sex-linked differences in the progress of some retinal diseases are, at present, hard to envisage on this basis.

R. A. Weale
Institute of Ophthalmology
University of London

References

Campbell, F. W. and Robson, J. G. (1968), 'Application of Fourier Analysis to the visibility of gratings', *Journal of Physiology*.

Davson, H. (ed.) (1976), *The Eye, vol. 2A*, New York, London and San Francisco.

Vocational and Career Development

The field of vocational and career development concerns itself with how and why individuals develop preferences for one or another type of work, how they eventually choose an occupation and proceed in their attempts to achieve satisfaction from their work. It has produced instruments and procedures to assist individuals via education, consultation and counselling to optimize their vocational and career potential.

The field cuts across many different domains. Thus, developmental psychologists are interested in the developmental antecedents of important vocational and career decisions; test and measurement specialists create instruments to measure such domains as vocational interests, personality, and vocational maturity; sociologists study the impact of family characteristics and the sociocultural environment on careers, and counselling psychologists develop methods to intervene in the vocational and career-development process.

The most significant theories in the field of vocational and career development have been formulated since 1950, and are summarized by Osipow (1983). The first of these emphasized that vocational development is more than a single decision regarding an occupational choice. It is a process, occurring over a number of years and consisting of several distinct periods during which the individual makes successive compromises between his wishes and the realistic opportunities present.

In 1953, Super presented his self-concept theory, which viewed vocational development as being inextricably linked to the development of a person's self-concept. Super extended his developmental approach to include not only the Exploratory Stage, during which vocational exploration and tentative decisions occur, but also the Establishment Stage, during which vocational decisions are evaluated and modified, leading to mature vocational behaviours and career decisions (see Super, 1982).

A third major theory is Holland's, initially developed in 1959. The basic feature of this theory rests on the assumption that there are a finite number of different work environments which attract different personalities. If the work environment 'matches' the personality of the person choosing it, this can lead to a successful career. Most research in this area has confirmed Holland's basic conceptualization (see Holland, 1973).

Other important approaches to vocational and career development since 1950 include Tiedeman's developmental theory (see Tiedeman *et al.*, 1978), Krumboltz's social-learning theory (see Krumboltz, 1979), and Roe's personality theory (see Roe, 1979). Interest in the field is growing rapidly, in part because of its recent attention to the vocational and career development of women and minorities, and in part because of its growing recognition of career development as a life-span process.

Fred W. Vondracek
Pennsylvanian State University

References

Holland, J. L. (1973), *Making Vocational Choices: A Theory of Careers*, Englewood Cliffs, NJ.

Krumboltz, J. D. (1979), 'A social learning theory of career decision-making' in H. Mitchell *et al.* (eds), *Social Learning and Career Decision Making*, Cranston, Rhode Island.

Osipow, S. H. (1983), *Theories of Career Development*, 3rd edn, Englewood Cliffs, NJ.

Roe, A. (1979), 'Confronting complexity', *Academic Psychology Bulletin*, 1.

Super, D. E. (1982), 'Self-concepts in career development: theory and findings after thirty years', Presented at the 20th International Congress of Applied Psychology, Edinburgh.

Tiedeman, D. V *et al.* (1978), *The Cross-Sectional Story of Early Career Development*, Washington, DC.

See also: *occupational psychology*.

Watson, John Broadus (1878–1958)

As the founder of behaviourism and as a publicist and popularizer of psychology, John B. Watson was perhaps the most influential American psychologist of his generation. Born in 1878 near Greenville, South Carolina, Watson grew up in a large and poor rural family. He attended Furman University, a small Baptist college near Greenville, and graduated with a Master of Arts Degree in 1899. Watson entered the University of Chicago in 1900, where he studied with John Dewey, psychologist James Rowland Angell, neurophysiologist H. H. Donaldson and biologist Jacques Loeb.

At Chicago, Angell had been instrumental in founding the functional school of psychology. Influenced by Darwin, William James and Dewey, the functionalists opposed the elementistic psychology developed by Wilhelm Wundt in Germany and espoused in America as structuralism by British-trained psychologist E. B. Titchener. Whereas structuralism attempted to discover the structure of mind by first isolating the basic elements of consciousness, functionalism was concerned with the mind in use and held that the function of consciousness was its capacity to enable an organism to adapt to its environment.

Although a protégé of Angell, Watson was later to reject both functionalism and structuralism. Even as a student he was particularly influenced by Loeb's insistence that all life processes could be explained in physiochemical terms. Watson's own interests lay in comparative or animal psychology. He was uncomfortable with human subjects and what he considered to be the artificiality of introspective methods, which required subjects to observe and record the sensations and perceptions of their own conscious experience. His dissertation, completed under H. H. Donaldson, was a study of the correlation between the learned behaviour and the neurophysiology of the white rat. In 1903, Watson received the first Ph.D. granted in psychology from the University of Chicago. With the recommendation of Angell and Dewey, he was invited to stay at Chicago as lecturer and director of the psychological laboratory and quickly gained a reputation as a leading figure in the relatively new field of comparative psychology.

In 1908, Watson was invited by James Mark Baldwin to develop a programme in experimental psychology at Johns Hopkins University. Less than a year later, Baldwin was forced to resign, leaving Watson as chairman of the department and editor of the *Psychological Review*. At Johns Hopkins, Watson became increasingly dissatisfied with the assumptions of both structuralism and functionalism. As long as psychology considered its subject matter to be the investigation of consciousness, he argued, it perpetuated a mind-body dualism that kept it beyond the pale of current scientific assumptions. Watson believed that he could resolve this issue by simply denying the existence of mind as a distinct entity. For years he had been investigating animals without referring to purely mental categories or functions. As early as 1910, he had become convinced that psychological investigations could be conducted exclusively through the observation of behaviour without any reference to consciousness. By 1913, he was ready to make his position public. In a lecture entitled 'Psychology as the Behaviourist Views It', Watson issued an open challenge to the established preconceptions of psychological method and theory.

Watson's behaviourism not only offered a new methodological approach to psychological investigation, but attempted to redefine fundamental assumptions of the profession itself. Claiming that psychology had 'failed signally' to take its place as 'an undisputed natural science', Watson placed the blame on the use of the introspective method and its underlying assumption of the existence of states of consciousness. Watson considered 'mind' and 'consciousness' to be as unverifiable as 'soul' and refused to make any assumption that could not be observed and verified from overt behaviour. Behaviourism, Watson argued, would at once enable psychology to become a 'purely objective natural science', with its 'theoretical goal' being nothing less than the 'prediction and control of behavior'. Watson hoped to ally psychology with the positivist trend in the natural and social sciences. He also sought to bridge the gap between experimental and applied psychology by claiming that behaviourism would enable psychologists to develop techniques that would be of direct use to 'the educator, the physician, the jurist and the business man'.

In 1914, Watson was elected president of the American Psychological Association. In his presidential address the following year, he consolidated his behaviourist theory by offering the conditioned motor reflex (as described by Russian neurologist, V. M. Bechterev) as an objective methodology that could be used to measure and control sensory responses. Watson then began experiments on human subjects which culminated in 1919 which his famous 'Little Albert' experiment, by which Watson claimed to have developed techniques to condition, at will, specific emotional reactions in infants. In the midst of conducting this experiment, Watson became romantically involved with his graduate assistant, and as a result, was forced to resign from Johns Hopkins in 1920 under the cloud of a widely publicized divorce scandal.

Watson then moved to New York, where he became a successful advertising executive until his retirement in 1945. During this period, he was a tireless promoter of the use of psychological techniques in business and industry. He also continued to teach at the New School for Social Research and sponsored psychological research on infants at Columbia University. During the 1920s and 1930s, Watson promoted behaviourism to a mass audience. His widely read *Behaviorism* (1924) was followed by an enormous output of popular magazine and newspaper articles. In *The Psychological Care of Infant and Child* (1928), Watson advised parents to raise children according to a strict regimen that discouraged displays of affection. Later writings included his utopian vision of a society ordered on behaviouristic principles and governed by a hierarchy of technicians.

Although few psychologists were willing to accept Watson's abandonment of consciousness wholeheartedly and came to reject the more radical aspects of his extreme materialism, behaviourism's objective methodology had a powerful impact on the direction of American experimental psychology. Moreover, the popular reception of behaviourism in America was not only a tribute to Watson's skill as a propagandist, but reflected a national preoccupation with order and efficiency in a society that was in the process of rapid urban and industrial expansion.

Kerry W. Buckley

Further Reading

Boakes, R. A. (1984), *From Darwin to Behaviorism*, Cambridge.

Buckley, K. W. (1986), *Mechanical Man: John B. Watson and the Beginnings of Behaviorism*, New York.

Watson, J. B. (1913), 'Psychology as the behaviorist views it', *Psychological Review*, 20.

Watson, J. B. (1924), *Behaviorism*, New York.

Watson, J. B. and Watson, R. R. (1928), *The Psychological Care of Infant and Child*, New York.

See also: *behaviourism; conditioning*.

Women's Studies in Psychology

Women as mothers have been, and continue to be, a major subject of interest to those working in developmental and abnormal psychology. Psychology's interest in women in their own right is of relatively recent origin. Prior to the late 1960s' resurgence of feminism, it was all too often assumed that generalizations about women's and men's psychology could be validly based on studies that included only male subjects. Now, however, it is generally recognized that the psychology of women may differ from the psychology of men. Indeed, some psychology journals even insist that their contributors control for the possibility of such differences.

Psychological sex differences have, in particular, been reported in the areas of aggression, visuo-spatial, mathematical, and verbal ability. Some seek to explain these differences in biological terms (Hutt, 1972). Much current research is guided by the view that men's aggressiveness is hormonally determined by the androgens and that sex-related cognitive differences are an effect of girls' brains being specialized earlier for verbal, boys' for visuo-spatial, processing.

Others seek to explain these differences, and sex-role development in general, as a consequence more of nurture than of nature. Two approaches currently dominate this perspective on gender development: (1) Social-learning theory, the approach of Walter Mischel (1966), views sex-role development as resulting from the child's imitation of those behaviours that parents, other children, education and the media convey as 'sex-role appropriate'. (2) The approach of Lawrence Kohlberg (1966) views gender development as crucially determined, not so much by external influence, as by the child's own ideas about sex and gender. These start with its ability (at about the age of two years) to categorize itself correctly by sex, then by its developing recognition that sex remains invariant through life. This process is accompanied, according to Kohlberg, by changes in the child's understanding of sex-role stereotypes which it regards first as given by biology, later as given by social convention, and which it finally comes to judge in terms of the conformity of these stereotypes with principles of equity and justice.

Social psychology has been more interested in sex differences in achievement – differences that are currently researched in terms of attribution theory. Women, unlike men, it is said, tend to attribute their successes to luck and their failures to lack of ability, and for this reason become easily disheartened from striving for educational and occupational achievement. Women's greater tendency to become disheartened and depressed has also become a focus of concern in abnormal psychology where it has been assimilated to the currently dominant behavioural model of depression, Seligman's 'learned helplessness theory'. According to this perspective the reason that women more often suffer from depression than men is that their social situation renders them less than able to control the sources of reward and reinforcement in their lives. Assertiveness training has been recommended as one way of alleviating this condition, and this technique has also been applied quite generally as a way of increasing women's self-confidence.

Behavioural approaches to the explanation and treatment of mental disorder have also been applied to other conditions that affect women more than men (such as agoraphobia, anorexia). Psychology's long-standing hostility to psychoanalysis has scarcely been affected by its recent interest in women's mental health, despite the fact that others are increasingly looking to psychoanalysis both as a means of understanding mental health problems in women and, more generally, as a means of understanding the psychological correlates of sexual divisions in society. One particularly influential theory in this context has been post-Freudian object-relations theory, according to which the infant is initially psychologically merged with the mother and only gradually comes to experience itself as individuated from her. It has been suggested by Nancy Chodorow that mothers, being the same sex as their daughters, identify more with them than with their sons and thereby foster in them a continuing sense of mergence in personal relations. On the other hand, being the opposite sex to their sons, mothers tend to relate to them as separate and different from themselves and thereby propel them relatively early into the separation-individuation process such that they grow up having a greater sense than women of their separateness in personal relations (Chodorow, 1978).

Whereas this use of psychoanalysis emphasizes psychological sex differences – women as more merged, men as more individuated in personal relations – others (for example, Juliet Mitchell, 1974) have used psychoanalysis to stress the psychological similarity between the sexes, to show that the traits associated with masculinity and femininity reside in both sexes. In this they draw on Freud's claim that girls and boys are initially 'bisexual', that they are both equally feminine and masculine in infancy, and on his view that even when girls become predominantly feminine (and boys predominantly masculine) following the Oedipus complex, masculinity remains present, albeit repressed and unconscious, within the female psyche (as femininity remains present in the male psyche).

The view that people are often psychologically feminine as well as masculine has also been propounded, although not in psychoanalytic terms, within mainstream psychology. Prior to the late 1960s it had been assumed that psychological health consisted, among other things, in conforming with the norms of one's sex – in being feminine if one was a woman, masculine if a man. The advent of the women's movement was accompanied, however, by a questioning of the adaptiveness of such sex-role conformity. And this resulted in the development by Sandra Bem of a test designed to measure the extent to which individuals adhere to masculine, feminine, or both masculine and feminine traits – a test now much used in conjunction with other measures to assess whether sex-role conformity is indeed adaptive or whether adaptiveness is instead a matter of 'androgyny', of combining both masculine and feminine traits (Bem, 1974).

Janet Sayers
University of Kent

References
Bem, S. (1974), 'The measurement of psychological androgyny', *Journal of Consulting and Clinical Psychology*, 42.
Chodorow, N. (1978), *The Reproduction of Mothering*, Berkeley and Los Angeles.
Hutt, C. (1972), *Males and Females*, Harmondsworth.
Kohlberg, L. (1966), 'A cognitive-developmental analysis of children's sex-role concepts and attitudes', in E. E. Maccoby (ed.), *The Development of Sex Differences*, Stanford, Calif.
Mischel, W. (1966), 'A social-learning view of sex differences in behaviour', in E. E. Maccoby (ed.), *The Development of Sex Differences*, Stanford, Calif.
Mitchell, J. (1974), *Psychoanalysis and Feminism*, London.

Further Reading
Sayers, J. (1985), *Sexual Contradictions: Psychology, Psychoanalysis and Feminism*, London.

Wundt, Wilhelm (1832–1920)

Wundt, a medically-trained German academic, was a professor of philosophy at the University of Leipzig and is remembered chiefly as a pioneer of experimental psychology. His establishment of modest facilities for experimental psychological research by some of his students in 1879 is conventionally regarded as marking the foundation of the world's first psychological laboratory. Wundt's innovation attracted a large number of students from all over the world, especially during the last two decades of the nineteenth century. In many cases these students attempted to found similar laboratories after they returned to their home countries.

A further contribution to the institutionalization of experimental psychology involved Wundt's publication of a journal, *Philosophische Studien*, in which reports of experimental psychological research appeared regularly, though still interspersed with philosophical papers. However, the major source of Wundt's reputation as an experimental psychologist was probably his textbook, *Grundzüge der physiologischen Psychologie* which first appeared in 1874 and grew to a monumental three-volume work in five subsequent revised editions.

It was Wundt's belief that the experimental method, which had proved so effective in physiological research, could be employed, with some modification, in the investigation of some of the problems which had been debated by philosopher psychologists. Two sets of problems were particularly important in this context: questions about the sources of our knowledge of the external world, and questions about the nature of voluntary action. This led to systematic research in the area of sensation and perception and in the area of reaction times.

While Wundt derived his experimental methodology from physiology, he took most of his theoretical concepts from philosophy. His central concept was 'apperception', a term which has its roots in the philosophy of Leibniz, was systematically developed by Kant and applied to psychology by Herbart. These were the men whom Wundt regarded as his intellectual ancestors. The concept of apperception referred to the active and synthetic qualities of the mind which were fundamental to all its expressions.

There is a double irony in the fact that posterity remembered Wundt mainly as the 'father' of experimental psychology. In the first place, his work in this area, extensive though it was, represented only a relatively small part of an enormously productive academic career. He published major works in all the main branches of philosophy, logic, ethics, metaphysics and epistemology. For him, though not for many of his pupils, the significance of psychological research very much depended on a philosophical context. Towards the end of his life, he strongly opposed both the notion of an applied psychology and the notion that psychology should cut its ties with philosophy. These were not the outcomes he had intended.

Moreover, this 'father' of experimental psychology had never seen this branch of the subject as more than a part of psychology as a whole. It was to be supplemented by another part, called *Völkerpsychologie*, a psychology of culture which would use a comparative and historical rather than an experimental methodology. Wundt devoted the last part of his life mainly to this subject. His ten-volume text with this title did not produce anything like the echo of his text on physiological psychology. It did, however, anticipate certain developments that took place long after Wundt's death, notably in the importance it gave to psycholinguistics.

In spite of his prodigious output and vast influence, Wundt founded no school and had no real disciples. He identified his psychological system as 'voluntarism' because he regarded the dynamic and affective aspect of psychological processes as fundamental. But there were no 'voluntarists' among his students, especially not among the strict experimentalists. By the time of his death in 1920, his version of psychology had become thoroughly unpalatable to the majority of psychologists, especially in the US, who saw psychology as a practical technology of behaviour and as a natural science like any other. By contrast, Wundt's vision for psychology had been that of a bridge between the natural and the humanistic sciences.

K. Danziger
York University, Ontario

Further Reading

Bringmann, W. G. and Tweenay, R. D. (eds) (1980), *Wundt Studies*, Toronto.

Rieber, R. W. (ed.) (1980), *Wilhelm Wundt and the Making of a Scientific Psychology*, New York.

Wundt, W. (1894 [1863]), *Lectures on Human and Animal Psychology*, 2nd edn, New York. (Original German edn, *Vorlesungen über die Menschen und Tierseele*.)

Wundt, W. (1897), *Outlines of Psychology*, Leipzig.